GENIUS
ON THE
EDGE

GENIUS
ON THE
EDGE

The Bizarre Double Life of
Dr. William Stewart Halsted

GERALD IMBER, MD

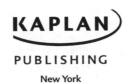

KAPLAN

PUBLISHING

New York

© 2011 Gerald Imber, MD

Published by Kaplan Publishing, a division of Kaplan, Inc.
395 Hudson Avenue
New York, NY 10014

Previously published in hardcover (ISBN-13: 978-1-60714-627-8)

Printed in the United States of America

10 9 8 7 6 5 4 3 2

Photographs reprinted with permission of the Alan Mason Chesney Archives of The Johns Hopkins Medical Institutions.

ISBN-13: 978-1-60714-858-6

Library of Congress Cataloging-in-Publication Data
Imber, Gerald.
   Genius on the edge : the bizarre story of William Stewart Halsted, the father of modern surgery / by Gerald Imber.
      p. ; cm.
   ISBN-13: 978-1-60714-627-8 (hard cover)
   ISBN-10: 1-60714-627-4
   1. Halsted, William, 1852-1922. 2. Surgeons—United States—Biography. I. Title.
   [DNLM: 1. Halsted, William, 1852-1922. 2. Physicians. 3. Biography.
4. General Surgery—history. 5. History, 19th Century. 6. History, 20th Century.
WZ 100 H1962I 2010]
   RD27.35.H36I43 2010
   617.092—dc22
   [B]

                                                            2009035525

Kaplan Publishing books are available at special quantity discounts to use for sales promotions, employee premiums, or educational purposes. For more information or to purchase books, please call the Simon & Schuster special sales department at 866-506-1949.

"Surgery would be delightful
if you did not have to operate."

W. S. HALSTED

CONTENTS

Prologue   ix

ONE   Tumultuous Times   1

TWO   Setting the Stage   9

THREE   Physicians and Surgeons   21

FOUR   Becoming a Surgeon   29

FIVE   New York   37

SIX   Cocaine   47

SEVEN   The Visionary   59

EIGHT   The Very Best Men   75

NINE   Baltimore   85

TEN   The Hospital on the Hill   95

ELEVEN   Finding the Way   101

TWELVE   William Osler   105

THIRTEEN   The Operating Room   111

FOURTEEN   The Radical Cure of Breast Cancer   117

FIFTEEN   Life in Baltimore   127

SIXTEEN   The Big Four   139

SEVENTEEN   Hernia   145

EIGHTEEN   Establishing the Routine   155

NINETEEN　Country Squire　167

TWENTY　The First Great Medical School　183

TWENTY-ONE　Teaching without Teaching　189

TWENTY-TWO　Residents　193

TWENTY-THREE　Changes　205

TWENTY-FOUR　Into the 20th Century　221

TWENTY-FIVE　Harvey Cushing　229

TWENTY-SIX　All Quiet on the Home Front　247

TWENTY-SEVEN　After Cushing　257

TWENTY-EIGHT　New Horizons　267

TWENTY-NINE　Addiction　277

THIRTY　Vascular Surgery　283

THIRTY-ONE　Scientist　287

THIRTY-TWO　A New Paradigm　297

THIRTY-THREE　A New Era　307

THIRTY-FOUR　The World Changes　321

THIRTY-FIVE　"My Dear Miss Bessie"　331

THIRTY-SIX　The Final Illness　341

THIRTY-SEVEN　Afterward　345

Epilogue　353

Acknowledgments　357

References　359

Index　375

About the Author　389

PROLOGUE

APRIL 1882.

Fresh, white sheets were brought down from the linen cupboard and laid over the kitchen table. A down pillow was placed under the head of the jaundiced 70-year-old woman. She was febrile, nauseated, crippled with abdominal and back pain, and clearly in extremis. Dr. William Stewart Halsted carefully examined his patient, working his way to an inflamed mass on the right side of her abdomen just beneath the rib cage. Pressing his fingers against it, he caused the woman to jerk away and cry out.

For more than a year, she had complained of a sour taste in her mouth, loss of appetite, and episodes of sharp pain penetrating through to her back, symptoms that confounded the finest consultants in New York City. Now, while the woman was visiting with her daughter in Albany, the pain had become unrelenting. The onset of high fever; rapid, shallow breathing; and the yellow cast of her eyes made those attending her fear for her life. A telegram had been sent summoning Dr. Halsted, who arrived by train from New York late that same evening.

By 2 A.M. the septic patient was on the kitchen table and prepared for surgery. What had been an elusive diagnosis was now clear: acute cholecystitis (an infection of the gallbladder); empyema (a collection of pus in the distended gallbladder); and gallstones, which blocked the egress of the bile and pus. Halsted realized that nothing short of emergency surgery could save the patient's life.

THE INSTRUMENTS HE brought with him were boiled and dipped in carbolic acid. He rolled his coat sleeves above his wrists, washed his hands with green soap, dipped them in the carbolic acid, and approached the patient, who was now breathing ether fumes and unaware of the impending surgery. With a scalpel in his bare hands, he cut through the tense skin and subcutaneous fat above the hot mass, then swiftly through rectus abdominus muscle and the peritoneum lining the abdomen, exposing the enlarged, pus-filled gallbladder. Halsted incised the inflamed organ, releasing a flood of purulent material and seven gallstones. He clamped the bleeding points with artery forceps and tied them off with fine silk ligatures. He closed the peritoneum and re-approximated the abdominal muscles. The skin, and the fat beneath it, were left open and packed with cotton gauze.

RELEASING THE ACCUMULATION of pus and removing the gallstones effectively relieved the acute problem. The patient recovered uneventfully and was symptom free for the remaining two years of her life. William Stewart Halsted had successfully performed the first known operation to remove gallstones, and in the process had brought his mother back from the brink of death.

CHAPTER ONE

Tumultuous Times

WILLIAM STEWART HALSTED WAS born in New York City on
April 23, 1852, in the decade of booming mercantile prosper-
ity and civic unrest preceding the Civil War. Immigrants seeking to
escape famine and poverty in their native lands poured into the city
at an astounding rate, often as many as 250,000 in a single year. The
new arrivals, then largely Irish, supplanted free blacks as an inexpensive labor source, and the slums were soon overrun. Only half the
children born in the entire country would live to the age of five. More
New Yorkers were dying from disease each year than were being born.
Two cholera epidemics in the 1830s and 1840s had claimed thousands
of lives, while earlier outbreaks of malaria and yellow fever had taken
many more. Within the filthy slums, especially the notorious Five Points
neighborhood, about which Charles Dickens said, "All that is loathsome,
drooping and decayed is here," the death rate was three times that of the
rest of the city. Without the new immigrants, the population of the city
would have been decimated. With them, the city was almost unlivable.

Tuberculosis was rampant. It was a scourge of greater proportions
than AIDS, influenza, and polio combined, and had run unchecked for
centuries, killing hundreds of millions of people worldwide. The disease
was not limited to the lung infection, or consumption, immortalized

in literature by Dumas's Marguerite in *Camille*, and later Violetta in Verdi's *La Traviata*. It was a generalized condition that also produced draining scrofulous abscesses of the lymph glands of the neck and axilla, and bone infections necessitating amputation. Little could be done other than drain the tumors and remove the festering parts.

Rich and poor lived in close contact, and resentment and unrest were everywhere. Riots in the first half of the century were common and usually reflected class and ethnic hostilities. Among these were the deadly Astor Place Riot in 1849 and the Klein Deutschland Riot of 1857. Earlier riots had erupted between Catholic and Protestant street gangs, and several were prompted by the city's efforts to remove some 20,000 feral pigs from city streets.

As mid-century approached, the gentry abandoned lower Manhattan and moved "uptown" to the wide-open spaces of Greenwich Village. Among them were the prosperous Halsteds.

By mid-century, 14th Street had become the epicenter of society. Broadway was the busiest shopping corridor in the world, and 200,000 horses plied the city streets, pulling stagecoaches, buses, delivery wagons, and cabs. Sanitation was nonexistent and health hazards were overwhelming. Each horse produced more than 15 pounds of manure daily, and there was no organized system for its disposal. Manure piles were everywhere, seeping into street-level rooms in heavy rain, drying in fly-infested piles in summer. Each year, 20,000 horse carcasses were dragged from city streets to the pier on West 38th Street to be shipped to rendering plants in Barren Island, Brooklyn, where the bones were turned into glue. New "brownstone" homes were built with high entry stairs to avoid the ubiquitous manure.

Human excrement was also a problem. There was no municipal sewer system, although more affluent neighborhoods could petition for the construction of sewers and share the cost among the residents. Elsewhere, chamber pots were still emptied from tenement windows into the street. Women used parasols to protect themselves and their finery from flying excrement. The exodus uptown provided some relief, but it wouldn't be until after the turn of the next century that electric buses and the automobile supplanted horses and eased the situation.

In the late 1830s, a professor of art at the University of the City of New York named Samuel F. B. Morse designed the first operable telegraph. Less than a decade later, private telegraph companies turned New York into a communications hub with lines connecting the nation. Financial institutions relished the quick transfer of information available in Manhattan, and the industry found a permanent home in the growing financial district around Wall Street.

By 1860, there were 30,000 miles of railroad track connecting the country. As railroads expanded westward, a key link opened along the route of the Erie Canal connecting the Great Lakes and the Atlantic Ocean. Manufacturing and transportation prospered. The Croton Distributing Reservoir was built far uptown, at 42nd Street and Fifth Avenue. A massive structure on a four-acre site, which is now home to the main branch of the New York Public Library, the reservoir held 150 million gallons of pure upstate water for the thirsty, growing city. Nearby, the Crystal Palace, a monumental exposition hall of cast iron and glass, was opened in the summer of 1853 to house the first World's Fair in America. Music and entertainment venues sprouted all over town. The city was in thrall to Jenny Lind, the "Swedish Nightingale," who was on a two-year tour promoted by P. T. Barnum. Tickets to her performances sold for as much as $650 at auction. Stephen Foster's popular songs, such as "Oh Susanna!" and "Camptown Races," were perennial favorites. Some, such as "My Old Kentucky Home, Good-night," stirred sympathy for the plight of America's slaves even as most northern blacks, while free, had achieved nothing close to equality.

The Halsted family had lived in and around New York City since the 1657 arrival of the Englishman Timothy Halsted in Hempstead, Long Island. By the mid-18th century the next generation of Halsteds had moved to Elizabethtown, New Jersey, where Robert and Caleb, the first physicians in the family, were born. Robert's son, William Mills Halsted, did not follow his father's calling and instead, with a partner, R. T. Haines, founded Halsted, Haines and Company, dealing in the wholesale importation and sale of dry goods. The firm was immediately successful, and the family was soon entrenched in the prosperous mercantile society of the city. William Mills Halsted became an elder in the University Place Presbyterian Church, a governor of the New York Hospital, which was then located at Broadway and Pearl Street, and a founder of the Union Theological Seminary. He also invested heavily in the rapid development of Chicago; the longest thoroughfare in that city is still called Halsted Street.

The family fortune grew, and in 1835 William Mills Halsted built a large, finely appointed home on the northwest corner of Fifth Avenue at 14th Street, soon adding three adjoining houses for his children. He was a picture of Presbyterian rectitude, constantly preaching to his children. One of his children, Thaddeus, became a physician. To another, William Mills Halsted Jr., then away at school, he wrote, "endeavor my son to qualify yourself in usefulness and responsibility." Young William learned his lessons and succeeded his father at the helm of Halsted, Haines and Company. He was a founder of the Commonwealth Fire Insurance Company, joined the board of governors of the New York Hospital and Bloomingdale Asylum, the board of the College of the City of New York, and the board of the College of Physicians and Surgeons. William Mills Halsted Jr. married his cousin Mary Louisa Haines, and together they raised a family in New York City, summered at Irvington, 25 miles north along the Hudson River, and were pillars of the community.

Frugal and strict, William Mills Halsted Jr. adhered closely to his father's Presbyterian ethic and demanded the same of his four children. Though he provided well for his children, he forbade them to bring friends to their home for meals. When his youngest son, Richard, disobeyed this rule, he presented Richard and his friends with a detailed bill for the food they consumed.

William Stewart Halsted was the eldest of the four children. Until the age of ten he was homeschooled by governesses, then a common practice among the affluent. Public education in New York City was inadequate, and those of means sent their older children to the numerous private institutions throughout New England, most of which had close church ties.

The Halsted family remained seemingly untouched by the Civil War raging in the South. In the summer of 1862, just a few months after the Battle of Shiloh claimed the lives of 24,000 Union and Confederate troops, William Stewart was sent off far from the fray, to a school at Monson, Massachusetts, run by a retired Congregational minister, the Reverend Mr. Tufts.

It was an unpleasant experience, and Halsted later wrote:

> There were about twenty boys in the school, all much older than I. I can recall very little of the method of instruction, but I must have studied Latin for I was given the choice of learning a lesson in Latin grammar or stirring soft soap in a great cauldron on Saturday afternoon when I was kept at home for misdemeanor, usually for swimming in the river. Sunday was a nightmare: we were driven to church two miles away and spent the entire day in the churchyard—Sunday school from nine to ten or ten-thirty, church until 1 P.M. luncheon from basket, Sunday school again at 3 P.M. and church say from four to five-thirty. In the spring of 1863 I attempted to escape, walked to Palmer, four miles, took train to Springfield twenty miles; was captured at Springfield and taken back to Monson.

In July 1863, the Draft Riots, the bloodiest riots in American history, were ignited at a conscription office on 47th Street and Third Avenue when poor Irish protested a new law that allowed anyone to buy their way out of military service for $300. The violence soon took on racial overtones, and many blacks were targeted and hanged. Over five days the mayhem claimed as many as 1,000 lives.

That fall, young Halsted, kept safe from all of this, was enrolled at Phillips Academy, a preparatory school in Andover, Massachusetts, north of Boston. The school, founded in 1778 by Samuel Phillips, is more commonly known as Andover, distinguishing it from its rival Phillips Exeter Academy, in Exeter, New Hampshire, founded three years later by another family member, Dr. John Phillips. The Phillips Academy, Andover, is rich with American history. Its great seal was designed by the silversmith Paul Revere. Two of its many distinguished graduates were telegraph inventor Samuel F. B. Morse and U.S. Supreme Court Justice Oliver Wendell Holmes. From its earliest days, Andover established a tradition of preparing its young men for enrollment at Yale. In 1868, of a senior class of 40 students, 25 went on to continue their studies in New Haven.

Even at this early stage of his life, Halsted was careful about his dress and always well turned out. A photograph from the period shows a good-looking young man in suit, waistcoat, and matching cravat—his blond hairline already rather high on his forehead, and prominent patrician nose turned up at a fairly high angle over a wide, smiling mouth and full lower lip. His ears stood smartly away from his head, a feature about which he was often teased. Later in life he defused comments by joking about his ears before others could call attention to them. Barely five feet six inches tall, Halsted was solidly built, with a surprisingly muscular upper body and a tendency to walk with his elbows out.

Not yet 17 years old at graduation in 1869, and thought too young to enter college, he was enrolled in a private day school in Manhattan and tutored privately in Latin and Greek prior to college entrance exams. Halsted was admitted "without condition" to Yale, along with numerous of his Andover classmates. At Yale, "[I] devoted myself solely to athletics," and his grades were in no way equal to his athletic achievements. Andover boys were well prepared for the first few semesters at Yale, and it set them off with a relaxed attitude toward college education.

Athletics remained central to his life. He joined the junior and senior class crews, was shortstop on the junior class baseball team, and in his senior year served as captain of the football team. This was the first year of modern, 11-man football in college athletics. The 160-pound Halsted also knocked his friend Sam Bushnell flat in a boxing match.

There is no record of Halsted ever having borrowed a book from the Yale library.

The class at Yale was organized into four academic divisions based on performance. Halsted spent most of his lackluster tenure in the second and third divisions, although classmates believed he could easily have been in the first had he cared. Finally convinced to apply himself to his studies, he worked hard and did well on mid-term exams. He abandoned the second division and assumed what he believed to be his rightful place attending first-division classes. Not finding himself registered among the division-one students, his irate inquiry was met by an instructor informing him he had been placed in the third division. The lesson that a perception once formed is difficult to alter was one he learned well.

Notably well dressed at Yale as he had been at Andover, Halsted and a friend paraded around campus for a time in tailor-made suits of mattress ticking. Sam Bushnell believed the outrageous fashion statement was clearly a Halsted prank, but "he did not have the courage to carry out his idea alone."

Halsted was a member of a number of college clubs including the Freshman Society, Freshman Eating Club, The Tasters, The Sophomore Society, Phi Theta Psi, the Junior Society, and Psi Epsilon. But only inclusion in the elite senior society, Skull and Bones, mattered to him. His father had been a member and had aggressively pushed his son to seek election. The society seemed so important to him that Bushnell offered to decline election if his friend was excluded, but

Halsted refused: "If you get an election, you take it; if I get an election I shall take it. I shall expect you to do the same by me."

In the end, he was not tapped for the society. The rejection was all the more devastating since his "Bonesman" father did not take it well, saying to Bushnell, "Why didn't you get him into Skull and Bones? You made it."

Halsted acted in plays, "did not go in for social activities," and did not drink. There is no mention of girls in any of Halsted's letters or reminiscences, or in the comments of friends. He continued to attend church regularly while at school but was increasingly dismissive of the strict religious fervor of his parents. The trip to New York was fast and convenient on the New Haven Railroad, and he came home frequently during the school year. He visited with the families of college friends and made several trips to Baltimore with his friend Henry James, son of a leading local financier. Summers were spent at the family home at Irvington, in the lower Hudson Valley, and the four children remained close with their parents and one another. Several of the family members were avid gardeners, and this became a passion that William Stewart shared as well.

In a totally uncharacteristic act early in his senior year, the unscholarly Halsted purchased copies of *Gray's Anatomy* and *Dalton's Physiology*. He had shown no interest in science previously, but now immersed himself in the reading. He spent his free time around the laboratories and clinics at the Yale medical school, asking questions of anyone who would speak to him. As his time at Yale came to a close, young Halsted told his father that he was not interested in joining the family business but would like to study medicine. It was a decision that would change the face of modern medicine.

CHAPTER TWO

Setting the Stage

PRIOR TO 1846, very little elective surgery was performed in either the United States or Europe. London was teeming with 2.3 million people in the most unsanitary conditions imaginable. New York City was home to 700,000 inhabitants in 1850, and more than 2 million by 1860. Disease and deformity were rampant, yet medical centers in New York and London reported no more than 200 operations a year, largely because the pain of surgery was so intolerable that the idea was rarely entertained. For centuries, little more than alcohol and opiates were available to ease the pain, and these proved inadequate for the horrors of amputation or the evacuation of a tuberculous abscess.

When catastrophic injury demanded surgery, the outcome was often as disastrous as if the injury had gone untreated. Limb amputation was the most frequently performed operation. Often the victim of an overturned wagon or a mill accident who was strong enough to withstand the pain of surgery would die from postoperative infection. During the Civil War, trained surgeons were so scarce that uneducated recruits were taught the basics of amputation and operated without supervision. Their results were often no worse than those of traditional surgeons in what passed for field hospitals. In the face of such predictably dreadful outcomes, it is not surprising that surgeons were not well regarded by their medical colleagues.

A century earlier the teachings of the great Scottish anatomist John Hunter established some level of respect for anatomical dissection, the understanding of surgical anatomy, and well-planned operations with reproducible results. But operations were performed in only the direst of circumstances. Drugged patients were held down by several strong men and restrained from thrashing about until they ultimately fainted away, but no one could tolerate this torture for very long. Operative time was measured in minutes. The best surgeons could remove a limb in five or ten horrific minutes. Another half hour was spent attempting to stop the blood loss, which was usually enormous. Neither blood transfusions nor intravenous fluids where yet available, and patients simply went into shock and died. Bleeding was controlled with large ligatures, usually thick strings made of sheep intestine or silk, sometimes held in the surgeon's mouth for easy access. The ligatures were hastily applied and crushed the bleeding arteries and veins, as well as the surrounding muscle. Flaps were closed crudely, and a perfect environment for infection was created.

The cause of infection was unknown, and many physicians still subscribed to the theory that an imbalance of the four humors—blood, phlegm, black bile, and yellow bile—was the root of bodily dysfunction. Doctors drained abscesses with little thought of cause or prevention. It was simply the thing to do, and it happened to work. As late as the mid-19th century, the germ theory was still unknown, and the idea of bacteria growing in the warm culture medium of devitalized human tissue hadn't yet been suggested.

* * *

PAIN AND INFECTION had to be conquered before surgery could advance beyond barbarism. The first of the missing links was provided two decades earlier at the Massachusetts General Hospital in

Boston. In 1845, Horace Wells attempted to demonstrate the technique of painless dental extraction using nitrous oxide gas. The level of anesthesia he used proved too light, and the patient cried out in pain. The students in the gallery at the Harvard Medical School stood, shouted "humbug," and left the room.

A year later, on October 16, 1846, a dentist named William T. G. Morton administered a substance called ether while surgeon John Collins Warren painlessly removed a small tumor from the neck of a sleeping patient. With the memory of the prior failure still fresh, the audience of doctors and medical students at Morton's demonstration were prepared for another discouraging failure.

Morton first impregnated gauze with the ethyl ether compound, then placed the gauze in a decanter-like blown-glass inhaler. The inhaler had an intake valve for air and a mouthpiece through which the ether fumes were delivered to the patient. Virtually nothing was known about dosage or the levels of anesthesia produced. Warren had taught his Harvard Medical School students that ether was far too dangerous a substance for use, but Morton, who had attended those lectures, was crafty enough not to identify the mysterious substance within the glass contraption. He had employed it in several extractions in the past, and had gained enough support among respected members of the medical community to convince Warren to take part in the demonstration.

Gilbert Abbott, the patient, was strapped tightly into the blood-colored, velvet operating chair, and attendants stood by to further restrain him if it became necessary. A bit agitated as he first inhaled the ether, Abbott thrashed around, then quickly fell off to sleep. The operation went on uninterrupted, with Abbott sleeping quietly. Upon waking, he reported no sensation of pain, nor any memory of the event. Warren, who was duly impressed, turned to the gallery, raised his arms, and said, "Gentlemen, this is no humbug."

Numerous similar demonstrations of the technique were attempted for more extensive procedures with equal success, and ether assumed its place in operating rooms around the world. Oliver Wendell Holmes, renowned physician, lawyer, poet, and father of the future Supreme Court justice, wrote in 1846, "The state of lack of sensation should, I think, be called 'Anaesthesia' . . . The adjective will be Anaesthetic. Thus we might say the state of Anaesthesia, or the anaesthetic state."

The era of painless surgery had begun.

Chemical variations on ethyl ether came in and out of vogue, including trichloroethylene, or chloroform, which had the benefit of being considerably less flammable than ether. When Queen Victoria gave birth to Prince Leopold under chloroform anesthesia, it became all the rage. But chloroform proved more toxic than ether and soon fell from popularity. The word *ether* became interchangeable with *anesthesia*. It was used well beyond the first half of the 20th century, only to disappear from operating rooms when safer, and more controllable, anesthetics were introduced.[1]

In 1896, the 50th anniversary of the first operation under ether was being celebrated in Boston. At the same time, Hugh Young, the urologist on Halsted's staff at Johns Hopkins, unveiled a series of letters and affidavits, as well as a paper in the *Southern Medical Journal*, which told a different story. The documents credited Dr. Crawford W. Long with having operated on patients under ether anesthesia in the town of Jefferson, Georgia, four and a half years before Morton's demonstration. History seems to have been happy with the Massachusetts General version of events. If nothing else, it was well witnessed, quite dramatic, and gave the process a name.

---

1 In many teaching hospitals the induction of anesthesia with ether was taught into the late 20th century, both for its historical value and to demonstrate the phases of anesthesia through which the patient passes during "induction." One of these, the excitement phase, was obvious to observers of Morton's early demonstrations. Modern anesthetics are much faster-acting, and patients are premedicated with intravenous agents to smooth the way to sleep without noticeable stimulation.

* * *

PASSAGE INTO THE anesthetic era relieved patients of unbearable pain. Surgeons could be more adventurous in approaching disease and trauma, and the entire profession benefited from a new image. Although speed was no longer necessary in order to spare the patient, surgeons did not easily change their ways. Surgery was still performed as quickly and brutally as before, with only the patient's pain removed from the equation. Little thought was given to a more strategic, tissue-sparing approach.

While patients could now be less fearful of the pain of surgery, serious procedures still carried a mortality rate of nearly 50 percent. Compound fractures were a particular problem. Fractures can be simple breaks in which the ends of the bones have not moved from their normal position and need only immobilization to heal. Fractures can also be displaced from their normal position, requiring the ends to be returned to the normal position, or set. These procedures could now be performed under anesthesia, properly and painlessly, and with vastly improved results. More serious fractures in which the bones are fragmented, or comminuted, require setting and immobilization as well, but they remain contained within the unbroken skin and without risk of infection. Compound fractures are those injuries in which the broken bone pierces the skin. This represents potential catastrophe. In this pre-antiseptic, pre-antibiotic era, these injuries would nearly always result in devastating and life-threatening infection, and were often treated by immediate amputation. The actual amputation could now be performed in a more measured and respectful fashion with the patient blissfully anesthetized, but, asleep or not, the injury meant losing the limb.

Doctors still believed disease, infection, and suppuration, or "laudable pus," arose from an imbalance of humors, or just materialized spontaneously, and there was nothing one could do about it. The same magical thinking had been applied to putrefaction and spoilage of food. The first step in the climb from this deep well of ignorance was taken long ago by Francesco Redi. In 1668, Redi conducted a series of experiments in which he disproved the concept of spontaneous generation of flies and maggots in meat. He placed fresh meat or fish in jars that were either uncovered or covered with fine gauze. Meat in the uncovered jars soon became riddled with maggots and swarming with flies. Meat in gauze-covered jars remained free of maggots in the flesh and flies on the surface, though flies could be found outside the gauze screen circling the prey.

This had great implications for the sanitary preservation of food, but the concept did not carry over to medicine, where infective materials were believed to materialize spontaneously from the wounds themselves. Little thought was given to the possibility of introduction of infection from the outside, or protection from it. Suppuration was thought to be a natural consequence of wounds and a step on the road to resolution. This could mean resolution of the infection or, at the other extreme, death.

The American Civil War provided two horrific examples of the inability to understand and control these events. The two most devastating wounds a soldier could sustain were being "gut shot" or stricken with hospital gangrene. In the first instance, being shot in the abdomen meant spillage of the bowel's fecal contents into the abdominal cavity, resulting in peritonitis, and a painful death within two or three days. In the second instance, a small non–life-threatening wound would become infected in the unsanitary conditions of the hospital, tent, or whatever rudimentary facility was available to house the wounded. The wound would turn black, enlarge, and burrow under the skin, raising a horrible stench from the rotting tissue. Black spot, or hospital gangrene, typically resulted in amputation or death. In both cases, events were predictable, unpreventable, and untreatable.

This changed in 1861, when Louis Pasteur, a chemist in Paris, showed that the souring of milk was caused by bacteria and could be prevented by heat sterilization. His work not only lay to rest the idea of spontaneous generation but also placed the blame squarely on bacteria, and offered a solution, Pasteurization.

In 1878, Pasteur delivered a paper outlining the steps he would take, were he a surgeon, to prevent wound infection. Particularly prescient were his suggestions for the heat sterilization of instruments, gauze, bandages, and water used in surgery.

While Pasteur moved on and achieved worldwide fame for developing the rabies vaccine, a German physician and scientist named Robert Koch was able to cultivate the long, rod-shaped anthrax bacillus. In 1877, Koch demonstrated its life cycle, including the dormant spore form in which it was able to maintain viability for long periods until conditions were proper for conversion into the infective bacillus. His findings were celebrated, but were not universally accepted until Pasteur arrived at the same conclusions while working on an anthrax vaccine five years later.

Koch continued his work identifying organisms and correlating them with various diseases. In 1882, he arrived at what have become known as Koch's postulates, the equivalent of the Commandments of medical bacteriology. They provide the basis for proving the relationship between an organism and the disease it causes:

1. The organism can be discovered in every instance of the disease.

2. When recovered from the body, the bacteria can be repeatedly produced in pure culture.

3. The initially isolated pure culture, or its successive generations, when introduced into experimental animals can reproduce the disease.

4. The organism can be recovered from the animal and re-cultured.

Koch's clear and concise rules for identifying the cause of various infections forced even the hard-core nonscientists among physicians to take note.

In 1882, Koch identified the tubercle bacillus as the cause of tuberculosis, creating an uproar heard in scientific circles around the world. The following year he added greatly to his exalted reputation by clearly identifying another bacillus, this time the one that had caused cholera epidemics in Egypt and India, and indicted contaminated drinking water as the vehicle through which the dreaded disease was spread.

While Pasteur and Koch were inventing bacteriology, the man who would bring these concepts to life in surgery, Joseph Lister, was at work in Edinburgh and Glasgow, Scotland. Born in 1827 into a wealthy family in Upton, a Quaker community in the suburbs of London, Lister spent his youth within the insular sect in what amounted to something a bit less confining than a ghetto. Members were part of the economic fabric of the city, but they tended to intermarry and live close to their roots. Educated in London, Lister was ineligible to attend either Cambridge or Oxford since he was not a member of the Church of England. He practiced surgery in Edinburgh and Glasgow for the most productive periods of his career, and later, after achieving fame and adopting his wife's Anglican faith, he was offered the chair in surgery at King's College Hospital, London, which he accepted. He went on to become a talented and imaginative surgeon, but nothing he did as surgeon or teacher would equal the impact of introducing antisepsis to surgery.

Aware of Pasteur's work, Lister began thinking of ways to destroy germs in surgical wounds. The revolutionary idea had occurred to others, and some, including Oliver Wendell Holmes in Boston (the same Holmes who coined the term *anaesthesia*), had spoken out on the theoretical value of antiseptics, but didn't act. Only Lister saw the future and dedicated his career to it.

Since human tissue could not be heated to kill bacteria as Pasteur had done in the process that came to be called Pasteurization, Lister searched for a chemical agent to do the job. He settled on carbolic acid. Carbolic acid killed bacteria in experiments, and in dilute solution was fairly well tolerated by human tissues.

In 1865, Lister began a series of surgical experiments to test his theory. He began treating compound fractures, the devastating injury in which broken bone penetrates the skin, with carbolic preparations prior to operating, during surgery, and after surgery as well. Theories varied as to whether the inevitable bone infection was caused by humors in the ambient air or was introduced by the environment of the injury, manure being a common cause. However, no thought was given to introduction of infection from the surgeon's hands or tools as a source of contamination.

Lister's first two attempts resulted in failure. The third compound fracture, in the leg of an 11-year-old boy, was a resounding success. Carbolic acid was used to cleanse the skin and the wound and to soak the dressings. The wound healed slowly, but cleanly and completely.

From that point on, success followed success, and in 1867 Lister published his series of cases in *The Lancet,* the leading British scientific journal. Though experienced surgeons were impressed with Lister's results, there was no groundswell, no rush to adopt his techniques. Even in Glasgow and Edinburgh, where he was professor and held in the highest regard, the theory and practice of antiseptic surgery was not readily adopted. In London, both the author and his technique were met with indifference, if not open hostility.

Lister continued to believe that bacteria were in the environment as well as in the wound, and that it was imperative to infiltrate the air with antiseptic. He soon developed a carbolic spray device, which he called the carbolizer. This was placed in the operating room, near the surgical field, covering surgeon, patient, and assistants in a fine carbolic acid mist. Unpleasant as this aerosol irritant made the work environment, the number of surgical infections decreased.

In addition to the carbolizer, surgeons dipped their hands into a phenol or carbolic solution before surgery. Lister did not encourage scrubbing one's hands beyond social cleanliness, believing the process of scrubbing forced germs into the folds, lines, and crevices of the skin. Decades would pass before this position was challenged.

For generations, surgeons had entered the operating theater, unbuttoned and rolled their cuffs to keep their sleeves clean, and begun surgery. Some removed their dress coats in favor of "working coats," already blood-stained and foul from prior operations, which were stored outside the operating room. The coats were donned, the sleeves rolled, and they set to work. Today, "surgeon's sleeves" remain an arcane fashion statement, and bespoke tailors still incorporate four working buttons on suit coats.

Antiseptic surgery was far better received in Germany than at home in England and Scotland. A lecture and demonstration trip to the United States in 1886 was met with interest, but the leading surgeons of the day were unconvinced, and resistance persisted. A few young surgeons, Halsted included, subscribed to the germ theory and Lister's efforts to combat infection, and did what they could to promote its acceptance.

The carbolizer, carbolic acid dressings, and hand dip were important steps. Killing the infective bacteria, which were assumed to be everywhere, was the goal of antiseptic technique. For the truly forward-thinking surgeon the goal would become asepsis, the absence of virulent bacteria in the surgical wound and environment.[2]

---

2 Eventually, steam sterilization of tools and dressings (as predicted by Pasteur), scrupulous hand scrubbing, sterile gloves, clean if not sterile operating clothing, sterile gowns, and the concept of not bringing bacteria onto the scene became the rule. But proper standards were not strictly enforced until well into the 20th century. Today, the simple expedient of hand washing or disinfecting is often ignored. Medical personnel still go from patient to patient without washing their hands or using antibacterial compounds; hospital personnel wear operating room scrub suits in corridors, hospital rooms, and coffee shops, potentially spreading infection.

By the time William Stewart Halsted entered medical school, these two leaps forward, anesthesia and antisepsis, opened the door to the future of surgery—a future Halsted envisioned to include true aseptic surgery.

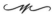

CHAPTER THREE

Physicians and Surgeons

HALSTED RETURNED HOME TO New York City in the fall of 1874 and became one of 550 young men to enroll at the College of Physicians and Surgeons at 23rd Street and Fourth Avenue. Although it was affiliated with the prestigious Columbia College, Physicians and Surgeons, like all medical schools in the country, was a business. They were in reality little more than trade schools, and the instructors benefited from the large enrollment by sharing in the revenue. Applicants did not need undergraduate degrees for entry. Lectures were poorly prepared and poorly attended. Students had little reason to take either lectures or lecturers seriously, and both jeering and snoring were common. The three-year course was almost purely didactic, and no laboratory or clinical work was required. Students did not examine patients and often did not see patients at all. Most of the faculty members were competent and high-minded, but the ultimate goal was to fill the seats and graduate doctors.

To fill the gaps in their education, most students enrolled in private tutoring sessions called quizzes. Participation in the quizzes was expensive, costing as much as $100 a year, the equivalent of more than $2,000 in current value. The annual medical school tuition of $140, or $2,800 in current value, was not much higher. Various experts, including some of the school's own lecturers, drummed facts into the heads of the medical students until they could regurgitate enough to pass their final examinations at the completion of the third year. Clinics, where students could observe doctors treating patients, were available but not required and so were infrequently attended.

Inadequate as this education was, Physicians and Surgeons was a cut above most medical schools across the country. Increasingly, schools like Physicians and Surgeons in New York and the Harvard Medical School in Boston were attempting to take science and education more seriously, but there was no consensus, no model to emulate, and they were struggling to find their way. The bacterial basis for disease was becoming clear, but most physicians were unwilling to abandon the faith of Hippocrates in the mystical balance of humors. Scientists were in the minority, and medicine was being taught largely as it had been for centuries.

Despite the dismal system that he entered, Halsted managed to ferret out the best teachers and role models. Each student at Physicians and Surgeons was assigned to a preceptor from among the faculty who would serve as his mentor. The mentoring was spread thinly, as mentors would oversee several students in each of three classes. It was up to the student to make the best of the opportunity. Halsted registered with Henry B. Sands, a surgeon and professor of anatomy, the subject that had sparked his initial interest in medicine.

From the beginning Halsted spent a great deal of time in the dissecting lab, both learning from Sands and doing his own work. Dexterous and diligent, he quickly became expert in the eyes of his fellow students and stood well above the others in the eyes of his preceptor. Sands took the opportunity to shift some of the demonstration and preparation work to his student.

John C. Dalton, whose textbook had inspired Halsted in his extracurricular reading at Yale, was also on the faculty at P&S. Dalton's interests were wide-ranging, and he studied everything from local-ization of brain functions to the physiology of digestion. The work itself was important, but Dalton's maverick scientific approach was a groundbreaking example of the experimental model. His students were taught to perform animal and human experiments and observe the physiological responses to stimuli. Traditionally, instructors would simply tell students what the expected response would be. Dalton taught the students to stimulate a muscle, measure the response, and learn cause and effect. This method would become the model for medical teaching in the future, and it made a lasting impression on young Halsted. He began spending increasing portions of his day in the physiology laboratory, ultimately becoming Dalton's primary assistant and an expert in the use of the experimental model.

It was a perfect beginning. In the nurturing hands of Dalton and Sands, Halsted was excited by his work. Attending lectures, reading, and doing dissections with Sands and experiments with Dalton was a full load, but he was energized by the demands. Intentionally or not, Halsted had the ability to associate himself with the important figures in his world. Later in life, when roles were reversed, Professor Halsted's radar would be finely tuned against young surgeons seeking his good graces, unfailingly cutting them off at the knees.

In his second year at Physicians and Surgeons, he began conduct-ing chemical tests in the office of Dr. Alonzo Clark. Clark was presi-dent of the medical school, a professor of pathology and of the practice of medicine, and the leading medical consultant in the city.

In the summer of 1875, Halsted befriended Thomas McBride. McBride, several years his senior, was already physician-in-chief at the Centre Street Dispensary, where Halsted spent the summer working in the pharmacy learning about the potions, plasters, pills, and tonics popularly used at the time. McBride was a fun-loving, handsome man-about-town, and very successful in his practice. He earned a great deal of money and spent it lavishly, and in some ways served as a role model for the younger man. They spent a great deal of time together, and their lives became closely intertwined.

With his interest focusing on anatomy and surgery, Halsted seized every opportunity for dissection, spending many hours at the table. Having access to adequate finances, he bought extra cadavers, which he dissected and studied well beyond the level required of students.

At the completion of his second year, the hard work and extracurricular activities were finally getting the better of him. Exhausted, he retired to Block Island, one of the rugged and isolated dots of terminal moraine off the coast of Rhode Island. There he spent the summer of 1876 recuperating.

Reinvigorated by sailing and fresh air, Halsted soon returned to his studies in the evenings and decided to prepare for the examination for an intern position at Bellevue Hospital in New York. The possibility excited him, but the rules for internship at Bellevue had just changed, and interns were now required to have already earned an MD degree. Despite this new requirement, Halsted decided to pursue the opportunity, and though he had some difficulty convincing his professors to allow him to sit for the examination, his dogged persistence won out.

"I had little expectation of being admitted to Bellevue for I was ineligible, not having a medical degree, nor had I taken the cram quiz," Halsted wrote. Tanned and fit from his summer in the sun, "I recall contrasting my physical condition with that of the other fellows who presented themselves for this examination. Most of them were pale and nervous having remained in town all summer for the cram Quizzes." He took the exam "as something of a lark," knowing that if he failed he could take it again in the spring. To everyone's surprise, he placed fifth, and though technically unqualified, he was offered the position, which he happily accepted. Halsted later said that the good news had resulted in one of the few sleepless nights of his life, which he spent contemplating the boundless opportunities of his future.

The internship at Bellevue began on October 1, 1876. Halsted was assigned to the fourth surgical division, although he "would have preferred the second surgical, on which Thomas A. Sabine was visiting surgeon." Sabine and Stephen Smith were among the few surgeons in New York who enthusiastically embraced Lister's antiseptic surgery. Halsted was convinced of the importance of the concept, if not of Lister's specific techniques, and working with believers was where he wanted to be. But the coveted position with Sabine went to Halsted's friend Samuel Van der Poel. One year ahead of Halsted at P&S, Van der Poel had done poorly in his first attempt at the Bellevue exam the previous year, but after intensive coaching by Halsted, he performed better than his tutor and won the prized position. The two young men were off to Bellevue.

The senior surgeons at Bellevue were a mixed lot. Halsted studied with many of the great ones, but he also encountered many who "left everything to the interns." His immediate superiors, led by famed Civil War surgeon Dr. Frank Hamilton, did not subscribe to Lister's antiseptic techniques, but they were open-minded enough to allow interns to adopt the new method. Those interns who did so noted a significant reduction in postoperative infection, but their findings had no effect on hospital policy.

Hamilton was one of the stars of Halsted's Bellevue experience. An army surgeon who had commanded the field hospital at the first battle of Bull Run, Hamilton cut a dashing figure in riding boots and spurs, arriving dramatically each day on a large, iron-gray charger. An expert in skin grafting, his primary interest was treating fractures, about which he had written a textbook. Surgical intervention to treat disease was not yet a reality and was limited to attempting to stem the damage of traumatic injury, and trauma meant fractures. Not quite convinced of the usefulness of Lister's new ideas, Hamilton examined patients and operated bare-handed, without washing or decontaminating his hands after his horseback ride to work.

Bellevue was a very busy place, and interns worked a grueling seven-day week. They were a small, close-knit group, helping one another, spelling one another to attend surgery, and spending what little free time they had talking surgery. Looking old beyond their years, they were generally men from affluent families and arrived at work dressed no differently than bankers. Halsted favored wing collars, waistcoats, and wide cravats. Most smoked, and those who did smoked freely at work. This was particularly true during anatomical dissections in the dead house, or morgue, where, before refrigeration, smoking provided a defense against the noxious odors of decomposing flesh. The only area off-limits for smoking was the operating theater, but this was only because of the explosive nature of gaseous ether.

During Halsted's seven-month internship, there were only 95 patients admitted to the fourth surgical division. Of these, 50 had simple fractures and dislocations. Few elective operations were attempted, for even clean surgical incisions were likely to become infected and result in death. Already contaminated wounds such as compound fractures were doomed to infection and amputation. The fear of infection loomed everywhere, and abdominal surgery remained so risky that even appendectomies had not yet been performed. The diagnosis of perityphlitis, as appendicitis was then called, was made clinically, but nothing could be done other than confirming it at autopsy. Under the best of circumstances an abscess developed around the infected appendix, which could be successfully drained. In some cases the natural body defenses and the large fatty apron in the abdomen called the omentum helped wall off the infection. These defenses, combined with prompt drainage, managed to control the infection and might allow the patient to survive. Often, when the appendix burst and overwhelming peritonitis developed, the less lucky patient died, as expected.

At the completion of his premature internship in May 1877, Halsted returned to finish his final year of medical school and prepare for examinations. He finished in the top ten students of the class, was graduated with honors, and qualified for the honors essay contest. Halsted spent the entire three hours on a single question: the description of the arteries of the neck. It was as if the young anatomist had written his own question. In a final coup for the student who had shown no academic aptitude before finding medicine, he won the contest and the $100 prize.

CHAPTER FOUR

Becoming a Surgeon

T O GAIN FURTHER EXPERIENCE, Halsted took a newly created
position as house physician at New York Hospital. It was not a
surgical post, but at least he would be able to learn more of the ins and
outs of a doctor's work in a hospital setting.

New York Hospital, chartered by King George III in 1771, was the
second oldest hospital in the nation. From inception it was an important local institution, and its governors were the leaders of the New
York business and social worlds. Halsted's father and grandfather were
members of the board of governors and significant financial supporters
of the hospital. An uncle, Thaddeus Halsted, had been an attending
surgeon at the hospital as well, so the Halsted name was anything
but unknown when the young physician sought employment. Halsted
always claimed to have taken a competitive exam to win the position,
but New York Hospital records make no mention of an examination
ever being offered. The medical wards of the new hospital building were
about to open, and based on a glowing recommendation from Dr. Henry
Sands, the board of governors ordered "Dr. William S. Halsted, late
house physician at Bellevue hospital," appointed without delay.

In March 1877, the new hospital opened. A six-story, neo-Gothic
brick building, it occupied the entire block between 15th and 16th

streets and Fifth and Sixth avenues. It was said to be at the cutting edge of hospital design. A decade earlier, the tragic conditions of the Civil War underlined the need for a sanitary environment, good ventilation, and adequate heating in hospitals. A report in *Harper's Weekly* said of the new building:

> Various appliances said to be available in no other public hospital in the world have been introduced, which add to the comfort of the patients and reduce at the same time the labor of attendants. Bell wires and speaking tubes are placed throughout the building, and two elevators run from the basement to the top story . . . . Bars will be placed over beds offering patients able to take advantage of them the means of shifting their positions without assistance.

Many of the faculty members of the College of Physicians and Surgeons used New York Hospital for their patients, and Halsted was happy to find himself among familiar faces. Though he was house "physician," he utilized the opportunity to attend conferences, observe surgeries that interested him, and continue his relationship with the professors he admired from his student days. Fascinated by the clinical and surgical challenges around him, he studied every aspect of hospital life and questioned everything he saw.

Clinical progress notes were made in longhand in the physician's recording book. All entries were made by the same man, and since hospitalizations were usually long, the notes read like an epic novel. There were no laboratory tests to scan daily, so the only recognizable signs of change were the patient's appearance and the chart of vital signs: pulse, temperature, and number of breaths per minute. Blood pressure monitoring would not be invented until the turn of the 20th century. This graphic record of vital signs was then made available on the bedside chart. While still a junior staff member, Halsted redesigned the patient's bedside chart to include color-coded graphs of temperature and pulse, marked by joined dots. This made changes in the pattern of vital signs quickly apparent. Halsted had these charts lithographed and provided them for use at the hospital.[1]

While he spent as much time as possible observing surgery, it became clear that little more could be learned under a stagnant system with no organized postgraduate training. He made it his business to read the flood of new surgical papers coming from the European capitals where the leading professors and practitioners held forth. Great strides were being taken in Germany, Austria, Switzerland, and Great Britain; barely the smallest steps were being made at home. Observing these great men at work was the most desirable training available. With the indulgence of his proud father, Halsted set off to spend two years traveling through Europe, availing himself of the best that surgery had to offer.

* * *

GIVEN THE RIGOROUS track of modern surgical training, it is difficult to imagine the haphazard state of higher education in Halsted's time. Formal surgical training simply did not exist in America. Young surgeons, at least those with the means, would seek out this or that great European surgeon, brush up on the language, study the written works of the master surgeon, present himself, and proceed to shadow the master through clinics and surgeries. Experiences varied. Sometimes the visitor could ask questions, sometimes he was permitted to assist at surgery, and sometimes he was lost in the gallery, unable to see much more than the surgeon's back and an occasional glimpse of the procedure.

---

1 Some evidence exists that the Halsted charts were abandoned shortly after his tenure, though they do show up later, both at the New York Hospital and at Johns Hopkins. Others believe that the now ubiquitous bedside chart is the direct result of Halsted's innovation.

Halsted had performed well and was fairly well connected in the New York medical establishment, and he was easily able to secure the proper letters of introduction for access to European surgical circles. Financed by his father, he sailed for France. Arriving in Paris in the fall of 1878, Halsted was met by several New York friends, including his P&S chum Samuel Van der Poel, who had been studying in Germany. The two young doctors planned to travel and study together for the next several months.

The trip got off to a bad start, and they aborted their stay in Paris after only a few days. The New York friends hosting them were anything but serious, intent only on squiring them to local hot spots. After a night in Montmartre, and too many bars and cafés, the new arrivals were already worn down. They had little interest in nightlife, and promptly packed up and left for Vienna.

Arriving by train on November 4, the two young men threw themselves into their studies. The first task was to become fluent in German. Halsted was capable enough in the scientific German needed for medical reading, but the living language was another matter. He engaged two tutors, took German lessons early and late in the day, and in between studied pathology; diseases of the eye, ear, and skin; and gynecology. His German was soon passable, and he took every opportunity to speak it instead of English whenever he could.

Still interested in anatomy, he studied with the notoriously standoffish Professor Emil Zuckerkandl. In a stroke of good fortune for Halsted, Zuckerkandl developed a painful inflammation of the epididymis, and asked the young surgeon to care for him. Halsted applied a poultice of iodoform ointment to the professor's scrotum, which brought relief. Thereafter, said Zuckerkandl, Halsted "was invited to do all my dissection in his private room to which no one else was admitted." Access to fresh bodies for dissection in the pre-refrigeration era was still a difficult hurdle, and he now had bodies available straight from the morgue, as well as the professor's full attention whenever he needed it. It was an anatomist's dream, and Halsted made the best of it.

Knowing little neuroanatomy, Halsted persuaded Professor Theodor Meynert to tutor him on the dissection of the brain. The sessions took place at 6 A.M., before Halsted's pre-breakfast German lesson. It was not a pleasant experience.

"He was always in bed on my arrival and the lesson was given in his unsavory bedroom," Halsted wrote. It was not long before Professor Meynert was "released from the contract."

Giving up on neuroanatomy, Halsted began work in the new science of embryology, which was attempting to explain the origin and relationship of body parts by studying the differentiation of fetal cells from fertilization through birth. The new science captured his imagination, but it did not supplant surgery.

He also made the acquaintance of two men with whom he felt instantly close: Anton Wölfler, whose work on surgery of the thyroid gland particularly interested Halsted, and Johannes von Mikulicz, a Polish-born contemporary of Halsted's who would gain great fame as a pioneer of abdominal surgery. Both were serving long assistantships under the acknowledged master, Professor Theodor Billroth, the most famous surgeon in Europe. Billroth was known as an accomplished musician as well and was the closest friend of Johannes Brahms, who dedicated two string quartets to him.

Among his surgical contributions were the first excision of a rectal cancer, the first laryngectomy, and the first successful gastrectomy to treat stomach cancer. Billroth was an early subscriber to Lister's antiseptic techniques, and pioneered abdominal surgery adventurously but with careful preparation. As a believer in long and intensive surgical training, his graduate doctors served two or three years as apprentices doing hospital care and anatomical dissections, followed by numerous assistant years during which they performed surgery and studied the surgical literature. Everything about the experience was stimulating, and Halsted found a regular place in the amphitheater observing the master at work.

The new discipline of abdominal surgery with attention to hemostasis (control of bleeding) and antiseptic technique, use of the animal lab, and Billroth's concept of surgical training left their mark on young Halsted. They would all resurface at Johns Hopkins a decade later.

IN THE SPRING of 1879 Halsted left Vienna to study embryology in Wurzburg, and then went on to Liverpool, where he would join his parents and siblings and travel with them for the summer. Halsted looked forward to the reunion and the respite from constant study. With his father's permission, he invited Samuel Van der Poel to join the family traveling party. The trip was a great success, and by summer's end Van der Poel had become engaged to marry the youngest Halsted daughter, Minnie.

Returning to Vienna in the fall, Halsted continued his studies with Richard von Volkmann, another proponent of aseptic surgery and a pioneer of joint and extremity surgery; Johannes Friedrich von Esmarch, a German military surgeon who instituted training in first aid for civilian and military personnel, and introduced the use of the first-aid bandage on the battlefield and a surgical tourniquet that allowed a bloodless field for extremity surgery; and Karl Thiersch, who is credited with having invented skin grafting. All three surgeons are still known for work they did more than 100 years ago. On his two-year learning tour, Halsted had yet again managed to find himself in very accomplished company.

He took up residence with two other men in a boardinghouse, where they took their meals. The arrangement forced them to speak German all day. Although he never mentions women in his journals and letters home, he referred to his Vienna housemate, George Dixon, as a very attractive man who became involved with numerous women and whose charm opened many doors for the trio.

Another American friend who had joined him in Leipzig soon fell ill with typhoid. One day Halsted was called to see him by the attending nurse, who anxiously reported the patient's pulse had risen to 200. Halsted was stymied. His friend looked well enough, and his pulse was quite normal. Apparently, the nurse, who didn't have a watch, held his wrist to count pulse beats while the patient was instructed to count out loud to 60, to determine the number of pulse beats in a minute. His German was halting and he counted very slowly. Halsted later commented, "This was beyond his powers and I have never understood why the nurse stopped counting at two hundred."

The final stop on the tour was to study with Karl Thiersch, who introduced the split-thickness skin graft in 1874. Halsted found most of Thiersch's operations "minor," and knowing that his friend Frank Hamilton of Bellevue had been performing skin grafts for years, he was unimpressed.

In early September 1880, Halsted sailed for New York, ready to begin his career.

CHAPTER FIVE

New York

THAT SEPTEMBER, HALSTED WAS 28 years old and in physically fine shape, though his muscular upper body was perhaps a bit broader from two years of heavy dining and little or no exercise. His fine, light hair, now thin to the point of baldness on top, was cut short at the sides, further accentuating his prominent ears. No longer clean-shaven, he sported a close-cropped beard and was, as always, immaculately groomed. He was charged with energy and ideas, and couldn't wait to get to work.

Not fully accepting the need for the carbolizer, or the idea that the danger of germs was in the ambient air, Halsted and a colleague worked hard to modify Lister's technique and institute the scrubbing and chemical decontamination of hands and tools before operating.

He renewed contact with his medical school preceptor, Henry Sands, who invited him to join his practice at Roosevelt Hospital. Sands was an important man in New York. He covered a busy surgical service at Roosevelt, had a large private practice, and was professor of private practice and anatomy at P&S. Having the tireless Halsted to share the load would be a great help.

Sands encouraged Halsted to operate on any cases that interested him and allowed him to purchase new equipment for the surgical service. The surprised staff had no idea what to do with the large number of fine artery forceps that soon arrived from Germany. The purchase had come about as a direct result of observing Billroth carefully clamping and tying blood vessels to prevent hemorrhage. This procedure amazed Halsted, as it seemed so logical and proper. Few American surgeons bothered with the time-consuming technique, but it soon became a religion to Halsted.

Although he spent long hours operating and assisting, it became apparent that Roosevelt needed a clinic to care for nonoperative cases, minor surgical cases not requiring hospitalization, and follow-up patients. Halsted suggested the idea to Sands, who helped convince the trustees of its potential usefulness. He was given rooms in the hospital basement, buried deep among the gas and water pipes. Early each morning, Sundays included, Halsted hailed a horse-drawn cab at 25th Street, where he had set up house with his friend Thomas McBride, and made the two-mile trip to 59th Street and Ninth Avenue. His outpatient clinic was an immediate success. Soon the hospital devoted an entire floor of a new building to it. Roosevelt Hospital's reputation was growing, and the physical plant was growing with it. Plans went forward to add two floors of opulent private rooms for wealthy patients above a new outpatient building. These rooms and suites would cost $25 to $75 per night, depending on size and furnishing, and they would help defray the cost of the primary mission of the hospital, which was the 180-bed charity ward.

Halsted worked in the hospital laboratory as well as in the clinic and operating room. There he devised a successful irrigation treatment for gonorrhea, washing out the infected urethra with dilute disinfecting solution, counting the reduced numbers of gonococcus organisms, and establishing a successful therapy for a ubiquitous disease. Half a century before the advent of antibiotics, any relief at all was welcome. The work did much to raise Halsted's stock at Roosevelt, but his procedure was not generally adopted by the medical community, where it was thought excessively time-consuming, a judgment that would be applied to much of Halsted's future work.

Sands thought enough of the 28-year-old to invite him to share his teaching responsibilities as well. He had neither the time nor inclination to prepare dissections for his lectures at P&S, so this fell to Halsted, who took great pleasure in the work. Throughout the school year he spent long hours strutting through the dissecting room among the partially dismembered bodies; in shirtsleeves, pince-nez glasses, and high hat, he inspired students with his knowledge and enthusiasm as he demonstrated the intricacies of human anatomy.

He took a position as visiting physician at the city hospital on Blackwell's Island (now Roosevelt Island) and at Emigrant Hospital on Ward's Island, both located in New York's East River. Most of his duties at these hospitals were carried out at night, since, as he later wrote, "few hours by day were unoccupied."

Halsted held these charity hospitals in high regard and was full of praise for the staff physicians. Allen M. Thomas, the obstetrician at Emigrant Hospital, was said to have reduced maternal mortality at childbirth from 25 percent to ½ of 1 percent. Most maternal fatalities were due to puerperal fever, a virulent infection spread by physicians with unclean hands performing bare-handed vaginal examinations and deliveries. It was not a new problem. In Vienna in 1847, Ignaz Semmelweis had noted that the maternal mortality rate at the Wiener Allegemeines Krankenhaus (Vienna General Hospital) was much higher in the wards where doctors coming from morgue dissections and surgery performed bare-handed exams and deliveries than they were on the ward where deliveries were done by midwives, who had no such duties. This was before Lister and Pasteur and germ theory, yet Semmelweis believed some sort of invisible infective particles were being transferred to the susceptible mother. He found that by having those on his service wash their hands with a chlorine solution, maternal mortality rates plummeted from 18.2 percent to 1.2 percent. Sadly,

Semmelweis's work was largely ignored until after his death in 1865. Prior to Thomas's precautions, the statistics at the Emigrant Hospital had been significantly worse than those in Vienna, and the eradication of puerperal fever in America similarly parallels the grudging acceptance of antiseptic techniques.

* * *

DURING THIS PERIOD Halsted shared a house with his friend Thomas McBride on 25th Street between Madison and Fourth avenues at fashionable Madison Square, just a short walk from his parents' home at 14th Street and Fifth Avenue. It was also conveniently located around the corner from the University Club, where he spent time with friends, frequently dined, and sometimes bowled ten-pins. The house was large, stylish, lavishly appointed for entertaining, and included medical offices for the wealthy young men. Together, they gave small dinner parties several times a week and entertained bright young professional men like themselves. There was always food and drink enough for unexpected guests, and visits were encouraged. Halsted's closest friend, William Welch—a pathologist at Bellevue, faculty member at Bellevue Medical College, and the man who had begun the nation's first pathology laboratory—was a frequent visitor.

Halsted was always central to the fun. Vivacious and amusing, he was unfailingly thoughtful and extremely well-mannered. He might have an occasional glass of wine, but he was anything but a drinker. His only vice, it would seem, was the endless stream of carefully rolled cigarettes he smoked in inexpensive white holders. These were purchased by the hundreds and disposed of the instant a sign of tarnish or wear appeared. The details of running the house were largely his concern, and everything was properly arranged for entertaining, even on those Sunday afternoons when the furniture was repositioned to accommodate an audience for concerts given by male singing quartets.

Madison Square was central to the changing city. New elevated railroad lines were running on Second and Third avenues, the latter even operating trains through the night. Electric lights were installed along Broadway from 14th Street to Madison Square, with the final light in the center of the small park. The area was a showplace for Thomas Edison, who purchased a four-story house on Fifth Avenue and 14th Street, a few doors from Halsted's parents. Edison outfitted the house with 100 electric bulbs, and kept it lit night and day to give the public a taste of the future. The first telephones became operational that year and boasted 252 early subscribers. Soon, new telephone companies cropped up to meet the booming demand.

* * *

HALSTED'S WORKDAY WAS staggering: early morning at the Roosevelt Hospital outpatient clinic, daily surgeries, patient care at several hospitals, instructing and dissecting in the anatomy lab, and frequent trips to the charity hospitals to consult and operate. Several of the hospitals he attended were within walking distance of Madison Square; others, particularly the charity hospitals, required time-consuming transportation. In addition to these responsibilities, he and several colleagues organized a quiz for P&S medical students. Students entering the quiz were required to have bachelor's degrees, making the standards for entry higher than those of the medical school. Determined to encourage real learning in addition to the rote memorization and regurgitation they had endured, Halsted and his colleagues began assembling a faculty interested in expanding the students' knowledge. Many of the quizmasters were P&S instructors, but they were chosen carefully and were primarily younger faculty members. Outside faculty was sought as well. The star among them all was William Welch.

Just two years older than Halsted, Welch had already earned a significant reputation. At the quiz he not only lectured the students on histology and pathology, but also allowed them access to his laboratory and freedom to observe his processes in action. Most important, he provided a wealth of autopsy material—cadavers—for study.

Some 25 or 30 medical students, and at one point up to 65, met several evenings a week. The locale was usually Halsted's office in his 25th Street residence, with side trips to Welch's pathology laboratory. As was standard, the fee for the course of study was $100 a person. The fee always struck Halsted as excessive, but they accepted the money.

Teaching anatomy and surgery, Halsted was a walking, talking *Gray's Anatomy* textbook. His knowledge was so encyclopedic that students made a game of trying to catch him in mistakes, but his command of the anatomy and near-photographic recall of *Gray's* always seemed to carry the day. On one occasion when he challenged a student's answer, they went to *Gray's*, where the student was surprisingly upheld.

"Wait a minute, I'm sure *Gray* gave it my way in the edition I studied," Halsted said. Out came the older edition of *Gray's*, which was exactly as Halsted had remembered.

He was idolized by the students and, in turn, was dedicated to seeing them succeed. Graduates of Halsted's quiz invariably did well in their exams and often occupied the first ten places in the medical school graduating class, a feat that brought him considerable joy and the quiz great popularity.

Halsted quickly earned a reputation as a bright and aggressive surgeon, and his practice prospered. He analyzed situations differently from those around him, acted quickly, and often followed an unorthodox course of action. In 1881, he made medical history by performing the first emergency blood transfusion, under extraordinary circumstances. He was in Albany visiting his youngest sister, Minnie, just as she was giving birth to her first child. Her husband, Sam Van der Poel, came happily downstairs from the bedroom to greet his old friend and announce the birth of a healthy baby boy. Normally following delivery, the stretched and torn muscles of the uterus contract, and bleeding ceases. Minnie continued to hemorrhage. Twenty minutes later, Halsted was called to his sister's bedside in consultation. Van der Poel, Halsted, and the attending physician tried controlling the hemorrhage with ice-water douches, pressure, and packing. Finding Minnie "ghastly white, quite pulseless and almost unconscious," Halsted drew blood with a syringe from his own veins and injected it directly into his sister's vein, possibly saving her life.

The identification of the ABO blood groups by Karl Landsteiner would not occur until 1900, but Halsted hinted at some early insight into the risk of blood group incompatibility, saying, "This was taking a great risk but she was so nearly moribund that I ventured it and with prompt result." He left no clue about the volume of transfusion. A small volume of transfused blood would have been unlikely to turn the tide, and a significant transfusion would have required more than simply drawing and transferring a syringe or two of blood. Minnie Halsted Van der Poel was a lucky woman, as mismatched blood might have killed her.

Halsted's interest in transfusion led him to focus his efforts on a common condition of the day, illuminating gas poisoning. The first residential electric lights became available in New York City in 1882, but consumers had to be within a one-mile radius of Thomas Edison's direct-current generating plant on Pearl Street in order to receive service. It would be another decade before alternating current, which could transmit current farther, became generally available. Meanwhile, homes, businesses, and streets continued to be illuminated with gas, and a by-product of burning gas was carbon monoxide. Workers exposed to illuminating gas were often acutely poisoned by it, particularly in confined spaces like the gaslit night boats plying the rivers. In the emergency ward at the Chambers Street Hospital, Halsted devised a procedure called centripetal transfusion, in which the patient's blood was removed, aerated, and returned to the donor. Aeration removed carbon monoxide from its combination with hemoglobin and allowed the hemoglobin to combine with oxygen from the air. Halsted believed it was preferable to retransfuse the blood into an artery rather than a vein, so that it would go "against the stream and not mix with other blood and cause gangrene of the extremity." Whether arterial retransfusion was of any particular value is debatable, but the blood's renewed ability to carry oxygen cleared the acute toxicity and patients recovered rapidly.

A year after transfusing his sister, Halsted received the telegram summoning him to Albany to see his moribund mother, whose condition had so mystified her doctors, including Halsted's housemate Thomas McBride, under whose care she had been. Dramatic as operating on his own mother on the kitchen table would seem, the finest surgical suites of the day were not much better equipped, and it was common for visiting surgeons to operate in patients' homes. Tools were rudimentary, sterility was in its infancy, and anesthesia was administered by untrained assistants or bystanders.

By 1882, things were beginning to change. Henry Sands was named sole attending surgeon to Roosevelt Hospital, and Halsted, assistant to the attending surgeon. For the first time, a single surgeon was given the responsibility of overseeing a department of surgery. Roosevelt Hospital had been founded with a bequest from James Roosevelt, an uncle of Theodore Roosevelt. It was privately funded and open to all patients regardless of their ability to pay. At the time it may well have been the finest hospital in New York City.

Halsted was soon named to the staff of both the Presbyterian Hospital, the New York Hospital, and the Chambers Street Hospital, and was now actively working at five hospitals, consulting, operating, and teaching. In 1883, he became visiting physician to Bellevue, the very busy city hospital where teaching was held in high regard. It was here that Welch had established the first surgical pathology lab. The availability of teaching material at Bellevue was perhaps the greatest in the city. For a young surgeon eager to innovate, operate, and teach, this was a significant career opportunity. Halsted had had Bellevue in his sights ever since the joyful, sleepless night he was accepted for internship.

Happy to return, but finding the operating conditions unacceptable, Halsted requested a modern operating room be built for his sole use. This was an outrageous request from a young man in practice barely three years. His proposal was promptly denied for lack of funds and conflict with the hospital charter.

Unwilling to abandon the idea, Halsted raised $10,000 from family and friends, secured a site on the Bellevue grounds, and had an elaborate tent constructed. Designed by an architect, the tent was large, fully enclosed, and heated. The floor was constructed with tightly laid maple, much like a bowling alley, and sloped gently toward gutters for drainage and cleaning. Skylights were built into the roof, hot and cold running water were provided, as was gas for light, heating, and sterilizing instruments. In 1885, this tent at Bellevue Hospital was perhaps the most modern operating room in the country.

However, Halsted would work in his new operating room for only a few months, as his life was about to take a drastic turn.

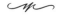

CHAPTER SIX

Cocaine

IN APRIL 1884, an impoverished young physician in Vienna named Sigmund Freud wrote the Merck Company of Darmstadt, Germany, to inquire about purchasing a gram of their newly available cocaine alkaloid. Shocked at the cost of three gulden, 33 kreuzer—ten times what he had expected to pay (about $1.27 U.S. at the time)—Freud was so excited about the experimental possibilities that he made the purchase anyway. He would worry about finding money to pay for it later. He had been reading a great deal about the unique stimulant properties of the drug, which was said to enable German soldiers to fight like supermen without sleep. Abstinence from food was possible for days without feeling hunger, and users reported a mild euphoria and general sense of well-being. The substance, long used by South American Indians in religious rituals, had recently been extracted from the coca leaf by Merck chemists and made available for sale.

Having only recently entered practice, Freud was constantly searching for a way to make his mark. He was engaged to marry his beloved Martha Bernays, and frustrated by his inability to earn enough money to support them. His fledgling neurology practice was not yet busy, and his experimental work, though significant, had not yet been noticed. As a laboratory scientist, he had already developed a method for staining nerve fibers with gold, which would later prove to be an important contribution to neuropathology. Meanwhile, Freud was suffering from depression, both psychological and situational.

As an alkaloid that lent itself readily to solution in alcohol, the new drug was fairly easy to deal with. Freud carefully calibrated dosages and reactions in animals and human volunteers, primarily himself. Astounded by the elation he felt shortly after using the drug, he praised it in letters to Martha and referred to it as a "magical drug" in conversation with colleagues. When feeling depressed he found that a small dose left him euphoric and exhilarated yet in every other way normal, and without a craving for more.

Among the friends he introduced to the new drug was Dr. Ernst von Fleischl-Marxow, who had developed a morphine addiction from the treatment of neurological pain. Freud's idea was to substitute cocaine for morphine and break the addiction. Fleischl began using enormous amounts of cocaine, often as much as a gram a day. These were massive doses by Freud's standards; he himself had been using occasional injections of 50 milligrams, one-twentieth of a gram. Fleischl became severely addicted and, to Freud's dismay, developed a full-blown cocaine psychosis: "white snakes creeping over his skin," paranoia, disorientation, and a full separation from reality.

But this was the only bad reaction Freud observed in the early days. Others, using smaller amounts, found the drug cured colds or at least dried up the sniffles, boosted energy levels, cured nervous exhaustion, and allegedly sharpened the senses. It became a pleasant recreational tool.

Freud, meanwhile, had noted that when taken orally the drug caused a numbness of the lips and tongue. He injected himself in an attempt to cause localized anesthesia, but because of his imprecise knowledge of the anatomy the experiments proved unsuccessful. He abandoned the idea of injection but remained steadfast in his belief that anesthetic possibilities existed. Freud mentioned his suspicions to an ophthalmologist friend, Leopold Königstein, and encouraged him to experiment with cocaine to relieve the pain of trachoma, a common agonizing infection caused by poor sanitation and hygiene that often led to blindness. Königstein found treatment with cocaine controlled the pain of trachoma as well as several other eye ailments, and the experiment was considered a great success.

Freud performed experiments with an ophthalmology intern to determine whether the sense of increased physical strength associated with cocaine was objective or subjective. The intern, Carl Koller, noticed, as had the others, that the drug caused numbness of the mucous membranes. While Freud and Königstein were dealing with the drug's various therapeutic properties, Koller began experimenting with cocaine as a topical anesthetic for eye surgery. He was not alone in understanding what might be possible, but he was alone in testing it, using it, and writing about it.

In July 1884, Freud published his quickly written but comprehensive paper on the history and properties of cocaine. In the last paragraph he mentions that "cocaine and its salts have a marked anesthetizing effect when brought in contact with the skin and mucous membrane in concentrated solution; this property suggests its occasional use as a local anesthetic."

By September, Koller was testing the anesthetic properties for surgery on the eyes of animals, and then humans. It worked. On September 15, Koller sent a communication to the Ophthalmological Congress meeting in Heidelberg, and on October 17 read a paper on his findings in Vienna. Freud and Königstein soon began similar testing of topical cocaine for eye surgery, but it was too little too late. Koller gracefully credited his interest in working with cocaine to Freud, but the great discovery and international fame went to Koller. Freud was surprisingly sanguine about the whole issue, blaming himself for missing the forest for the trees, and for laziness in not pursuing every avenue.

ON OCTOBER 11, Dr. Henry Noyes, who attended the congress in Heidelberg, published a report of Koller's work in the *New York Medical Record*. Reading this, Halsted saw the possibilities for the use of cocaine as a local anesthetic in surgery.

As was his routine, each morning Halsted attended the "outdoor clinic" at Roosevelt Hospital, the equivalent of today's ambulatory or outpatient clinic. Chatting with his first assistant, Frank Hartley; second assistant, Richard J. Hall, with whom he had studied in Vienna; and third assistant, George Brewer, he suggested they conduct some experiments. Coca extract was already in everything from tonics to Coca-Cola. In America, the Parke, Davis and Company had begun extraction and distribution, and was selling coca-leaf cigarettes, elixirs, nasal sprays, and injections. Cocaine powder was being used as snuff and in dilute solutions as a tonic. The talk of superhuman strength crossed the Atlantic. An apocryphal story circulated about a confrontation between a group of southern blacks and police in which the rioters were so supercharged on cocaine that they could not be brought down by the .32-caliber bullets routinely used by police. Police forces around the country switched to .38-caliber pistols for their greater stopping power based on an incident that never occurred.

There were some anecdotal reports of addiction, but Halsted's decision on that morning in late October 1884 to begin experimenting with cocaine was neither rash nor without a reasonable possibility of success.

The human nervous system is made up of two portions. The central nervous system which is comprised of the brain and spinal cord, and the peripheral nervous system comprised of sensory and motor nerves. Motor nerves receive impulses from the central nervous system and relay them to the muscles, initiating movement. Sensory nerves bring sensations such as pain, heat, and cold from body parts such as skin, teeth, or joints to the brain for interpretation. Scratch your cheek, and the sensation is read by a sensory nerve ending that carries the sensation along its branch to its trunk, through the cheek-bone and ultimately to the brain for interpretation. It's just a scratch, and so it feels benign, like a scratch. But if a surgeon cuts through the same skin of your cheek with a scalpel, the sensory nerve carries the sensation to the brain, where it is interpreted as pain.

Halsted, like Freud before him, postulated that if one could inject a numbing substance into a sensory nerve it would block sensation in all the skin served by the branches of that nerve. Cocaine numbed the conjunctiva and cornea of the eye; Koller had just proven that. Why then would it not numb the branches of peripheral nerves?

Halsted knew the anatomy. He had memorized *Gray's Anatomy* and dissected out all the little nerve branches on all those bodies in the morgue. He knew where to find the accessible sensory nerves. He would inject cocaine into the sensory nerve and block the transmission of the pain sensation to the brain. No sensory transmission, no pain.

Koller's paper had been delivered on October 17. Within two weeks, Halsted acquired a supply of 4 percent cocaine solution from Parke, Davis and Company, and began testing his hypothesis with a group of 25 or 30 medical students from P&S. The students were easily enlisted, since Halsted was their preceptor. The experiments began in the early evenings, during the quiz at the Madison Square house. Halsted systematically injected every nerve he could locate. He quickly discovered that cocaine injected into a large nerve trunk on the leg would induce anesthesia everywhere below the injection, along the distribution of the nerve, but caused no change in sensation above the point of injection. When the needle was inserted accurately and struck the nerve, the subject felt a sharp shooting pain from the point of entry down the extremity encompassing the area from which the nerve delivered sensation. An injection made through the skin into the subcutaneous tissue near the nerve but not into the nerve itself would not cause the shooting pain, but did result in anesthesia for several inches below the site of injection. The results were predictable in the arm, leg, face, and wherever the path of a sensory nerve was known.

Their success at inducing local anesthesia exceeded all expectations, but there were side effects. Several minutes after a trial injection, Hall reported feeling giddy. He soon became disoriented and nauseated, his skin dripped with perspiration, and his pupils dilated widely. The symptoms persisted for 20 minutes and abated at about the same time the anesthesia wore off. The predictable combination of unpleasant symptoms was observed repeatedly during the first few weeks of experiments, and strategies were considered to make the process less forbidding.

In succeeding trials, Halsted decreased the concentration of the cocaine solution and was able to achieve equally potent, and predictable, local numbness of the tissue without the profound side effects. Carrying this to the ultimate dilution, he began injecting water into the skin. When the skin was fully distended with water, it became briefly numb. Halsted attributed this to the effect of volume blocking sensation in a small area of skin. He also found he could increase the duration of anesthesia by using a tourniquet to prevent the cocaine being flushed away by the circulating blood. The technique also lessened generalized symptoms by keeping the drug localized.[1]

Halsted postulated that blocking the inferior dental nerve, which was easily located as it exited the jaw, would provide a pain-free field for dental work on the lower jaw. Blocking the infraorbital nerve branches, which exited from the cheekbone beneath the eye, could provide anesthesia to the upper teeth. Armed with this extrapolation

---

1 Today, when surgeons use local anesthetics such as lidocaine, a small amount of epinephrine is added, which constricts the local blood vessels, reduces blood supply, and keeps the anesthetic in the area longer. Less lidocaine can be used for a more extended period of effectiveness.

from earlier tests on other nerves, he planned to test his hypothesis and present his findings.

Dentistry in 1884 was in an unhappy state. Extractions and serious dental surgery could be performed under general anesthesia, but the state of the art was crude. Inducing anesthesia, breathing, and access to the teeth all needed control of the same small space, the open mouth. These operations were dangerous. Dental work such as simple extractions and fillings was done without anesthesia of any sort, making the procedures agony. If Halsted could anesthetize the specific nerves carrying sensation from the teeth and jaws, he would revolutionize the profession. He didn't have to wait long to put it to the test.

On November 26, Hall developed an excruciating toothache. Visiting Dr. Nash, his dentist, he brought along a syringe of cocaine solution. Hall convinced the dentist to inject the nerves exiting the infraorbital foramen, under the eye, to try to deaden the pain. Nash inserted the needle from inside the upper lip at the gum line and aimed toward the cheekbone. Hall felt no pain on the introduction of the needle or from the injection of the cocaine solution. "In two minutes there was complete anesthesia of the upper jaw." Hall went on to detail the dental work done on the previously exquisitely painful tooth, all without pain.

Halsted was elated by the news. He spent the next two weeks injecting cocaine in and about the dental nerves of the medical students until he could reliably reproduce the desired area of anesthesia. The cocaine tests began to consume a great deal of the evening quizzes, and animated talk carried on late into the night. Reduced concentrations of cocaine had resulted in significant numbness, with fewer frightening symptoms, and an increasing sense of strength and pleasure.

While these experiments were going on at Madison Square, Halsted brought his new discovery to the Out Door Department at the Roosevelt Hospital. There, Halsted and his assistants successfully performed more than 1,000 minor surgeries under cocaine local anesthesia.

Thomas McBride, though not an active part of the team, was aware of the new discovery, and referred a wealthy and prominent woman suffering from facial pain to Halsted's care. Localizing the neuralgia to the trigeminal nerve, Halsted set up for the surgery in his home office. Assisted by Hartley and Hall, he injected the nerve with cocaine, totally anesthetizing the area in the otherwise alert patient. Using a finger to guide a large clamp into an incision made in the mouth, he found the nerve trunk, clamped and cut it, and was met by "a great gush of arterial blood." Unable to reach the large, bleeding artery, and fearing the patient would drown in her own blood, the unflappable Halsted firmly packed the open cavity with gauze. McBride, not wishing to be present for the demise of his patient, left the room when the hemorrhage seemed uncontrollable. Halsted's quick action stopped the bleeding, but the pressure of the tight packing created the additional risk of crushing and devitalizing the surrounding tissue. Two nurses were hired from the Presbyterian Hospital to attend the patient, and after two stable days she was transferred to Presbyterian and recovered. Eight days after surgery, the packing was removed and the patient discharged. Though the whole episode was more dramatic than expected, it proved to Halsted once again the value of cocaine local anesthesia.

By December 1884, Halsted was barraged by surgeons and dentists interested in his new local anesthesia. On January 20, 1885, the regular meeting of the New York Odontological Society was held at the East 43rd Street home of Dr. W. E. Hoag. The subject was cocaine local anesthesia. Halsted was called in to inject the inferior dental nerve of Dr. John Woodbury, who was about to have a "very sensitive cavity" evacuated and filled. The introduction of local anesthesia was accomplished without difficulty. The lower jaw became numb, the tooth senseless, and the entire procedure painless. Glowing reports followed, and the technique was widely adopted to the delight of both patients and dentists.

Meanwhile, the medical students and their teachers came to enjoy the sense of exhilaration they experienced in the experiments, and began to use cocaine snuff and injections in social circumstances. It enhanced their appreciation of theater and music, helped ward off drowsiness, and generally made their days more enjoyable. They began using it more regularly and in increasing amounts. Gradually, doctor by doctor and student by student, they became addicted. The students began to drop from sight. The doctors' behavior grew increasingly erratic. They slept less, talked endlessly and excitedly, and eventually performed less surgery and ignored their duties.

By September, when Halsted finally set about writing a paper on his findings, he was himself lost in the netherworld of drug addiction and unable to communicate in anything approaching a clear and concise manner. His paper, published in the September 12, 1885, issue of the *New York Medical Journal*, began:

Neither indifferent as to which of how many possibilities may best explain, nor yet at a loss to comprehend, why surgeons have, and that so many, quite without discredit, could have exhibited scarcely any interest in what, as a local anesthetic, had been supposed, if not declared, by most so very sure to prove, especially to them, attractive, still I do not think that this circumstance, or some sense of obligation to rescue fragmentary reputation for surgeons rather than belief that an opportunity existed for assisting others to an appreciable extent, induced me, several months ago, to write on the subject in hand the greater part of a somewhat comprehensible paper, which poor health disinclined me to complete.

The long-winded, rambling article was impossible to follow and made it obvious to all who knew him that something was terribly wrong. Some, including McBride and Welch, understood the nature of the problem. Although the use of cocaine was a relatively recent phenomenon, scientific papers and newspaper articles had begun to appear warning of its "debasing and enslaving of the will."

The drug was taking command of Halsted's life. He began to miss morning sessions at the outdoor clinic and was erratic in meeting surgical responsibilities, to say nothing of the embarrassment and whispering caused by his unreadable paper. But his addiction had just begun, and he was unable to fully comprehend the chokehold it had on him. He made excuses to himself and others, lied when he had to, and tried to carry on with both his increasing cocaine habit and his busy life. It proved impossible. He had passed the point of exhilaration, heightened sensibility, and "super human strength." His hands shook, he often became suddenly drenched in perspiration, and he lost focus. His need for the drug grew. Claiming failing health due to overwork, Halsted said his "breakdown necessitated a trip abroad" to recover his strength.

The most comfortable destination for him would be Vienna. He was fluent in German, had influential friends in the surgical community, and was anxious to spread the word of his new discovery. The drug was readily available in Europe, through Merck, and there was no stigma associated with its purchase.

Much of Halsted's time in Vienna was spent with Anton Wölfler, Billroth's former assistant, with whom he had developed a warm friendship during his visit five years before. Both men had achieved a great deal during the hiatus, and they had exchanged letters and maintained their relationship over the years. Halsted and Wölfler expressed great joy to see each other, dined together, and caught up. Halsted's personal grooming, dress, and manners remained elegant, and Wölfler had only laudatory comments about the visit. Halsted, for his part, was excited to show Wölfler his new technique for injecting the cutaneous nerves. He had last been to Vienna to observe and learn, and now he was proud to be teaching the teachers. Wölfler did not believe that cocaine anesthetic would work and had previously told Halsted as much. But Halsted successfully demonstrated its use in a number of surgical procedures, and Wölfler was suitably impressed. The following day he published a laudatory paragraph about cocaine anesthesia in the Vienna morning newspaper, neglecting to credit Halsted's role.

In a formal demonstration, Halsted taught the technique of injecting the inferior alveolar (dental) nerve to a Dr. Thomas, a well-known American dentist practicing in Vienna. He spoke of the new technique to anyone who would listen and demonstrated it to whomever would watch. Before cocaine, Halsted had never sought credit for his achievements, never promoted his contributions, and never talked about himself. He was now clearly under the influence of the drug, and off balance.

Although he was in Vienna, where the whole cocaine story had begun, Halsted did not meet with Freud. One wonders whether Freud, who was already familiar with the characteristics of cocaine abuse, would have recognized Halsted's aberrant behavior.

Returning home in January 1886, Halsted resumed his heavy workload. George Brewer, who worked with him in the outdoor clinic, described a conversation in which Halsted spoke constantly, excitedly, and endlessly, "about everything under the sun." Halsted was losing control.

* * *

WILLIAM WELCH HAD left his position at Bellevue in March 1884 to become professor of pathology at the new Johns Hopkins University in Baltimore, and part of the team chosen to build the institution from the ground up. He had spent a year in Europe immersed in the latest experimental techniques before settling in Baltimore in 1885. Alerted by McBride to the rapid deterioration of his friend, Welch immediately returned to New York to help. He hired a sailing vessel with captain and crew, and planned to take Halsted on a long sailing trip to the Windward Islands off the coast of South America. The trip was to last through February and March—long enough, he hoped, to gradually wean Halsted from his drug, watch over him, counsel him, and help him break the habit.

It did not end well. Halsted had brought a two-week supply of cocaine aboard. Either Welch had miscalculated how much to allot or Halsted had not shared with him the increasing dosage necessary to satisfy his need, but in mid-passage Halsted ran short of cocaine. In desperation, he broke into the captain's medicine locker. In the most dramatic retelling of the story, he was caught in the act of stealing cocaine and restrained by the crew. However, it is unlikely that a sailing ship would have any reason to carry cocaine, unless the locker was the repository for Halsted's personal supply and some had been withheld as part of the process. It is far more plausible that the drug stolen from the captain's locker was morphine, which would have been carried on board for emergency medical situations. In either event, Halsted's desperation had transformed him overnight from a model of patrician rectitude to a thief.

UPON RETURNING TO New York, Halsted continued using the drug. Welch returned to Baltimore, where he was immersed in his laboratory work and building the team for the Johns Hopkins Hospital.

CHAPTER SEVEN

The Visionary

W HEN JOHNS HOPKINS DIED in 1873, Baltimore was a city of 267,000, not yet fully recovered from the economic hardships of the Civil War. Divided by the tensions of Union loyalty and southern ethic, it had not fared well during the war years, and the economic strife that followed for a decade was sharply exacerbated by a financial panic that swept the nation that year. The city was an unprepossessing industrial seaport of endless row houses, each typically built with three stone entry stairs at front and a small yard behind. Squalor and poverty surrounded the port. The city had neither a cultural nor an academic center, and social and commercial opportunities were limited. Little existed to attract newcomers, and the city did not benefit from the postwar population surge seen elsewhere in the East.

Johns Hopkins had spent his lifetime in and around Baltimore, never traveling farther from home than Cape Ann, New Jersey. It was the world he knew, the city where he had amassed his wealth, and it was not surprising that the millionaire bachelor would earmark the bulk of his fortune for the civic good.

Hopkins was born in 1795, at Whitehall, his family's 500-acre tobacco farm in Anne Arundel County, Maryland. His early life of rural southern ease was interrupted in 1807, when his abolitionist Quaker father freed hundreds of slaves and radically changed the family's economic circumstances. Johns's formal education ended immediately, and the 12-year-old was sent to work in the tobacco fields alongside his siblings. There was little he enjoyed about tending tobacco, and his father arranged for him to move to Baltimore when he was 17 and work in his Uncle Gerard's wholesale grocery store. An ill-fated, youthful romance with his cousin Elizabeth ended with Johns being denied her hand. His religious uncle considered the romance incestuous and ousted his nephew from both his home and his grocery. But Johns had learned his financial lessons well. Backed by his family, including $10,000 from Uncle Gerard, he set out on his own and had little difficulty building a thriving mercantile business. Johns was soon supplying dry goods and tobacco to the surrounding states, often bartering for whiskey, which he marketed under the name Hopkins' Best. Trading in alcohol caused his temporary expulsion from the "Meeting," his Quaker religious order, but this was soon resolved and he retained a long, if not close, relationship with the sect. By all accounts, Hopkins was a hard-driving businessman—so much so that his original partner, Benjamin Moore, left the successful firm saying, "I just don't love money as much as he does."

Hopkins bragged to a nephew that in his first year of business, "I sold $200,000 worth of goods."

He soon enlisted three of his brothers as salesmen in the thriving business, renaming it Hopkins Brothers. He remained at the helm for 25 years, and at age 50, as his business interests expanded, he ceded the company to his siblings. He remained close to his extended family, and his home was always filled with relatives, including his old flame, cousin Elizabeth, who had, like Hopkins, honored their pledge never to marry others.

Hopkins had invested wisely and had become a very wealthy man. In addition to being a director of the Baltimore and Ohio Railroad during a period of rapid and successful expansion, he became its largest individual stockholder, with holdings exceeded only by those of the State of Maryland and the City of Baltimore. Among several of his banking interests was the Merchant's National Bank of Baltimore, where he held the presidency. His influence in business and civic circles was substantial and, Hopkins being in a position to come to the aid of the city he loved, Hopkins lent $500,000 to Baltimore to bridge a financial crisis brought about by the Civil War. After the war, railroads expanded the reach of economic life and were often a source of great wealth for investors and operators. But the opportunity for enrichment also fostered a highly competitive, often cutthroat environment. The fortunes of the highly leveraged railroad industry were subject to many variables, not the least of which were competition for routes, rising interest rates, and financial gossip. In this volatile environment, great fortunes were made and lost quickly.

In the fall of 1872 an equine viral epidemic, called the Great Epizootic, infected nearly 90 percent of the horses in the country. Four million horses died before the disease ran its course, leaving the country at a virtual standstill. Every industry was affected. Goods could not be produced or delivered, and financial panic engulfed the nation. Coal could not be transported from the mines to power the locomotives, and the railroads were forced to shut down. Income for the already financially extended railroads ceased; all were hit hard and many were forced into bankruptcy. Hopkins, who remained financially stable through diversified investments, was able to advance the B&O large sums of money to meet its interest obligations, thereby averting disaster for the company and solidifying his already lofty position in Baltimore business circles.

During the war, Hopkins's sympathies lay strongly with the Union. Remaining true to the Quaker faith's opposition to slavery, Hopkins was a "peaceful abolitionist," and he employed all peaceful and legal means at his disposal to end the practice. He communicated with President Lincoln and openly supported Union causes. He encouraged the encampment of Federal forces in Baltimore and placed the facilities of the B&O railroad at the disposal of the Union Army. When the war ended, feelings among Baltimore's citizens, which were already frayed by partisanship, became hardened by economic strife. Hopkins remained successful during and after the struggle, and attempted to heal the wounds and divisions while doing what he could to help undo the wrongs done the blacks.

Unmarried, with no direct heirs, and his extended family on firm financial footing, Hopkins planned to use the bulk of his fortune "for the good of humanity." His initial charitable bequest was $1 million for the establishment of the Johns Hopkins Colored Children Orphan Asylum. The same trustees named to oversee the orphanage would also lead the university to be built bearing his name. On April 24, 1867, he incorporated both The Johns Hopkins University and The Johns Hopkins Hospital. That year Hopkins spent $150,000 to purchase 13 acres on Loudenschlager's Hill, the site of the Maryland Hospital for the Insane, which was to be moved elsewhere. The purchase was predicated upon the city's closing the streets within the site so that the new hospital and medical school could be self-contained.

At his death, on Christmas Eve of 1873, the *Baltimore Sun* estimated Johns Hopkins's wealth at $8 million, the equivalent of $160 million current value. His estate consisted of $2.25 million in Baltimore and Ohio railroad stock, $1 million in bank stock, and the remainder in real estate and commercial paper. Of this sum, $7 million had already been earmarked for the university bearing his name. It was the largest single philanthropic bequest in the history of the United States, and The Johns Hopkins University became the most richly endowed university in the country.

Hopkins's plans were farsighted and proudly utopian but grounded in the plain words and vision of a successful businessman. The cause of higher education would benefit from the creation of the first true university in the country, offering both undergraduate and graduate courses of study, including law, medicine, and the humanities. Though initially organized under a single board of 12 trustees, the university and medical school would be financially separate from the hospital. Half of the $7 million would go toward construction of the hospital; the other half for the university, including the medical school. Hopkins had stipulated in his will that the capital for the hospital would be invested in stocks and real estate, and the interest from these investments would fund construction, staffing, and operation, without invasion of the principal.

In an 1873 letter to the trustees, written nine months before he died, Hopkins outlined the principles of his hospital. The plan would consist of an initial building, with symmetrical additions, that would "ultimately be able to receive four hundred patients" and "compare favorably with any other institution of like character in this country or in Europe." The hospital would treat the "indigent sick of this city and its environs without regard to sex, age or color." The indigent would be admitted and treated without charge, and the trustees were obliged to secure the services of "surgeons and physicians of the highest character and greatest skill." Hopkins continued, "In all your arrangements in relation to this hospital, you will bear constantly in mind that it is my wish and purpose that the institution shall ultimately form a part of the Medical School of the University for which I have made ample provision in my will."

Despite the rich endowment, The Johns Hopkins Hospital would not open until 1889, and the medical school in 1893, 20 years after the grand plan was unveiled.

In 1874, the presidency of The Johns Hopkins University was offered to Daniel Coit Gilman, then president of the University of California. Gilman was a Yale graduate, born and educated in the East, who had spent the last three years overseeing the expansion of the University of California. He was 44 years old, a family man, and an ambitious and forward-thinking educator who compensated for his sharply receding hairline with wildly luxuriant side whiskers and mustache. Gilman saw the mission to build a university devoted to research and scholar-ship as a unique opportunity, and immediately accepted the position. He assumed office the following year and would remain at the helm for more than 25 years.

The university opened its doors in 1876, and while this part of the dream had come to fruition, Gilman and the trustees wrestled with plans for the hospital. In order to build the finest facility possible, there was much to learn. They began by seeking out the leading hospital and sanitation authorities of the day. A decade beyond the Civil War, and two decades since the Crimean War, the great lessons linking sanitation and survival in hospitals were to be applied in planning the physical plant.

Among the candidates for medical and construction advisor was an army colonel, Dr. John Shaw Billings. As medical inspector of the Army of the Potomac, Billings had become expert on issues of sanitation and the prevention of epidemics. Having established his considerable reputation during the war, he was put in charge of building the Library of the Surgeon General. In seven years at the job, Billings reorganized and transformed a minor collection of 2,253 medical volumes to one with more than 25,000 books and 15,000 pamphlets, and established the index medicus to catalogue all known medical publications. Before his retirement in 1895, the Library of the Surgeon General would further expand to 116,000 volumes; it would ultimately become the National Library of Medicine, the greatest medical library in the world.

The new thinking in hospital construction would, for the first time, incorporate public health concerns into the design. To prevent the spread of disease, patients were separated from one another. Those with contagious diseases were isolated in quarantine quarters. Adequate ventilation, clean water, and sanitation were provided through-out the hospital. However, these steps were based on the erroneous theory of the presence of a miasma, or pollution of the air by some sort of putrefaction, which was believed to be responsible for everything from cholera to the black plague. As measures to improve environmental cleanliness decreased the prevalence of disease, supporters of the theory gained strength. There was something bad in the air, and proper ventilation and adequate private space could avoid it.

The true bacterial origins for disease were not yet proven, and methods of person-to-person transmission of disease remained unclear. Though ambient air was rarely responsible for disease, and certainly not without the presence of microorganisms, cleanliness, separation of individuals, and sanitation had been shown to stem the growth of epidemic disease. Billings, believing in the theory of contaminated air, did not incorporate elevators for fear of contamination through the shafts. Others had moved on. The New York Hospital, erected in 1877, was built to a full six elevated stories, no longer adhering to the same, unproven, principles. The Billings plan consisted of a main building from which branched separate, two-story wards, or pavilions, surrounded by a number of outbuildings. Covered outdoor walkways connected the buildings and all stairways were outdoors. Patients admitted to the pavilions were carried up the external stairs. Amenities of the new hospital included central heating, hot water, fresh cold water, adequate ventilation, and electric lighting. The complex consisted of 17 buildings, including an isolation building, a pharmacy, a bathhouse, a nurses' dormitory, the pathological, and the four primary ward buildings. The large main building from which the pavilions flowed was topped by a stately dome, which was later renamed to honor its designer. Billings's careful renderings of the Queen Anne–style buildings were not actual architectural elevations, and the Boston firm of Cabot and Chandler was contracted to provide working drawings.

The $3.5 million willed to the hospital was made up primarily of Hopkins's commercial real estate and his bank stocks. These proved to be stable but yielded only about $125,000 annually, hardly enough to move full steam ahead. Forbidden to augment this sum by invading the principal or borrowing to finance construction, the process, dependent entirely on the available funds, was painfully slow. Construction was finally completed in 1889 at a total cost of $2,050,000.

It was necessary for the men chosen to lead the hospital departments to be in residence by the time the hospital opened. They would be professors at the university and the medical school, and would command all aspects of their respective departments. This was a revolutionary concept. Elsewhere, medical school faculties were made up of local practitioners not employed by the university. For the new plan to work, they would have to enlist the very best men possible. These individuals would have to share the devotion to excellence, be willing to adapt and innovate, and be substantive enough to add weight to the new endeavor. To accomplish this task, Francis King, president of the hospital board of trustees, and Daniel Coit Gilman, president of the university, turned once again to John Shaw Billings. Billings traveled widely and was very well connected in medical circles. During the early stages of hospital construction, he was busily acquainting himself with both the laboratory-centric German model and the clinically based British model. Billings thought the two systems could be joined and that the result would be superior to all others, and he set out to find professors who shared his views.

In 1877, Billings visited Ernst Wagner's laboratories in Leipzig, where the fledgling pathologist William Welch was studying. That evening the two Americans met to drink beer and talk medicine at Auerbach's Keller. Sitting in the very room where Faust was supposed to have struck his deal with Mephistopheles, the discussion ranged widely over a very long evening. Billings left with the impression that the young man might well fit into the future of Johns Hopkins, and Welch left believing that Johns Hopkins would be the future of medicine. Faust was said to have left flying on a wine barrel powered by the devil.

Seven years later, Billings initiated the series of events that resulted in identifying Welch as the philosophical and scientific heart and soul of The Johns Hopkins Hospital and School of Medicine.

William H. Welch was the son and grandson of physicians from Norfolk, Connecticut. Born in 1850, he was two years older than Halsted. Their years at Yale and the College of Physicians and Surgeons overlapped and they were acquainted, but not yet friends. Like Halsted, Welch won the Bellevue internship competition in 1875. There, he studied with Francis Delafield, one of the noted "dead house" men and a pathologist to the hospital. Delafield was renowned for entries in his little book, in which he correlated patients' clinical diagnoses with his findings at autopsy. He was among the first to remove tissue specimen at autopsy, prepare slides, and stain them with hematoxalin dye to study the abnormal pathology under the microscope. Pathology itself, the study of disease with the naked eye or under the microscope, was a new science, and dedicated pathology laboratories did not exist. More an avocation than a recognized specialty, the study was restricted to a few interested physicians who earned extra income performing autopsies in the dead house for other doctors. The more academically driven internists performed their own autopsies as the final examination in the quest to understand the natural progression of disease. Some, like Welch, under the spell of Delafield, became fascinated with the subject. With no facilities or professors to expand their scientific education in America, interested young men traveled to Austria, Germany, and France, where pathology and histology (the microscopic study of normal tissue) laboratories were flourishing.

Welch spent the summer of 1876 in Strassburg, initially studying histology under Wilhelm Waldeyer. He became adept at using the microscope, which he had been unable to master in New York. His primary impetus for visiting Strassburg was to study pathological anatomy under F. D. von Recklinghausen. Von Recklinghausen was the first to identify the leukocyte, the infection-fighting white blood cell, and he described a condition called neurofibromatosis, which bears his name. He was a man of wide interests and towering intelligence, and was overly confident of his knowledge and judgment. Von

Recklinghausen was an early master of microscopic pathology, but he vehemently resisted all evidence for the bacterial basis of disease. He was particularly vocal about Koch's identification of the tubercle bacillus as the cause of tuberculosis, claiming it was no more reasonable to come to this conclusion than to ascribe the piles of horse manure on the Viennese streets to sparrows. Still, despite this major lapse, his contributions were significant, and he had much to teach. But von Recklinghausen accepted only students with strong microscope skills, and initially Welch did not qualify.

In September, Welch moved from Strassburg to Leipzig, where he studied with the physiologist Carl Ludwig and the pathologist Ernst Wagner, and where his first encounter with Billings took place. Welch was acutely aware of the plans afoot at Johns Hopkins and eager to learn all he could. Though he had not met Billings before, this was not his first brush with the new institution. The previous summer his closest friend, Frederic Dennis, had encountered Johns Hopkins University president Daniel Coit Gilman during an Atlantic crossing. Dennis openly promoted Welch to Gilman, but was met with enough courteous disinterest for Welch to later say it was "folly for me to aspire to attaining such a position when there are so many distinguished men in the country who have already acquired great reputations as pathologists."

In April he traveled to Breslau, where Julius Cohnheim was conducting important work in experimental pathology and bacteriology. One of Cohnheim's many contributions was explaining the nature of the reaction that created pus. The thick, yellow-green substance was obviously associated with infection, but little more than that was known. Cohnheim found it was composed of white blood cells, leukocytes, and cellular debris. The process, he found, was set in motion by infection, to which the body responded by depositing leukocytes in the area and creating pus, thus clearing up a mystery that had confounded physicians for centuries. Noting the predictable presence of white blood cells in inflammation, he categorically stated, "no blood vessels, no inflammation."

Welch learned a great deal from Cohnheim, particularly the elements of bacteriology, a science unheard of at home. It was in Cohnheim's laboratory that Welch first met Robert Koch. Welch also worked closely with Cohnheim in experimental pathology. In the most celebrated of these adventures he was assigned to study the collection of fluid in the lungs, known as pulmonary edema, which was due to more blood being pumped into the lungs than was being pumped out, leaving the fluid behind as pulmonary edema, the essence of heart failure. Blood is delivered to the lungs from the right side of the heart, via the pulmonary artery, aerated in the lungs, and returned to the left side of the heart by the pulmonary vein, and then pumped into circulation by the left ventricle. Welch opened the chests of rabbits and dogs, and immobilized the left ventricle by squeezing that portion of the beating heart between his fingers. The left ventricle stopped pumping, blood backed up, and pulmonary edema resulted. This simple exercise illustrated the nature of pulmonary edema and was a major career milestone for Welch.

When he returned to von Recklinghausen's laboratory it was as a seasoned scientist adept at the use of the microscope. Much of his time was spent confirming Cohnheim's theory of inflammation against the intuition of his supervising professor.

RETURNING TO NEW YORK full of enthusiasm for his new profession, Welch convinced the authorities at Bellevue of the importance of instituting an independent department of pathology. With three small rooms, a $25 furniture allowance, and a few microscopes, he opened the first pathology laboratory in the United States.

In addition to pathological anatomy and general pathology, Welch taught the first laboratory course in the country. His course was enormously popular with the students at Bellevue Hospital Medical

College, and soon medical students from all three medical schools in the city attended his sessions.[1]

The College of Physicians and Surgeons, where Welch had been rebuffed when he presented the idea for a pathology laboratory, soon realized their blunder and tried to win their star alumnus back to the fold. Welch resisted their offers, helped in their search for a substitute, and continued on with his work at Bellevue. To earn a living, he performed autopsies, continued to see private patients, and served as a lecturer at Halsted's quiz, where he welcomed interested students to his laboratory. He was much revered for his "hands on" method of teaching, relying increasingly on laboratory demonstration and discussion.

Billings had followed Welch's progress. He often traveled to New York City and sat in on Welch's classes whenever possible. He attended a session on March 1, 1884, that Welch remembered clearly, not merely for Billings's presence but because much of the day's discussions centered around syphilitic lesions of the testicles. In the Victorian manner of the day, even physicians were uneasy with frank discussion of sex-related topics.

AFTER THE SESSION, Billings quizzed Welch on his goals and how his methods could fit into a new university setting. Both men saw an opportunity, and the discussions advanced further when Billings returned to New York a week later. The next day, Welch traveled to Baltimore to meet with President Gilman and was offered the professorship in pathology.

Returning to New York, he discussed the offer with his medical friends, including Halsted, McBride, and particularly his friend and housemate Frederic Dennis. All counseled him against moving.

---

1 There were three medical schools in Manhattan at the time: Physicians and Surgeons, associated with Columbia University; Bellevue; and New York University. The latter two would combine in 1898.

Dennis, who seemed to take the defection personally, set in motion a counter-offer from Bellevue. The Bellevue proposal was built around a $50,000 pledge from Andrew Carnegie to build a new laboratory for Welch on a site for which the trustees hurriedly appropriated another $45,000.[2] The general feeling was that exchanging an unlimited future in New York for a position based on the German laboratory model at a new, unknown university, and in Baltimore at that, was pure folly. But Welch believed in the vision of Gilman and Billings, and three weeks later he accepted the offer. At a going-away party in New York his friends, by now resigned to losing him, offered the following thought: "You may become a connoisseur of terrapin and Madeira, but as a pathologist, good-bye."

The search committee at Bellevue believed they had secured an adequate replacement for Welch in a distinguished German pathologist with a long, black beard named Otto Lubarsch. At one of numerous farewell dinners for Welch, Halsted was seated opposite Lubarsch and they were eating corn on the cob. The German remarked to Halsted, "I wish I had a picture of you eating corn on the cob."

Halsted's retort was intentionally spoken quickly and wasn't translated into German: "I wish I had a picture of you, Dr. Lubarsch, combing your beard with your fork."

A good deal of laughter followed, and Lubarsch never learned what Halsted had said.

Despite all temptation to stay in New York, it was the right position at the right time, and Welch would become the prime mover in the American medical revolution—the first professor named to The Johns Hopkins medical school, its first dean, and later, the founder of the first school of public health in America. He was instrumental in choosing

---

2 According to Donald Fleming, in *William Welch and the Rise of Modern Medicine*, the Bellevue offer required Welch to continue outside work to meet his personal financial needs. When the offer was declined he became estranged from the irate Dennis.

the core medical faculty of the fledgling institution, free to pursue his research as he wished, and with an annual salary of $4,000, he would no longer need to practice general medicine to supplement his income.

With the encouragement of the trustees, Welch returned to Europe to keep abreast of recent medical progress. Much had transpired in the laboratory sciences in the eight years since his last visit, and virtually all of it in Western Europe. Bacteriology had taken giant leaps forward in Koch's labs with the startling cultivation of the tubercle bacillus and the isolation of the cholera bacillus. The focus of investigation of disease abruptly shifted from the pathology laboratory to the bacteriology laboratory. Those who did not run for the speeding train would be left behind.

In 1882, the noted physician and skeptic Alfred L. Loomis said, "People say there are bacteria in the air, but I cannot see them." When the comment was passed on to Welch, he replied, "That's too bad. Loomis is such a nice man."

Such was the dynamic state of affairs. In a mere 20 years, the height of disease awareness and control had passed from fresh air and isolation to the study of bacteriology and the promise of control of bacterial disease.

Welch spent a year working in the laboratories of several of Koch's distinguished students and a month with the master himself. Before returning to America and his new position, Welch visited Louis Pasteur in Paris. Though he did not have the opportunity to actually study with Pasteur, it was a significant moment for him. Later, Welch proclaimed, "I shall never forget the circumstances of my visit when he put aside his test-tubes and showed me around his laboratory." [3] This

---

3 Fleming states that Welch was passing through Paris in May of 1885, and did not stop to see Pasteur, saying, "There is nothing special of a scientific nature to lead me there." This is at odds with the quote above, from a stenographer's report of a speech given by Welch at the New York Academy of Medicine in 1930, on the occasion of his 80th birthday.

was early 1885, and Pasteur was already an international celebrity. He had already formulated his germ theory of disease; pasteurization; a vaccine against anthrax, the great killer of sheep; and another against cholera in chickens; and had been working on the rabies vaccine for dogs. Pasteur and Koch had been anointed as the great microbiologists and leaders of the new world of laboratory science, and Welch had become part of the inner circle. And so the stage was set for the new professor to install himself in a new institution with the lofty mission of transforming and elevating American medicine. The reality was nothing so impressive as the promise.

CHAPTER EIGHT

The Very Best Men

IN SEPTEMBER 1885, William Welch arrived in Baltimore and installed himself in two large, well-furnished rooms at 20 Cathedral Street, a fashionable address. There he was well cared for by the proprietor, Mrs. Thomas Simmons, the widow of a former Civil War major, and her daughter. In this setting Welch established a routine, which included familiarity, caring, and occasional comfortable chats without the need for intimacy. Never seeking grander accommodations and never buying a home, he lived in this modest fashion throughout his life, surrounded by his enormous personal library and close to his work.

Thirty-five years old, short and plump, with receding dark hair, a generous beard, and a benign demeanor, he brought with him an appetite for conversation as insatiable as his appetite for food. As an interesting newcomer to a stagnant society, numerous attempts were made to introduce him to the available young women in Baltimore society, but it was soon apparent that Welch would not pursue these relationships. Consumed by his work, and gracious and amusing even when demurring, he remained a much sought-after guest long after his disinterest became apparent.

THE JOHNS HOPKINS UNIVERSITY had been functioning on the under-graduate level since 1876. Its small graduate programs within the faculty of philosophy included the professors of the sciences. Welch was the first professor appointed to the medical faculty, but the hospital did not yet exist and the medical school was still a distant dream. Welch established himself in borrowed space in the laboratories of the British physiologist H. Newell Martin, who had been appointed the first professor of biology, until the Pathological was ready for occupancy, which paved the way for several years of fruitful research by the two men.

The pathology building, referred to by a generation as the Pathological, was the first building in the hospital complex, and it was hastily completed to accommodate Welch. A small, rectangular, two-story redbrick building, it had six tall, thin windows on the long side and four on the short side, two central chimneys, and a basement. Originally meant to house only the hospital morgue, it was quickly reconfigured. Within it were the bacteriology laboratory, experimental pathology laboratories where experimental animal surgery was performed, a surgical pathology laboratory where surgical specimens were examined, and the morgue, or dead house. Bodies were brought from elsewhere for autopsy until the hospital was completed. Here, Welch oversaw the department of pathology and the first institute for experimental medicine in the country.

Welch was given autonomy in selecting his staff and students, and his uncanny ability to recognize men of great promise would serve Johns Hopkins well. His first appointment was his assistant, William T. Councilman. Locally bred and educated, Councilman was a graduate of the University of Maryland Medical School. Trained in pathology in Europe, he had already established a fine reputation in Baltimore, and his appointment did much to defuse the seething resentment within the local medical community against the new academics who were threatening to upset their system and challenge their primacy.

Welch appointed Franklin P. Mall as a fellow in pathology. Mall, then only 23, was a slight, pugnacious, and sharp-tongued man who would become an important, often difficult, and famed professor of anatomy. He had a habit of stammering when he was excited, and with his tiny frame and argumentative nature, he became the most outspoken proponent of learning by doing. This was very much the same position of Welch, whose laissez-faire attitude at the Pathological helped solidify Mall's stance. The insensitive enforcement of this attitude would soon make Mall the most disliked of the Hopkins professors. Often refusing to lecture, and voicing his visceral dislike of anatomy books such as *Gray's*, he would provide his students with body parts and a scalpel and leave them to their own devices.

Few would ever accuse Mall of laziness. A prodigy, he was brilliant, opinionated, and obdurate. A graduate of the University of Michigan School of Medicine, he trained with Ludwig in Leipzig, where he first met Welch. There, Mall had produced an experimental model of the intestinal blood supply composed of segments of intestine served by individual vessels. Using this model, he and Welch expanded upon his work, producing experimental occlusion of intestinal vessels in order to understand the sequence of events resulting in infarction, or tissue death, in the intestinal segment deprived of blood supply. The work added significantly to the knowledge of the phenomenon at a time when surgeons had just begun attacking intestinal problems and needed a clear understanding of the complex anatomy.

With no hospital, no medical school, and only Mall and Councilman aboard, Welch accepted 16 graduate students to study at the department of pathology. Of the 16, more than half were doing original research, making the Pathological the first institute of experimental medicine in America. Included among them would be a fully trained surgeon named William Stewart Halsted.

* * *

WITH WELCH A DAY'S journey away, Halsted had had no monitor other than his housemate Thomas McBride, who attempted to support and counsel him. But McBride, thought to have become addicted himself, began suffering lapses in his own health.

Halsted remained unwilling or unable to reach out to his family for help. The constant preaching by his father, William Mills Halsted Jr., seemed to have driven the two apart, although the younger Halsted was still supported by his father's largess. Then, in a turn of events worthy of a Victorian novel, Halsted, Haines and Company, the 80-year-old firm begun by William Mills Halsted Sr., suffered complete financial collapse and bankruptcy. Not only did the family fortune disappear, but William Mills Halsted Jr., the strictly moral Presbyterian, was accused of deceptive business practices and self-dealing. The *New York Times* reported on August 4, 1884, that the firm was insolvent, and on May 7, 1887, printed a virtual indictment of the W. M. Halsted Jr.:

Halsted, Haines, and Co., the old dry goods firm that failed in July, 1884, was built on a solid foundation away back in 1804. The founders established an enviable reputation and amassed fortunes. One by one they died or retired and new blood was infused into the concern. Modern methods of business and habits of living are different from the old fashioned way, and the insolvent firm seems to have floated along of late years largely on its reputation. The junior partners never bothered about the books or the general business, but left everything in the hands of the senior, who manipulated them apparently to his own satisfaction, and regardless of the creditors.

Questions were raised about the senior Halsted having secured loans using worthless stock as collateral. In the end, the creditors suffered severely. There was apparently no legal remedy for the debt nor punishment for the perpetrators. William Mills Halsted issued preference notes in favor of his children and his brother, which were paid out of existing assets before the creditors were considered. The young surgeon benefited from a questionable "preferred loan" to the tune of $24,800, the equivalent of more than $500,000 today.

Somehow, Halsted managed to continue his routine as surgeon and teacher, and apparently was able to discharge his duties. His state of constant excitement did not go unnoticed, though few understood its nature, and no one questioned him about it.

In April 1886, it was announced that Dr. William S. Halsted was among three men being considered for the chair of surgery at P&S. The other candidates were Dr. William T. Bull, the well-respected surgeon at the Chambers Street Hospital, and Dr. Richard J. Hall, Halsted's assistant at Roosevelt. The candidates were to write and deliver a series of papers, after which one of the three would be awarded the position. Halsted wanted the position but was unable to write the papers. By the time this became evident to him, he had already spent $1,000 on charts and pictures for his lectures. Again, he blamed failing health for his poor performance. Halsted withdrew from competition, and the job was offered to Hall. By then an addict himself, Hall declined the position and moved to Santa Barbara, California, to recover. He corresponded with Halsted over the years and often alluded to his illness, though neither ever mentioned cocaine by name.

Halsted withdrew from all of his professional responsibilities when he could no longer disguise the extent of his disability. Welch, McBride, and Halsted's younger brother Richard, an alcoholic himself, convinced him to seek hospitalization. Though drug addiction was still relatively uncommon, alcohol abuse was not, and private mental hospitals accepted patients for the treatment of alcoholism. A few hospitals had begun treating drug addiction as well. Butler Hospital, in Providence, Rhode Island, was one of these.

Halsted arrived in Providence by train, was driven to Butler, and registered anonymously as William Stewart. Dr. Sawyer, the head of the hospital at the time, was well thought of and well connected, and took great interest in his new patient. Despite Halsted's having registered anonymously, the staff knew his identity. Halsted had a number of visitors during his months at Butler. He was friendly with Dr. Fred C. Shattuck, an intern at the hospital who would later become a distinguished professor of medicine at Harvard, and a Dr. Folsom, who became a well-known psychiatrist. During Halsted's hospitalization, Dr. Sawyer became seriously ill. The three physicians—Halsted, Shattuck, and Folsom—gathered around Sawyer's bed to hear his dying words, which were an appeal to Halsted to abandon his drug addiction.[1]

HALSTED REMAINED HOSPITALIZED for seven months. His treatment was based on encouraging a healthful lifestyle, with emphasis on diet weighted toward vegetables, outdoor exercise, meetings with alienists (as psychiatrists were then known), and a gradual reduction in his cocaine dosage. Various sedatives were employed to mitigate withdrawal symptoms, but the backbone of the treatment for cocaine addiction was substitution with morphine. This, if successful, produced addiction to a different drug with a different set of symptoms.

Apparently, the strategy was not entirely successful. Halsted bribed hospital employees to procure cocaine for him even as he was receiving morphine. One drug produced heightened sensations and a feeling of omnipotence, the other a peaceful release from the world. They created a balancing act that became central to the rest of Halsted's life.

---

1 Here things get a bit fuzzy. The information about Butler comes from a 1952 recollection of Halsted by a Hopkins pediatrician named Edwards A. Park. Park, who had lost the notes of his interviews with Shattuck, states that Sawyer died in December of 1885, which, if true, would make the episode temporally impossible.

* * *

WELCH HAD BEEN at Hopkins for less than six months when he returned to New York to help deal with Halsted's deteriorating condition. The unsuccessful sailing cure and the seven months at Butler did not end the cycle of addiction. Halsted left Butler in November 1886. By then his housemate and great friend Thomas McBride had died prematurely of kidney failure. Many who knew him believed his demise was complicated by drug addiction. Halsted found himself alone, isolated from the medical community, bereft at the loss of McBride, and now addicted to both cocaine and morphine.

Recognizing that Halsted needed a friend and a controlled environment, Welch made the problem his own and invited him to Baltimore. Halsted had been among the leading surgeons in New York when his star crashed. In addition to his personally costly discovery of local anesthesia, he had begun work on an operation to cure breast cancer, campaigned for cleanliness and asepsis where there had been filth and death, and was thought by all to be the great young teacher of surgery. But he had lost control, and Welch was taking a great risk with his own future to help his friend. In December 1886, Halsted was on the train to Baltimore.

Welch counted Halsted among his few close friends, and most of the medical world in which he freely circulated as friendly acquaintances. He spent a great deal of time reading, and had an extensive library and Catholic tastes. He became the de facto medical ambassador from Johns Hopkins, and was in constant demand as a lecturer and visiting professor. Welch dined almost nightly at his club, usually in the company of Halsted and two or three nonphysician friends, and whiled away the evenings chatting by the fire in the intimate little chess room.

Halsted was good company. He was outgoing, always attentive, full of good humor, ready with an amusing remark, and every bit

Welch's match. His disposition in the evenings stood in sharp contrast to the quiet, reserved, often acidic demeanor for which he was known at work. The comfort of being with friends substantially contributed to his ease and confidence. In the late afternoon, Halsted sequestered himself behind locked doors and emerged after 90 minutes refreshed and in high spirits. Productive mornings, midday letdown, occasional sweats and shaking chills, followed by afternoon seclusion and strong evenings lead to obvious conclusions.

Halsted traveled a great deal during his tenure at Johns Hopkins, just as he had before. Medical meetings and clinic visits in Germany and Austria, small hotels on the English coast, and quiet places in France all called to him. His long itineraries were mostly unannounced, and he invariably traveled alone.

Welch also traveled alone. But unlike his friend, who favored isolation, Welch was enamored of the seashore, rest cures, and garish resorts such as Atlantic City. Little of what occupied him on these holidays was known, but he wrote frequently, socialized freely, and was happy to see a friendly face. There were no women in his life. Harvey Cushing, in his Pulitzer Prize–winning biography of William Osler, suggests that Welch was homosexual, though no evidence was offered beyond personal suspicion. The private Welch was something of a mystery to everyone at Hopkins. Lovingly referred to as Popsie, a limerick popular among the students tells the story:

Nobody knows where Popsie eats,
Nobody knows where Popsie sleeps,
Nobody knows whom Popsie keeps,
But Popsie.

William Welch was the least physical of men. Never known to indulge in any form of sport, he suffered from gout, and was always overweight and under-exercised. As a celebrated elder statesman,

H. L. Mencken described him as a "two hundred pound eighty year old" who had been up late into the previous night at a banquet. At lunch the following day, Mencken reported that he ate a large portion of ham and greens washed down with several mugs of beer, and followed by "an arc of at least 75 degrees of lemon meringue pie, after which Welch smoked a six inch panatela, made a speech in English and finishing in German, and ambled off to attend a medical meeting and to prepare for dinner." Mencken wisely concluded "that pathology is still far from an exact science."

CHAPTER NINE

Baltimore

I N 1886, SOUTHBOUND TRAINS from New York were boarded at the Baltimore and Ohio terminal in Jersey City, less than two miles across the harbor from the tip of lower Manhattan. Wind-driven snow and frigid air had plagued the Northeast for days, and the crossing was rough early that December morning. The rail trip to Baltimore took nine hours along the well-traveled line between New York City and Washington. The old steam locomotive pulled slowly up the grades, and the cars rattled and screeched around every turn, but it was far more comfortable than the ferry crossing. The food was good, there were gas lamps for reading, and all the proper amenities were provided for first-class passengers.

Halsted had pleasant memories of Baltimore and had remained in contact with his Yale chum Henry James, the son of a prominent Baltimore banker. But he was no longer a college student and his circumstances had changed. At 34 years of age, he was both fragile and hopeful, and was attempting to outrun the cocaine addiction that had left his professional life in ruins. This was a chance for redemption and a new start, and he was determined to make the best of it.

Welch welcomed Halsted with the warmth and good fellowship that only a truly close friend could provide, and arranged accommodations for him in the Cathedral Street rooming house where he himself resided. There, Welch could watch over him, and he would be well cared for by Mrs. Simmons. Halsted appeared healthy and self-confident, and exhibited none of the excitability and nervous energy that had characterized his plummet. Still wearing a neatly trimmed mustache and beard, his immaculate figure and shambling gait soon became familiar sights at the laboratories on the second floor of the Pathological. Halsted cut quite a figure in the winter streets, his silk top hat sitting jauntily on his head above his jutting ears. Men in Baltimore typically wore homburg or derby hats, and the topper was a New York affectation to which he continued to cling.

Halsted was immediately comfortable in the laboratory. He and the men around him were intellectually connected by their devotion to the scientific method that had germinated in Europe. Projects quickly materialized, and the atmosphere was electric with ideas. From the earliest days, it was clear that this might well be the best group of young medical scientists ever assembled in America. Welch, ever the sounding board, thoughtfully considered the ideas presented to him, advised when asked, and never interfered. His new teaching method was finding its sea legs. Learn by doing was the rule from the start, and most of the early group were self-motivated and able to thrive under the lax but nourishing conditions.

A bit removed from the hubbub around him, Halsted often walked past colleagues in the corridor without greeting them, as if he were elsewhere. For the most part, his detachment was attributed to immersion in his work, but severely compromised vision and his unwillingness to update his glasses added a physical aspect to the isolation.

From the beginning, even during his New York years as a harried, old-school surgeon, Halsted was able to step back and question why things were done the way they were and wonder how they could be done better. Now distanced from the pressure of patient care and teaching, he was able to concentrate on the whys and wherefores of surgery and confront the issues standing in the way of progress. At the Pathological, he developed a manner of dealing with animal experiments that soon became the national standard. Physiological experiments were usually performed on small animals, which were abundant and inexpensive, but surgical procedures demanded larger subjects, usually dogs. With the growth of experimental science, the use of the dog laboratory increased. Animal experimentation, whether humane or callous, whether performed on frogs or dogs, drew the wrath of the increasingly powerful antivivisectionists.

Halsted, not in the least bending to pressure, and perhaps not even mindful of it, demanded that all surgical procedures performed on the experimental animals were to be conducted with the same care and humanity afforded hospital patients. He set these standards for himself, lived by them, and demanded nothing less from others. Dogs were properly cared for. They were fully anesthetized for surgery, which was carried out under stringent aseptic conditions using sterilized surgical instruments and proper technique. The dogs were the patients. They were treated carefully and humanely, their pain promptly relieved by opiates, their diets nutritious, their environment sanitary, and their surgical findings recorded as thoroughly as in any hospital chart. Halsted took great pride in entrusting the responsibility of overseeing the dog lab to his favored assistant. This scrupulous attention to detail yielded rich dividends.

At the Pathological, Halsted worked alongside Franklin Mall, Welch's 23-year-old wunderkind and fellow in pathology, who was continuing his own studies of intestinal anatomy and physiology while working on projects with Welch. Mall and his new laboratory mate got on well from the start. Halsted focused on anatomy as it related to surgery, while Mall concentrated on the uncharted fine points of anatomy. His prior work had identified the repetitive arch pattern of intestinal blood supply as discrete segments integrated into a functioning organ. He was interested as well in the role of the microscopic finger-like villi in the absorption of intestinal contents. Recently, Mall had become aware of the tough submucosal coat between the outer muscular layer and the inner mucosal layer of the intestine, and he was puzzled by its seeming lack of function. Halsted's interest was piqued. Surgeons had been wrestling unsuccessfully with the problem of reconnecting two ends of surgically separated intestine, or intestinal anastomosis, for years, unaware of any possible role for the submucosal coat.

The intestine is a long, squirmy tube filled with food and rapidly multiplying bacteria digesting that food. The contents are more liquid in the small intestine near the entry of food and water from the stomach, and are propelled through the intestine by muscle contractions called peristalsis, where nutrients and liquids are absorbed. Farther along the 25 feet of intestine as water is absorbed in the large intestine, or colon, the contents become increasingly fecal through bacterial proliferation until they ultimately become stool.

Typically, the excision of a cancer or the correction of an intestinal obstruction requires the removal of a section of intestine. The surgeon was then faced with both the need to avoid spilling bowel contents into the abdomen and to find a method of joining the two ends of intestine together in a manner that could withstand the movement and pressure of peristalsis. Careful handling could minimize the initial problem of spillage, but the frequent late breakdown of the anastomosis was catastrophic, spilling feces throughout the peritoneal cavity. Half a century before the advent of antibiotics, this often resulted in death. Abdominal surgery was in its infancy, and surgeons used thick sutures to sew the two ends of the tubes together, intestinal muscle layer to intestinal muscle layer. They tied the heavy sutures tightly and hoped for the best. More often than not, the muscle was devitalized, and when the catgut sutures dissolved, or tore through, the muscle-to-muscle anastomosis broke down, spilling intestinal contents into an abdomen compromised by devitalized tissue.

Mall's curiosity about the submucosal layer seemed worth exploring for its surgical implications. Halsted set about suturing cut intestines together, incorporating various suturing levels and techniques, and ultimately coming to believe the key to a strong anastomosis was, in fact, in the mysterious submucosa.

Halsted wasted no time. The first experiments were completed one week after his arrival in Baltimore. Ensconced in a small room on the southeast corner of the second floor of the Pathological, close by Mall and Welch, he worked feverishly. Total immersion had always been the way he approached new projects, and in that regard intestinal anastomosis was no different from the cocaine experiments, but now the stakes were higher. He had to fit in, justify Welch's faith in him, and keep control of his private life.

The work went well and it soon became clear that the hypothesis was correct. Intestinal anastomosis using fine silk sutures incorporating the submucosal layer withstood the pressures of normal function. To reinforce the point, Halsted devised a demonstration measuring the force needed to pull apart intestines sutured by the various methods. Invariably, an anastomosis including the submucosa was stronger and more difficult to separate. According to Councilman, Welch's assistant pathologist, he was also "fond of demonstrating that when a loop of small intestine was clamped in the handle of a scissors and pulled through, both the muscularis and mucosa were stripped, but a stitch caught in the submucosa still held." The graphic evidence was undeniable.

Sixty-nine experiments were carried out through the winter. They were completed on April 1, 1887. On April 5, only four months after arriving at Johns Hopkins, Halsted delivered an important paper on his findings at the Harvard Medical School.

Among his remarks were the following:

The current ideas among surgeons are not only incomplete, but absolutely incorrect as regards some important details in the structure of the intestinal coats. My experiments have led me to attach great weight to an accurate knowledge of the thickness and physical characters of the submucosal coat of the intestine. I am not aware that the importance of this coat in connection with this operation has hitherto been emphasized.

Typical Halsted. Direct, severe, and gentlemanly.

OTHER SURGEONS SOON corroborated the importance of the submucosal layer in intestinal anastomoses. In short order, the maneuver was generally adopted. Combined with the growing application of aseptic precautions and gentle handling, it provided the link necessary to make intestinal surgery safe and predictable.

Halsted's surgical work was performed only on laboratory dogs and not tested on humans. The dog lab was his life, and he often referred to these years as his happiest. Perhaps more important than discovering the use of the submucosa was the methodology: rigorous animal testing in a controlled surgical environment prior to human trials.

Before this, surgical advances were the fruit of a surgeon's following his idea to the operating room. Sometimes, the inspiration appeared subjectively correct and found its way into other operating rooms. If it was incorrect, the outcome could prove fatal for the patient on whom the experiment was carried out. What was necessary was a method of developing objective evidence of efficacy without a cost in human life. Halsted had replaced trial and error with investigative method.

His technique, his laboratory protocol, and his new career were off to an admirable start. But things were not all they seemed to be.

* * *

IN THE THREE YEARS following his arrival in Baltimore in December 1886, Halsted lived a thoroughly different life than he had in New York. Far from the elegant surroundings of his fine home off Madison Square Park, his private space was restricted to a room in

Mrs. Simmons's house at 506 Cathedral Street. He did no entertaining at home, took his lunch with his laboratory mates at the tavern across the street from the Pathological, did no exercise or sports, and most unusual of all performed no surgery on humans. His laboratory was his clinic and the dogs were his patients. Halsted saw the replication of proper operating room conditions as both a sign of respect for the animals and a means of eliminating as many variables from the equation as possible.

But the overriding reason for his isolation in a laboratory was that Halsted was a surgical pariah. He had wrecked his career in New York and was at Hopkins on trial and under scrutiny. Though the issue of his addiction was not commonly known or openly discussed, it weighed heavily on Welch. He had shared his knowledge with Gilman, the trustees, and very likely Billings, who was intimately involved in staffing the new medical center. Billings was also well connected in New York medical circles, where the cocaine stories were well known. To the few with whom he discussed it, Halsted declared himself cured of his addiction. This, sadly, was fabricated of whole cloth. Not only was it likely he had continued using cocaine, but he had become increasingly dependent on morphine since "taking the cure" at Butler.

Halsted did well at hiding his addiction from experienced professionals, including several aware of his history. Welch was apparently unaware of any recurring difficulties, and although Halsted seemed distracted and introverted, he was able to function at an extremely high level. He was good company when he appeared for lunch, and he was in great spirits in the evening for dinner and socializing. To combat the flagging energy and irritability he experienced in the afternoon, he chose late afternoon for part of his morphine dose. Restored, he was able to function well for the remainder of the day and into the evening.

For the first six months in Baltimore it all went according to plan. He worked hard, produced significant work, and gave no hint of losing control. But addicted to two powerful drugs, he was performing a precarious dance. Shortly after delivering his paper at Harvard, he voluntarily returned to Butler Hospital.

Again he registered under an assumed name, but this time he didn't bring cocaine, or money to bribe hospital employees to procure it for him. Records of this hospitalization went missing, and virtually nothing is known about the episode other than the sparse reports he made in letters to Welch. He also corresponded with Mall but begged off writing extensive letters, claiming weakness. There is no evidence that he ever told Mall the whole truth.

Halsted remained hospitalized for nine months and returned to Baltimore in December 1887. To those who knew the nature of his indisposition, including Welch, Halsted declared himself completely "cured." But Welch was protective of his friend and toyed with the truth. Halsted continued his clandestine life. Whether he believed he had control of the situation is unknown. He guarded the truth carefully and continued to successfully juggle two seemingly conflicting aspects of his life.

He behaved normally, made few excuses, lied when pressed, and went on with his life. In the early winter, he returned to his lodging on Cathedral Street and resumed full-time work at the Pathological. His biographers, who were either students or acolytes, trumpeted Halsted's heroic determination and willpower in conquering his demons. No one knew the whole truth but William S. Halsted, and he was keeping his own counsel.

When Halsted returned to the Pathological, the closely held secret was protected. There was no talk of drug addiction, nor was there ignorance of his important discovery of cocaine as a local anesthetic. The world that had taken note of his achievement was largely unaware of the suffering and loss of life associated with it. Halsted shied away from discussing any aspect of the cocaine episode, but when the need arose, his colleagues sought his expertise.

When Councilman suffered great pain from an infected inferior molar, he walked across the hall of the Pathological and sought help from Halsted. An injection of cocaine brought "complete relief, followed by a painless extraction." Over several years, the use of cocaine as a local anesthetic had become thoroughly integrated into surgical practice and was no longer automatically associated with Halsted. He was happy to be distanced from a subject he did not wish to discuss, and he did not seek credit for his discovery. Having paid dearly, he had lost all enthusiasm for the use of cocaine anesthesia.

Life returned to normal on Cathedral Street, and Halsted resumed his role as if there had been no interruption. He participated in the scientific chatter at lunch with colleagues from the Pathological and dined, as usual, among friends at the Maryland Club. The club, located in a fine old mansion at Franklin and Cathedral streets, had seen better days. Welch was a constant presence, and under his sponsorship Halsted became an active member. The run-down, rat-infested building was steeped in local history, and its proximity appealed to the ease of the two bachelors living down the street. Neither man was involved in a relationship with a woman, nor did they profess any interest. They saw a great deal of each other, as well as a number of Baltimore and Hopkins friends. Days were filled with the excitement of discovery, evenings with intelligent talk and easy banter in convivial settings.

Back on the second floor of the Pathological, Halsted turned his attention to the thyroid gland, a complicated endocrine organ in the neck whose unexplained functions appeared responsible for dramatic physical manifestations. So little was known of endocrine function at the time that every new finding made unscrambling the mystery more difficult. The very nature of endocrine glands was not yet understood, and 30 years of study began, which would lead to Halsted's publication of the definitive tome on the subject.

Things at the Pathological were braced for change. The days of a few good comrades sharing their love of pure research with similarly inclined graduate students were winding down, and the Pathological was about to be integrated into a larger whole. There was still no medical school, but the hospital was finally set to open in May 1889. A full team would need to be assembled. The task fell to Welch and Billings, and they were scrambling to put together the finest medical staff in the country. The previous fall, William Osler had been lured away from Philadelphia to become physician-in-chief, but as yet no one had been chosen as surgeon. In fact, there was only one surgeon associated with Johns Hopkins, and it was barely a year and a half since he had been hospitalized for drug abuse.

CHAPTER TEN

The Hospital on the Hill

J. M. T. FINNEY WAS a short, solid, round-faced New Englander with jet-black hair and a thick mustache, and had arrived from Boston just before the opening ceremonies for The Johns Hopkins Hospital. It was May 7, and this was his second visit to the new hospital in just a few weeks. Baltimore was in the middle of an unusually cool and rainy spring, but that Tuesday the city awakened to a perfect morning. In the bright sunshine the hospital looked decidedly different. Plantings were in bloom on the grounds, and the harsh red brick of the sprawling, ungainly structure was softened and relieved by copious bunting and colorful flags that continued into the grand rotunda. Garlands of similax hung from the chandeliers, great bowers of carefully arranged cut flowers were everywhere inside, and a crowd of elegantly dressed men and women enhanced the festive atmosphere. A marble bust of Johns Hopkins watched over it all from a corner of the rotunda. He, too, was festively draped in similax. The rows of seating erected for the occasion were still sparsely filled, save for the third tier, where a 25-piece band practiced the musical numbers they would be playing between speakers.

Previously, Finney had come armed with letters of recommendation from his seniors at the Massachusetts General Hospital, where he was house surgeon. Seeking out Dr. Halsted, he had been eager to present his credentials in hope of becoming part of the new world of scientific surgery. As luck would have it, Halsted had not yet returned from a European trip. Looking for someone in charge, Finney was sent to see Welch, who was working at home. Never having met the famous pathologist, he screwed up his courage and called on him at Cathedral Street. Welch, in typical fashion, welcomed the young man, hustled him into one of the old-fashioned bob-tailed Monument Street horse cars, and rode with him back to the hospital. Throughout the ride Welch asked about Finney's experience, interests, and aspirations in such a pleasant and offhand manner that only later did Finney realize he was being interviewed. Bidding him farewell and promising to relay the information to Halsted, Welch deposited Finney at the hospital with Franklin Mall, who provided the full tour.

Finney returned to Boston even more enthusiastic about Johns Hopkins than before. A week before opening day a letter arrived from Halsted with an invitation for a personal visit, and to witness the formal opening ceremonies for the hospital.

Six hundred attendees were expected for the long program, which would include remarks by Francis King, president of the hospital's board of trustees; Daniel Coit Gilman, president of the university; and John Shaw Billings, the man who conceived the structure. Mingling with the assembled dignitaries, Finney once again anxiously sought out Dr. Halsted. The hospital would not be receiving patients until the following day, and visitors had free run of the huge, open wards, each nearly 100 feet long and dramatically sheltering 28 empty beds under ceilings 27 feet high. Unable to locate Halsted in the throng, he spied Welch, who once again welcomed him and accompanied him through the hospital corridors. The portly pathologist chatted up the young man and put Finney at ease until Halsted surfaced among the crowd. Hastily introduced before the ceremony began, the nearsighted Halsted peered disarmingly over his pince-nez glasses at Finney for what seemed to him an eternity, before he finally spoke.

"Big crowd, isn't it?"

"Yes, sir."

"Nice day, isn't it?"

"Yes, sir."

Halsted looked away in silence, then after a few seconds turned back to Finney.

"I'll have to ask you to excuse me, as I have an appointment in the laboratory in a few minutes. What time can you report for duty?"

Finney had no idea how to respond.

"I beg your pardon, sir."

"I want you to come down here and work in the surgical dispensary. When can you begin work?"

"I'm not yet through at the Massachusetts General Hospital, not until July first, but I suppose they will let me off a bit earlier."

"Oh, I fancy they'll let you off all right. You come down just as soon as you can. I shall expect you. Good morning."

Pleased, and confused, Finney had just been hired in some capacity, to do he knew not what. No questions were asked in the three-minute interview, and Dr. J. M. T. Finney had begun a 33-year association with Dr. William Stewart Halsted in which he never received a single word of orders or instruction, and only once in 33 years, a compliment.

HALSTED HAD BEGUN seeing patients and operating at local hospitals during the winter of 1889. He was the only surgeon associated with Johns Hopkins at the time, and although his status was clouded by the knowledge of his drug history, he was doing remarkable investigative work. Since the hospital was to be up and running by early May, they needed to appoint a surgeon. President Gilman, Billings, and Osler had been charged by the trustees to seek a proper chief of surgery. They finally settled on Sir William Macewen, successor to the great John Lister in Glasgow, but the deal unraveled when Macewen insisted on including his entire nursing staff in the bargain. Whether the trustees reacted to his haughty attitude or if the wholesale importation of staff already set in their ways was felt to be at cross-purposes with the philosophy of the new institution, is not clear.

Whatever the case, The Johns Hopkins Hospital was about to open without a surgeon. As impossibly shortsighted as that situation seems, the surgical world of 1889 was unrecognizable from today's perspective and did not command the highest priority. So little surgery was being performed that there were fewer than ten physicians in the United States whose practices were restricted to surgery. The shutters condemning the world of surgery to darkness had only begun to creak open. The advent of anesthesia and antiseptic technique had made elective operations possible and survivable, but innovation and innovators still lagged behind opportunity. The appointment of Macewen, had it come to pass, might well have relegated Hopkins to an era of surgical stagnation. But, in February of 1889, in a decision with implications far beyond their imaginations, the executive committee of the hospital trustees invited William Stewart Halsted to be surgeon-in-chief to the dispensary and acting surgeon to the hospital.

Knowing what they did of Halsted's history, the trustees were hedging their bets. His colleagues, particularly Welch and Osler, threw their support strongly behind him and very likely helped secure the position. Osler, who had recently been appointed professor of medicine but was still at work in Philadelphia, wrote university president Gilman on March 6, "Halsted is doing remarkable work in Surgery and I feel that his appointment to the University and Hospital would be quite safe." The following October, Halsted was appointed associate professor of surgery at the university, and in March of 1890 he was made surgeon-in-chief to the hospital as well as the dispensary. It would be two more years before he was named full professor.

There was no staff, no assistants, no dedicated surgery ward, no specialized operating room, and no residents. Indeed, there was no such thing as a resident. The closest approximation was the German system, where young doctors lived in the hospital for an extended period but training was not formalized. Osler and Halsted proposed to expand on that principle for their departments. Halsted envisioned total immersion in the problems and practice of surgery until a superior level of competence and maturity was reached. The rigors of the work would demand that men be unmarried, live in the hospital, and be available for duty 24 hours a day, seven days a week. In keeping with this radical new idea, the hospital set aside a floor for residents' living quarters. The number of years of service required to be deemed "sufficiently trained" were not specified and would vary with the resident. There would be a system of graduated responsibility, with junior assistant residents, assistant residents, and at the top of the pile, the resident.

Not every man who began the program would reach the pinnacle. Some would continue to work as assistant resident, waiting their turn while another man served as resident year after year. For others the impossibility of succession would be made plain, and they would leave. But in 1889, there was very little surgery, very few patients, and only a single resident was hired. The first man to become a resident was Fred W. Brockway. A short time later, George E. Clarke was hired for the position of assistant resident.

Brockway was a New Englander and already a competent surgeon. He, along with the newly hired assistant surgeon to the dispensary, J. M. T. Finney, would be Halsted's assistants. They would be responsible for all patient care, perform all surgery that Halsted didn't care to do, and assist at all the operations he did. They would be responsible for all laboratory work, such as blood and urine analyses, and for keeping daily records of the progress of the patients. As the department took shape, and later when the medical school opened, the responsibilities greatly increased to include research and teaching, as well as overseeing junior residents.

As casual as the hiring of Finney and Brockway may have seemed, they were the cream of a limited crop. From the day the hospital opened it was understood that only the most qualified men would be hired. For the time being, that meant hiring as resident men who had already had surgical training elsewhere. The onerous task of spoon-feeding the new surgical resident would be unnecessary. Halsted's job was to set an example for them, and that he was ready to do. Thereafter, the junior men would learn from the senior men, and the senior men would learn from Halsted. The first residents, and their successors, were young, anxious to go where surgery had never been, and willing to dedicate a decade of their youth to get there. No one had ever attempted this adventure before, nor had there ever been a structured environment in which to offer such an educational opportunity.

CHAPTER ELEVEN

Finding the Way

I N THE EARLY DAYS of 1889, less than six months before the hospital was scheduled to open, little was in place beyond bricks and mortar. Francis King, president of the hospital board of trustees, found himself facing the enormous task of filling out the medical staff, organizing the internal organs of the organization, and selecting appropriate leaders for the many interconnecting departments who would transform the parts into a functioning entity. Realizing he needed help, the aging King called on university president Daniel Coit Gilman to assume the additional post of director of The Johns Hopkins Hospital.

Gilman was a man of enormous energy, organizational ability, and panoramic vision. He immediately exhibited his brilliant unorthodoxy by telegraphing Osler, who had only recently signed on and had not yet left Philadelphia, to meet him at the Fifth Avenue Hotel in New York on the following day.

At breakfast, Gilman announced, "Between an hotel and an hospital there is no difference, and knowing Mr. Hitchcock I thought I would first find out how the Fifth Avenue Hotel was managed."

In a few days' time Gilman learned the intimate details of hotel operations, and was immediately able to transfer that knowledge to hospital organization. He began with the search for department heads and asked Osler to call on his contacts from the hospital world. For the post of matron, what would now be called the head of housekeeping, Osler recommended Miss Rachel Bonner, a Quaker he described as "shrewd, business-like, and practical, but with a large warm heart always on the alert and doing daily, numberless little acts of kindness." Soon warmly referred to as Sister Rachel, she made the interns and residents her personal project, often dining with them, pleading their cause with the administration, and counseling them on affairs of the heart. It was generally agreed that she lived up to her advance billing as "a bond of peace."

For a time, Sister Rachel, who was described by Finney as "a quaint little Quaker lady," lived in a secluded apartment in the administration building. The house staff lived together on a separate floor. As the staff increased in size she was required to take up residence on an integrated floor, causing discomfort for all. The residents, who were about to lose what passed for an uninhibited lifestyle, convened an emergency meeting and arrived at a brilliant solution. For their part, they would add ruffles to their nightshirts, and Miss Bonner would wear a bell around her neck. Even the teasing of her crew of young men was part of the familial atmosphere.

The position of head of the nurses' training school was an important one, as it included not only the training of nurses but the position of head nurse of the hospital as well. The four leading candidates appeared, and were interviewed by Billings, King, Osler, and Gilman. The first three—Miss Louisa Parsons, a severe Englishwoman who had served with Florence Nightingale in the Crimean War; Miss Annie McDowell, an Irishwoman trained in England; and Miss Caroline Hampton, a daughter of southern aristocracy who had only recently completed nurses' training at The New York Hospital—were all well received. But the fourth candidate was the winner. Isabel Hampton (no relation to Caroline) was a Canadian who had been superintendent of nurses at Cook County Hospital in Chicago. With a beautiful face and figure, a sweet voice, and a commanding personality, she so charmed her interviewers that when she left the room they smiled broadly at one another as Osler whistled the first two bars of "Conquering Kings their titles take, from the foes they captive make." Little was made of her excellent practical experience and fine references.

Isabel Hampton was offered the lead position but could not begin until the following September. Miss Parsons became interim director, Miss McDowell took charge of the private ward, and Miss Caroline Hampton took charge of Halsted's surgical ward.

Joseph Hopkins, a favorite nephew of Johns Hopkins, was put in charge of the dispensary. L. Winder Emery, a local man and former hotel manager with a tough style and good instincts, was made purveyor. Emery's responsibilities included purchasing and catering, and the resident staff made it their business to befriend him as well as Ben and Gus, the two "colored" waiters in the doctors' dining room.

The last of the important executive appointments was Dr. Henry M. Hurd, a psychiatrist who had been in charge of a mental hospital in Michigan and was chosen to replace Gilman as permanent director of The Johns Hopkins Hospital. He was a slightly built man in his late 40s who favored starched wing collars far too large for his thin neck. He arrived shortly after the hospital opened, was formidable-looking but well liked, and soon became known as "Hank" among the house staff. Hurd was a generally good-natured man but known to suffer headaches, digestive ailments, and foul moods. As the entire institution was new, there was a great deal of trial and error in the evolution of routines, and the house staff would often petition Hurd for changes. Always more kindly disposed to requests when he was feeling well, they learned to send a scout out to take his temperature before making their approach.

CHAPTER TWELVE

William Osler

O N MAY 3, 1889, William Osler was two months shy of 40 years old. He arrived at his new job just three days before The Johns Hopkins Hospital was scheduled to open. By opening day everyone was aware of his presence. Word of his achievements as diagnostician and pathologist at McGill University in Montreal, and then at Pennsylvania, had preceded him. Welch believed that in Osler they had acquired "the best man to be found in the country."

Billings had visited Osler at his apartment on Walnut Street, in Philadelphia, in the early spring of 1889 to recruit him for physician in chief. Without sitting down, Billings asked, "Will you take charge of the medical department of The Johns Hopkins Hospital?"

"Yes," Osler replied.

"See Welch about the details: we are to open very soon. I am very busy today, good morning."

The position would pay $5,000 a year, and offer Osler the unique opportunity to reshape medicine.

He discharged his final duties in Philadelphia, attended a round of farewell dinners, and gave his immortal address, *Aequanimitas,* a primer for young physicians on the necessity of maintaining an even keel in the face of adversity. He wanted nothing more than to be the chief at Hopkins, and proudly arrived for the opening ceremonies stylishly dressed in a Prince Albert coat with a fresh flower in his lapel. Osler was fairly slightly built but not short. He had dark hair thinning on top and graying at the temples, wore a full mustache, and a grin from ear to ear.

An inveterate jokester, he always had a kind word or quip for student and patient alike. It was not unusual to see him walking the hospital corridors with his arm over the shoulder of his resident, sharing a confidence, enjoying a story, or discussing the elements of a case. He was as kindly and interested as Welch, but he positioned himself with the residents as a friend rather than a distant uncle. The doors to his home and office were always open, and Osler quickly became the most popular man at Johns Hopkins.

In April 1889, shortly before assuming his new post, Osler delivered a scathing address before the Medical and Chirurgical Faculty of the State of Maryland on the sorry state of medical education:

It makes one's blood boil to think that there are sent out year after year scores of men, called doctors, who have never attended a case of labour, and are utterly ignorant of the ordinary everyday diseases which they may be called upon to treat; men who may never have seen the inside of a hospital ward and who would not know Scarpa's space[1] from the sole of a foot. Yet, gentlemen, this disgraceful condition which some school men have the audacity to ask you to perpetrate; to continue to entrust interests so sacred to hands so unworthy. Is it to be wondered, considering this shocking laxity, that there is a widespread distrust in the

---

1 Scarpa's space, also known as Scarpa's triangle, is an anatomical area of the upper thigh, below the inguinal ligament. It is bordered by the sartorius and adductor longus muscles, its floor composed of the iliopsoas and pectineus muscles. Branches of the femoral artery, vein, and nerve pass through it.

public of professional education, and that quacks, charlatans, and imposters possess the land?

The indictment was met with a great deal of squirming, nodding, and looking at one's boots. The entire medical establishment was guilty, and the system had to be changed. Culpability aside, his statement could not have done much to defuse the festering town–gown schism. Osler was committed to improving medical education. He had just spent years at one of the most highly acclaimed institutions, which in reality was not much more than another proprietary school, and he was chomping at the bit for change. On this front, Johns Hopkins Hospital and Johns Hopkins School of Medicine were to make several momentous breaks with the past. The medical school would not be a "for profit" institution. The owners of the medical school would not be the teachers. The teachers would not share in tuition fees, and for the first time the preclinical sciences would be taught by full-time faculty. Hitherto this task had fallen to local practicing physicians. For the first time, the chief of service would be a medical school professor and not an independent operator. Medical education would no longer be a business, and the measure of success would no longer be the number of tuition-paying students enticed to enroll.

Postgraduate medical training was poised to take a major turn for the better as well. In a few short months, Osler and Halsted would institute the graduated responsibility residency system and forever change the way doctors were trained. Four years later, when the doors of the medical school finally opened, they would accept only qualified students who had already earned undergraduate degrees. It spelled the beginning of the end for proprietary schools, where unqualified students could enroll, were poorly instructed, and could pay their way to a medical degree.

Medicine was still largely in its diagnose-and-wait phase, and Osler was among the great diagnosticians. Patients followed him, even to this new southern outpost of Baltimore. Osler had little belief in most of the medications being freely prescribed, and it was often joked that he prescribed few medicines, all of which were poisons. Aware of the public's abuse of useless and often dangerous medicines, he wrote, "One of the first duties of the physician is to educate the masses not to take medicine." His blanket opposition was, in fact, flexible and guided by his desire to alleviate suffering.

Osler had attended the Toronto School of Medicine, a proprietary school, for two years and ultimately graduated from the McGill University School of Medicine in Montreal. He studied in England and on the Continent, and married the English and German systems into his teaching. With immense confidence in the value of laboratory work, he believed above all else that learning and teaching must take place at the bedside.

"He who studies medicine without books sails an uncharted sea, but he who studies medicine without patients does not go to sea at all." This became the basis for education in internal medicine at Johns Hopkins, and in tandem with laboratory science made it unlike anyplace else in the world.

Osler was a fixture on the medical wards. He could be seen quietly listening to patients and pointedly asking questions about the individual, not just the disease. But learning about disease did not end at the bedside or the laboratory. Osler had been one of the few physicians who understood the value of following patients to the dead house. The truth would be found on the autopsy table. In Philadelphia, as at Montreal General Hospital, he not only did the postmortem examination of his own patients, but working as a pathologist he had performed a total of 948 autopsies. This was both a source of income and a means of satisfying his immense curiosity about the nature of disease. At Johns Hopkins he remained a firm believer in the value of postmortem examination but was now strictly an observer, as Welch and Councilman were the pathologists. Setting the example for his residents, he not only attended the postmortem examinations of patients who expired on his service, but insisted on following any interesting and perplexing problems he became aware of to their ultimate clarification.

Unmarried, Osler lived in hospital quarters and spent long hours at work. His rooms, near Halsted's, were in a section shared by residents and interns. Osler's immediate neighbor was a resident, who noted that he could pretty much set his watch "at 10 P.M. each night when I heard him place his boots on the floor outside his bedroom door."

As an early devotee of surgical intervention, Osler was fascinated by the changes Halsted was bringing to surgery. As a man experienced in bacteriology, he was duly impressed by his new colleague's meticulous adherence to aseptic technique. This was a welcome change after the Philadelphia years, where little stock was held in its importance.

* * *

WITH THE FANFARE and ceremony behind them, the small, select staff of The Johns Hopkins Hospital set out to fulfill the mandate of the gift. Henry Hurd had replaced President Gilman at the helm; the nursing staff, made up of experienced leaders and enthusiastic newcomers, was quickly integrated into the daily routine, and a spirit of camaraderie was palpable throughout the institution. Much had been made of the quest for excellence at the new hospital, and the public, long-suffering and wary, was heartened by the promise to bring the best of European medicine to America. Despite the awful history authored by generations of surgeons, patients were willing to believe the new discipline would be different, and Halsted's service was busier than expected. Osler's reputation as the finest physician in the country immediately drew the rich and famous to Baltimore, and he did not disappoint. Howard Kelly was enlisted to head gynecological surgery, and his practice followed him, and Welch's reputation as pathologist and spokesman drew doctors and dignitaries alike to see the new phenomenon for themselves. The four young men, Welch,

Osler, Halsted, and Kelly; their assistants; and their residents arrived on the scene at a run.

The only dissenting voices were from within the Baltimore medical community. Not only were their patients being poached, but they were being relegated to an inferior position in the eyes of their community. The University of Maryland Medical School was the backbone of the local medical community, and the incursion of an elite institution, made up almost entirely of outsiders, was perceived as a threat. The possibility of elevating the profession and benefiting mankind did not enter into the equation. In the end it turned out to be a simple question of saving face.

Welch, Gilman, and the trustees were increasingly aware of the resentment building in the medical community, and made an effort to integrate some of the local medical leaders into their organization. The earlier appointment of Councilman, a Baltimore native, as Welch's assistant had had a salutary effect in the preclinical days, but now patients were added to the mix, and another gesture was necessary. This was found in the creation of a board of consultants. The eleven-man group, made up of prominent local physicians, went far toward defusing the situation, but how much their consultation was sought remains unclear. Additionally, seven influential members of the medical community were asked to head the Johns Hopkins outpatient clinics, which were based on the successful outpatient dispensary Halsted had devised at Roosevelt Hospital. The clinics were instantly popular with the indigent population, and becoming co-workers did much to smooth relations.

CHAPTER THIRTEEN

The Operating Room

B Y 1889, MOST LEADING surgeons were committed to antiseptic technique, and many sought to implement some level of aseptic surgery. Halsted's surgical service at The Johns Hopkins Hospital was dedicated to the concept of aseptic surgery from the very beginning, even while the goal remained out of reach. It had been easy, in fact a relief, to abandon the antiseptic precautions of Lister. Carbolic acid spray and dressings were unwieldy, irritating, and less than satisfactory for infection control. Halsted had rejected the Listerian idea of dangerous germs circulating in the air. The real threat were the bacteria harbored on instruments and on surgeons' hands, and all sorts of antiseptic solutions were employed in the effort to control the contamination.

Not long after it opened, The Johns Hopkins Hospital began sterilizing instruments by boiling them. But the withdrawal from carbolic was not complete. Following boiling, the sterile instruments were submerged in tubs of carbolic acid, awaiting use at the operating table. Bichloride of mercury and carbolic acid were still in favor for preparing the patient's skin for surgery. It was a thoroughly unpleasant experience for the patient. Preparation began the evening prior to surgery with shaving of the skin in the area of the incision and the application of antiseptic soaks, so that by the time of surgery the next morning the skin was uncomfortably, and sometimes painfully, irritated.

Carbolic acid, commonly known as phenol, was the primary antiseptic for maintaining the sterility of the surgical instruments. Its effectiveness as an antiseptic had been well known since its introduction by John Lister. One of its advantages was that it did not corrode the surgical instruments, but it did not make for a safe, worker-friendly environment. Patients were only occasionally exposed to these agents, but the operating staff was in constant contact with potentially troublesome substances. Carbolic acid, even in dilute solution, is a very toxic agent. In addition to direct local toxicity in the form of irritation, burning, and ultimately coagulation and destruction of skin, it is toxic to the liver and can cause severe cardiac arrhythmias, and possibly death.

For the first 15 years all surgical procedures were performed in a makeshift area best described as functional. The single, small operating room was located in the basement under Ward G. Getting patients into the operating room was a considerable task. Patients were first placed on the removable operating tabletop at their bedside, then the long board and its heavy human cargo were wrestled down the outside stairwell and into the basement and the operating room. Adjoining the operating room was a still smaller room used for the induction of ether anesthesia. Billings's initial plans for The Johns Hopkins Hospital were a reflection of the low regard in which surgery was held in the aftermath of the Civil War. Halsted made few demands, making do with what was easily available, knowing his needs would evolve over the first few years, as would his concepts of the proper surgical environment. The very basic suite had an open plan and was reasonably well lit. It had running water, which was not available on the wards; waxed hardwood floors; and adequate equipment storage in large wood cabinets in both the operating and anesthesia rooms—everything required for modern, aseptic surgery in the year 1889.

Halsted felt no need for so elaborate an exercise as the isolated tent he built at Bellevue to comply with the Listerian concepts of a decade earlier. The need for cleanliness at surgery was not debated at the new, forward-looking Johns Hopkins. The debate, if there was one, was within Halsted alone, for he had begun striving toward true aseptic technique. It was the moment for an open mind, trial and error, and change.

In the center of the room was an old German operating table first used during the Franco-Prussian War. The design of the table accommodated the copious amounts of caustic solutions used in wound preparation. It consisted of a strong wood frame into which was set a shallow trough, two and a half feet wide and six feet long. On the wooden table sat a stretcher, two feet wide and eight feet long, which served as the actual operating surface. A drain within the basin could be opened to collect the antiseptic fluid in a bucket beneath the table. It was a messy operation, and the surgeons often wore rubber aprons over their white operating suits to keep from getting soaked by the splashing antiseptic.

For the surgeons, preparing their hands for surgery was an unpleasant but necessary evil. Orange sticks were used to clear debris from under their fingernails, after which they scrubbed their hands for five minutes with green soap and scalding water. Then they dipped their hands and arms up to the elbows in permanganate solution, an oxidizing agent, which turned the skin a dark brown color. This was followed by an oxalic acid soak, which neutralized the permanganate and decolorized the skin. The process was completed with a final five-minute dip, fingers to elbows, in corrosive sublimate, now known more commonly as mercuric chloride, the most toxic substance of the lot. Mercuric chloride has a health rating of "4-poison." It is potentially fatal if ingested, causes redness and pain when applied to the skin, may cause allergy, is readily absorbed through the skin, and can cause neurological damage and kidney failure. Otherwise, it was a safe and useful tool.

For a time open wounds were irrigated with corrosive sublimate as well, but observation of the toxic effects led to the discontinuation of its use. Sterile instruments were stored before use in a dish of carbolic acid beside the operating table. The combination of mercuric chloride and the carbolic acid in which the sterile instruments were stored caused frequent painful rashes and red pimples, which were often debilitating. Weaker solutions of corrosive sublimate were tried, and soon it was replaced entirely with less irritating substances and reduced rituals, but until the advent of sterile rubber gloves the process of preparing for aseptic surgery remained decidedly unpleasant.

Traditional black, fitted Prince Albert coats had been in favor as operating garb since the 1876 visit to America by Albert, consort to Queen Victoria. Knee length, and with a full skirt, instead of being "cut away" the coats had notched velvet collars in single- or double-breasted styles. Before surgery they were pulled from pegs in the operating room where they hung, caked with old blood, tissue detritus, and pus from previous surgery. Using these filthy coats saved the surgeon's street clothes from becoming soiled, and the cumulative signs of battle on the coats became something of a badge of honor. In Halsted's operating room they were shed in favor of white duck operating suits, consisting of short-sleeved shirts, trousers, and a little round skull cap. In the final touch, the traditional short, rubber boots worn over street shoes were replaced by white tennis shoes.

While steadfast in his belief in aseptic technique, Halsted was willing to experiment with any modality to improve operating conditions and patient safety. Nurse Caroline Hampton fell victim to severe dermatitis of her hands, assumed to be caused by constant contact with mercuric chloride. Halsted sought a solution for the painful rash, which threatened to drive her from his operating room. On a trip to New York he met with representatives of the Goodyear Rubber Company, and arranged for them to produce two pairs of fine rubber gloves with wrist gauntlets. These were not unlike the rubber gloves

Welch had brought from Germany, and that he wore at autopsy, but Welch's gloves were very thick and dulled sensation far too much for use in surgery. The Goodyear gloves were thin enough to cause only modest loss of sensation, and after a bit of experience caused no appreciable tactile deficit. The gloves protecting Caroline's hands were sterilized by boiling and dipped in carbolic solution. They were sturdy and reusable, and allowed Caroline to continue to function as Halsted's surgical nurse.

By the end of 1889, rubber gloves were regularly worn by the nurses who squeezed out the gauze sponges soaked in bichloride of mercury, as well as the intern who passed instruments and was constantly fishing them from the carbolic basin and threading carbolic-soaked needles.

The introduction of rubber gloves to surgery began as simply and unremarkably as protecting a nurse's skin from irritation. No one, it seems, saw this innovation as anything more than that. Halsted had inadvertently set into motion the single greatest advance in the history of sterile technique.

Several months later, when Caroline Hampton left the operating room, rubber gloves were abandoned other than for optional use by the intern. Over the next six years, sterile rubber gloves were worn only when surgeons opened clean joints, which required the utmost sterility. Once a joint was seeded with bacteria, the infection was almost impossible to uproot. Why the enormous potential of sterile rubber gloves was missed for so long after being introduced remains a mystery. Halsted's seminal bacteriology work had proven the impossibility of sterilizing hands by scrubbing and immersion in bichloride of mercury, or other antiseptic solutions. The use of gloves by the nurse was ultimately ordered because Halsted felt that handling, dipping, and squeezing out sponges carried an additional risk of infection when done bare-handed. And yet he did not expand the use of gloves to include the surgeon. One would have expected a bell to go off long before 1896, when his resident, Joe Bloodgood, in a conversation about the gloves quipped, "What's sauce for the gander is sauce for the goose," and began wearing rubber gloves for every operation. Soon afterward, the entire team followed suit, and the days of bare-handed surgery came to a close as a sterile rubber barrier was placed between the surgeon's hands and the wound.

Soon the rubber gloves were heat sterilized, too, and the circle of sterility was complete. With routine use of sterile operating gloves the story of aseptic surgery was changed forever. Prior to this, Halsted had established an admirable record of clean, infection-free wounds, which was justifiably attributed to his technique. He insisted on scrupulous asepsis, gentle handling of tissue, careful control of bleeding, the use of fine silk sutures to minimize tissue damage, and subcutaneous silver wire closure to eliminate contact with the unsterile skin by tunneling under, rather than piercing, it.

Halsted's rate of infection after hernia repair was a very respectable 9 percent. After introducing the use of sterile surgical gloves, it dropped to less than ½ of 1 percent.

CHAPTER FOURTEEN

The Radical Cure of Breast Cancer

FINNEY SAT AT THE patient's head with the ether apparatus set in a box on the floor at his feet. The task was new to him, but he managed the inhaler well, keeping the patient unconscious without asphyxiating her. He had been enlisted for his free hours before the 10 A.M. opening of the dispensary, and though it wasn't what he chose to do, at least it brought him into the operating room. When the woman was fully asleep, her skin was washed with green soap, painted with mercuric chloride, and draped with sterile white sheets, exposing her lumpy, battle-scarred left chest. Thirty-eight years old and the mother of ten, she was fully occupied at home, and had waited until the pain in her breast and arm became severe enough to drive her to the hospital. The mass had been present and growing for at least six months, and the pain and infection under her arm could no longer be ignored. The tumor now occupied virtually her entire left breast. The nipple was retracted, and the infected, cancerous lymph nodes in her axilla had developed an abscess, which Halsted and his team had drained 17 days earlier. On the surgical table, her axilla was no longer inflamed, but it remained rock hard.

It was mid-June of 1889, and this was the first surgery for cancer of the breast to be performed at Johns Hopkins. Caroline Hampton, the scrub nurse; Fred Brockway, the newly minted surgical resident; and his assistant resident scrubbed their hands as directed with green soap and a stiff brush, rinsed in scalding water, and disinfected their hands and arms with the same caustic solution of mercuric chloride used on the patient. Dressed in the new operating uniforms of short-sleeved, white cotton operating suits and sterile gowns, they took their positions. Halsted inscribed an extensive incision from the axilla, near the old abscess site, counterclockwise down and along the sternum, under the breast, encompassing the entire breast, and up the lateral aspect, meeting the original swipe and forming a giant, bloody teardrop.

Hardened by infection, the skin near the axilla was unusually difficult to reflect upward, and the lymph nodes under the arm couldn't be reached. The recent abscess had matted them down. Common sense dictated returning to the axilla on another day. Dissecting with a scalpel, Halsted mobilized the entire breast and much of the underlying pectoralis major muscle. He applied artery forceps to arteries and veins as they appeared, and secured the vessels with fine silk sutures to minimize blood loss and crushed tissue. He removed the anatomical specimen in its entirety and carefully examined it at the operating table. Having taken great care to avoid cutting into the tumor for fear of spreading the cancer, Halsted now rolled the mass between bare fingers, and cut through its substance, making careful mental notes of its consistency and appearance before sharing his thoughts with his assistant. He placed numerous suture tags on areas of interest before sending the specimen to Welch's pathology laboratory, where microscopic sections would be prepared for later examination.

Halsted had performed the 12th operation at the new hospital, and the first for breast cancer. He had previously performed this new, extensive technique in New York more than five years earlier, and he had been determined to expand on it. Over the last decade, surgeons had searched in vain for a procedure to halt the ineluctable mortality from cancer of the breast.

European surgeons like Volkmann and Billroth were advocating radical removal of the breast for every cancer. For tumors that seemed particularly deeply invasive, the pectoralis muscle beneath the breast was removed as well. The concept of cancer of the breast spreading through microscopic lymphatic channels draining tissue fluid and lodging in lymph nodes was generally accepted, but the idea of the removal of all the regional lymphatic channels and the lymph nodes was not. Volkmann postulated that the fibers of the pectoralis muscle propelled the cancer cells along by muscle action, so he stripped off the fibrous facial coating of the muscle, sometimes including muscle fibers as well. Little thought was given to the possibility of distant spread of the cancer through the bloodstream. The success of surgery was determined by the presence or absence of local recurrence of the cancer. In the best hands, the rate of local recurrence—the reappearance of the cancer in the previously operated area—exceeded 50 percent. Distant metastases were universally lethal, and preventing their spread was not even considered.

Excluding death by distant metastases from the measure of success was not surprising. One changes what is changeable; impossible tasks come later. The idea of preventing distant metastases was simply impractical. Knowing what we know now, this seems insanely pessimistic, and the idea of a 50 percent local recurrence rate, unthinkable.

This abysmally poor performance was a direct consequence of how advanced the disease was at the time of detection. Though the first rudimentary mammography was performed in Germany in the late 19th century, it did not come into general usage until the 1960s. Public health information was negligible, and usually restricted to epidemic problems such as containing the spread of cholera and influenza. Self-examination of the breasts was unthinkable in the shadows of Victorian morality, and certainly not a topic of conversation. Breast cancers grew unimpeded and undetected, noticed only when they couldn't be ignored and treated when they couldn't be tolerated. Routine checkups didn't exist, and doctor visits were restricted to serious illness or injury. Most breast cancers grew larger than a lemon, ulcerated through the skin, retracted the nipple, or massively involved the axillary lymph nodes before they were treated. In all likelihood the advanced disease had already spread unseen to other parts of the body. Small wonder success was judged by reduction in the incidence of local recurrence. Radiation and chemotherapy were decades away, public awareness was negligible, and regular medical care was out of the reach of most women. Understandably, surgeons measured success in small increments.

ON THIS DAY, Halsted was frustrated by his inability to complete the operation. He had come to believe that the best chance at containing cancer of the breast was full removal of the tumor, the surrounding tissue, overlying skin, underlying muscle and fat, and all the regional lymphatic tissue into which the area drained. Giving the tumor a wide berth was essential. When he explained the extent of his radical surgery, he made it clear that he had weighed the efficacy of extensive excision of involved tissue against the added morbidity and discomfort to the patient. He always underscored the fact that "getting around" the tumor was crucial; one had to avoid cutting through tumor-infiltrated tissue. Halsted was certain that violating this premise would spread the cancer. The very knife used to remove the cancer would "infect" clean tissues with cancer cells if one cut through any involved area.

In the late stages of breast cancer commonly seen in clinics at the time, the tumor frequently grew into the undersurface of the skin, and sometimes through it, presenting as a fungating mass on the chest. The lymph nodes in the axilla, around the clavicle (collarbone), and even along the sternum (breastbone) were frequently enlarged, and were found to contain tumor at postmortem examination.

The cancer can spread its tentacles in every direction—most frequently through the lymphatic channels, as suggested by the presence of cancer-free tissue between the original mass and the lymph nodes into which the lymphatics drained. It burrowed deeply as well, sometimes onto the fascia covering the pectoralis major, the large muscle that makes up most of the substance of the chest; sometimes into the muscle itself; and often into the fat between the pectoralis major and the smaller, underlying muscle, the pectoralis minor.

Halsted studied all this. He examined every patient in painstaking detail, asking, touching, moving, and smelling. He examined every surgical specimen with Welch or Councilman, correlated his impression of gross appearance with microscopic findings, and ultimately followed those who succumbed into the dead house.

The conclusion was obvious: the only way this awful disease could be contained was to be more aggressive than the disease itself. Halsted postulated that removing the breast, including all the skin above it; the pectoralis muscles, major and minor, beneath it; the lymph node–rich axillary fat; the lymph nodes beneath the clavicle; and even removing a section of the bone itself to reach the lymph nodes above would encompass the most frequently involved sites. This he did "en bloc," or in one mass, never detaching pieces, cutting through possibly involved tissue, or excising separate segments. The large teardrop incision made through the skin and fat surrounds the breast. The insertions of the pectoralis muscle near the sternum are cut, and the entire specimen pulled upward until the axillary contents are dissected free and removed, hanging like a tail from the large bloody specimen.

Throughout the procedure, assistants applied dozens of fine artery forceps to every artery and vein in the field, taking care to cross-clamp, divide, and tie them with fine silk thread before they could be accidentally cut and bleed. Each vessel was cleanly identified, and care taken to grasp only the blood vessel, and not surrounding tissue, in the jaws of the fine instruments Halsted had designed after those brought back from Germany. Some 250 clamps hung from the wound and the specimen, this at a time when most hospitals owned a half dozen clamps, if any at all. Halsted demanded the silk tied around the vessels be applied with just enough force to stem the hemorrhage, and not enough to crush the tissue.

Anatomically correct dissection and compulsive attention to detail were required. It was not the province of the slash-and-dash surgeon. In fact, it was not then the province of any other surgeon in the world, and it fell to Halsted and his diaspora of residents to preach this gospel and make the surgical world believe.

If Halsted's examination of patients was lengthy, his operations seemed interminable. Some years after the first operation, Will Mayo, one of the famed Mayo brothers of Rochester, Minnesota, came to watch Halsted perform his by then famous breast operation. After watching for two hours, Mayo left the operating room and said, "I have never seen a wound operated at the top while the bottom was already healed."

Visiting colleagues who had known Halsted as one of the fastest, slickest surgeons in New York City were amazed by the transformation. In Baltimore, he had become a thinking surgeon who sacrificed speed and style for scrupulous care and anatomical integrity.

His blue-gray eyes were fixed on the surgical field, and he stared down transgressors over his pince-nez glasses when his attention was diverted. He spoke little during surgery, and expected the same of others. Once during a procedure he turned to an assistant and said, "May I ask you to move a little? You've been standing on my foot for half an hour."

Nothing took place in Halsted's operating room without study and planning, yet the hospital staff had nicknamed him "Jack the Ripper."

Much of the joking must have stemmed from how busy the surgical service was from the day the hospital opened its doors, and some may have arisen as a result of the magnitude of his new procedure. The apocryphal dark joke in the hospital was of the orderly asking Halsted which part of the patient was to be returned to the ward.

In the seven months from the hospital's opening in early May to the end of 1889, 316 patients were admitted to the surgical wards. Not all of these admissions culminated in surgery, but the sheer volume kept Halsted, Finney, Brockway, and the assistant resident, George Clarke, very busy. Five of these early patients had carcinoma of the breast. As word spread of Halsted's new operation, and its apparent success, women in need were drawn to Johns Hopkins for treatment.

To the uninitiated, the sheer magnitude of the procedure must have been seen as terribly brutal, despite its being devised to save, or at least extend, lives. Other surgeons were experimenting with similarly extensive procedures. One English surgeon summed up the new philosophy by saying that doing anything less was "a mistaken kindness to the patient." Osler and the other clinicians were impressed with the new surgical service, as well as the new attitude toward surgery, and began suggesting surgery for patients where previously they would have shunned the idea. Halsted quickly became a star.

In time, the "Jack the Ripper" sobriquet disappeared, and "The Professor" took its place. The new nickname originated with the father of a young patient who kept referring to Halsted in conversation as "professor" this, and "professor" that. Halsted turned to the man and said, "Oh, don't call me professor. I'm no dancing master."

That was enough for the residents and students, and "The Professor" it was. Welch was "Popsie," and Osler "The Chief." Halsted was "The Professor" for the remainder of his life. He endured the name in silence, and it was never uttered to his face.

In April 1894, Halsted presented a paper before the Clinical Society of Maryland, in which he reported that of "50 cases operated upon by what we call the complete method, we have been able to trace only three local recurrences."

Three local recurrences of 50; 6 percent local recurrence with the Halsted method, against more than 50 percent for surgeons employing older, less "complete" methods. Once the paper was published, surgery for cancer of the breast changed. Surely, the astounding difference in local recurrence was worth the extra effort. The Halsted mastectomy became the gold standard for care until the mid-20th century.

Halsted was seen as a formidable and eccentric figure. He was now using a great deal of morphine, and had become enigmatic and detached. He became increasingly fragile as the day progressed and his morphine level ebbed, yet he maintained a bruising schedule, rushing from operating room to dispensary, afternoon lectures to graduate students, and finishing the day in the experimental laboratory. By evening he was once again the Halsted of old.

HISTORICAL NOTE: By the 1960s, proponents of both more radical surgery and less radical surgery were challenging the Halsted mastectomy. Confusing and counterintuitive as this seems, it was the state of affairs. The ability to detect breast cancer using X-rays was demonstrated in 1913 by a German surgeon who studied 3,000 mastectomy specimens and was able to show a distinctive X-ray pattern associated with the cancers, making them identifiable within normal tissue. By the mid-1950s mammography was being used as a diagnostic tool, and by the mid-1960s it was generally available, and far more sophisticated and accurate. Breast cancers were being detected much earlier, and the huge tumors presaging florid disease became less common. Cure rates improved—not simply local recurrence rate, as in the Halsted years, but actual and complete cure as measured by five- and ten-year disease-free survival. As mortality figures plummeted with the mastectomy, some surgeons felt more aggressive surgery would save more lives. They encouraged wider dissection of lymph nodes, including chains within the chest. In effect, they were proposing super-radical mastectomies. These procedures were encumbered by longer hospitalizations and greater postoperative morbidity. They may, or may not, have increased cure rates in more advanced cases. With no clear statistical evidence of superior results, the super-radical mastectomy was not generally adopted.

From the other flank, a few well-regarded surgeons dared to suggest that with the disease being discovered so much earlier, perhaps smaller, less mutilating surgery would suffice to treat the much smaller tumors being incurred. By the 1970s, the surgical community had rallied behind the muscle-sparing modified radical mastectomy, which replaced the Halsted operation. Meanwhile, others were studying the possibility of doing even less extensive procedures. Leading the charge were Oliver Cope of Boston and George Crile Jr. of Cleveland, the latter the son of an esteemed contemporary of Halsted's. The medical community was fairly unanimous in their damnation of less radical surgery, calling the concept a step backward. But survival rates for "lumpectomy" and radiation for smaller tumors were the same as for the similar tumors treated with mastectomy. Growing pressure from women encouraged larger-scale trials resulting in similar outcomes within the early-diagnosis groups. With early diagnosis and the advent of effective adjunct therapy, lumpectomy with radiation and/or chemotherapy has replaced the radical mastectomy in the majority of breast cancers.

One hundred years ago the breast cancer patient was virtually doomed. Halsted changed all that. His actual cure rate was very likely depressing, given the advanced stage in which his patients were seen. However, he dramatically reduced the incidence of local recurrence, ensured an apparently disease-free period, and very likely cured a large number of previously incurable cases. He established a protocol for removing cancers and developed a more effective operation against which all others had to be compared. As diagnostic tools improved over the years, and smaller tumors were being detected and treated, the overall cure rates rose to nearly 90 percent. In smaller, early-stage cases the cure rate now approaches 100 percent.

CHAPTER FIFTEEN

Life in Baltimore

URING THAT FIRST HECTIC year, Halsted took his leave of Welch and the Simmons house on Cathedral Street. Johns Hopkins had made provisions for in-hospital living accommodations for interns, residents, and senior nursing personnel. For the young doctors under the new teaching regime, there would be little time for life beyond work. The in-hospital quarters not only implied total commitment, but facilitated it. Staff nurses were not lucky enough to have hospital housing. As a group, they felt themselves underpaid and overworked. In addition to learning nursing skills, the Training School taught them to cook and clean. Part of their uniform included brown oxford shoes. These, the nurses called their "duty bootie," and felt signified their underclass treatment and "second class citizen plight."

Both Halsted and Osler wished to be as close as possible to their still-evolving responsibilities. They chose to live in rooms not far from each other, on the third floor of the hospital. Halsted, far more particular about his surroundings than Osler, found time to furnish his small, two-room apartment with fine antique furniture and good carpets. Continually dissatisfied with the overall look, Halsted had the walls repainted a number of times until he found the proper shade.

One day in the spring of 1890, he entertained three young women in his suite. His guests were his surgical nurse, Caroline Hampton; her sister, Lucy Haskell; and their old friend, Sally Carter. The rooms had a Victorian air, with stuffed furniture, antique tables, and a large photograph of the Sistine Madonna over the mantel. There, in front of the open fire in the sitting room, Halsted and his guests chatted and drank black Turkish coffee, which he had carefully prepared.

The nature of Halsted's relationship with Caroline Hampton was immediately apparent to the two other women, and upon leaving the hospital they drew the obvious conclusion. Despite what she witnessed, Lucy Haskell knew her sister, and their upbringing, and could not imagine her marrying anyone but a southern planter. Certainly not a doctor.

WITHIN THE HIERARCHY of the antebellum South, few families had earned the distinction and power of the South Carolina Hamptons. Caroline Hampton was the daughter of Frank and Sally Hampton, granddaughter of Wade Hampton II, and great-granddaughter of the first Wade Hampton. By 1860, the Hamptons were among the wealthiest families in the South, holding vast cotton estates in South Carolina and Mississippi, and more than 3,000 slaves.

Caroline's mother, Sally Baxter Hampton, died of tuberculosis in 1862, and her father, Frank Hampton, was killed on June 9, 1863, at the Battle of Brandy Station, leaving the children in the care of his three unmarried sisters. The family fortune did not survive the war either. With the loss of slave labor and destruction everywhere, economic recovery for an agricultural dynasty was soon found to be all but impossible. Millwood, the ancestral family home, was directly in the path of Sherman's march to the sea and had been burned to the ground.

Land rich and cash poor, the remainder of the family struggled along as impoverished aristocracy. Apparently enough money was available for the children to be sent off to school. Caroline and her sister Lucy were educated at Edgehill, near Monticello, run by Miss Randolph, a great-granddaughter of Thomas Jefferson. Caroline returned home as young woman of 18, and for a number of years spent her time with her dogs and horses until the need to strike out on her own brought her to New York, where her maternal grandmother and aunt lived. Initially, Caroline enrolled in nursing school at Mount Sinai Hospital, but quickly transferred to New York Hospital, where she earned her degree and some nursing experience before relocating to Baltimore and her new job at The Johns Hopkins Hospital.

Caroline Hampton was a solidly built woman, perhaps a bit masculine in appearance, and accustomed to being treated with the utmost respect she believed due her station. From the start she drew mixed reviews. Efficient, patrician, and mechanically minded, she was well suited to work with the patrician, introverted, and sarcastic Halsted. Though she proved capable of discharging the responsibilities of head surgical nurse, she continually clashed with her superior, Isabel Hampton. Halsted, searching for an agreeable solution, made Caroline his scrub nurse, thereby removing her from Isabel's supervision, while keeping her close at hand.

A few weeks later, Caroline resigned her position at the hospital and she and Halsted announced their engagement. Osler was among the few who saw it coming; he had witnessed his colleague sitting close by Caroline, explaining the fine points of anatomy at a table strewn with human bones. It seemed so sudden and out of character that Osler composed a few lines gently mocking the surgeon. Halsted was capable of enormous charm and generosity of spirit, qualities that were rarely in evidence in the clinical setting but touched the few he welcomed into his world. To them, his engagement was cause for celebration. Welch and Osler gave dinners in his honor, as did others including the James family, Halsted's old Baltimore friends. There was a genuine sense of happiness for him among the hospital staff. Putting things into proper prospective, Sister Rachel Bonner, the hospital matron, spoke for most when she explained how well matched the new couple were, calling them both "a little odd."

After Welch, Halsted's closest friend was the anatomist and embryologist Franklin Mall.

By the time of Halsted's marriage, Mall had decamped to Clark University, and then became professor of anatomy at the forward-thinking University of Chicago, before he was lured back to head the department of anatomy when the Johns Hopkins medical school opened. Upon the occasion of his engagement, Halsted wrote to Mall:

My dear Mall:

I know that you will be amused to know that I am engaged to be married. A good joke for you I know. I wish that I could see your chuckles. Miss Hampton reminds Booker & me very much of you. I suppose that is the reason that I proposed to her.

Yours,
Wm. S. Halsted

Both amusing and confusing, one is unsure exactly what to make of the letter. For a period Halsted was very close to both Mall and Welch. The three were bachelors at the time, though Mall married a medical student four years later. Some, including Harvey Cushing, saw Halsted's friendship with Welch as more involved than was ever admitted by either man, but Cushing was the only contemporary to actually write that he believed a homosexual relationship existed between the two.

No evidence, offhand remarks, or writings have been uncovered to suggest anything more than friendship between Halsted and Mall. The letter stands alone as a successful attempt at humor. If the relationship was more intimate than we are aware of, then it would have a different significance indeed.

CAROLINE'S ATTITUDE TOWARD her impending marriage was decidedly different from that of her intended. Three months before the wedding, she wrote to her aunt Lucy Baxter:

> My life had very little ahead as matters stood before—now I do not see why I should not be happy. It is very pleasant to be the first with someone and be taken care of .... and tho' of course a good deal of that will wear off I still think we are enough alike to make each other happy ... One thing I am sure of is that I will never find Dr. Halsted anything but considerate and respectful ... Some time in April I am going to N. Y. for clothes and we will be married in June. We are going to take a furnished house for a year and take time to get some nice house that can be well fixed up ... Dr. H. is the most fussy of men and nothing suits him unless it is a little better than someone else's which means considerable extravagance. Still if he makes the money he might as well spend it and I luckily am very moderate in my tastes.

It is a revealing picture. From the first line, "My life had little ahead ...," one sees the marriage through the eyes of a woman of few prospects and little prior happiness. The idea of a financially secure existence with a sympathetic partner seems to be aspiration enough for Caroline Hampton. The sad pragmatism of the young woman conjures a disturbing picture, which would seem more appropriate as a retrospective rationalization of a decades-old marriage.

The statement "Dr. H. is the most fussy of men ..." quickly summarizes what many anecdotes illustrate. Halsted was a fussy and obsessive youth, and became more so with age. A man intolerant of a speck of dust on his hat and dressed by the finest English tailors and Parisian shirtmakers was about to marry a woman who paid little attention to her appearance; cared not at all for fashion; favored plain, dark dresses and sensible, sturdy flat shoes; and wore her hair tied back simply in a bun.

CAROLINE HAMPTON AND William Stewart Halsted were married on June 4, 1890. Festivities were held at the former Millwood estate—the Hampton family seat—and wedding services at the Trinity Episcopal Church in Columbia. William Welch served as Halsted's best man. Welch was pleased to see his old friend joyful and optimistic about his marriage. To Welch, Halsted confided his amazement that a woman of Caroline Hampton's stature could be interested in so unworthy a fellow like himself.

For their honeymoon trip, the couple went off to the Hampton family lodge in the Cashiers Valley of the Blue Ridge Mountains. The old house and the dramatic land around it meant a great deal to Caroline. They represented the best part of her youth, and she was instantly at home in the country surroundings. Halsted was unfamiliar with the hunting-lodge lifestyle. He neither hunted nor fished, but he was charmed by the place, as he had been with all the traditions of the southern gentry. Their first visit as a couple extended from their early June wedding until the early fall and began their custom of lengthy absences from Baltimore.

The Cashiers Valley, in the westernmost extension of North Carolina, lies at the center of an equilateral triangle bordered by Tennessee, South Carolina, and Georgia. The newly married Dr. and Mrs. William Stewart Halsted made the 180-mile trip from Columbia, South Carolina, by rail to nearby Lake Toxaway. The final leg, from Lake Toxaway to the Hampton lodge, was fewer than 20 miles, but made by wagon over very difficult terrain, the trip was long and arduous. Poor roads and switchbacks through the mountains, with frequent obstacles and washouts, were the price of escape. The land was nestled between angular granite peaks of the Blue Ridge range and commanded vistas of startling, pristine beauty. The elevation of 3,600 feet in a southern latitude made for sunny days and cool nights; 80 inches of annual rainfall provided deep, lush green, bountiful lakes and cascading waters. The remote environment was a paradise for Caroline and William Halsted.

For Caroline it was a triumphant return to the scene of her youth. For William, the initial interest was to escape the oppressive heat and humidity of the Baltimore summer. But the mystique of his wife's southern heritage and his new role as loving husband brought an enthusiastic, if skeptical, attitude toward this new environment. He was a thoroughly urban creature, but the remote beauty of the setting immediately captivated him as well.

Halsted, who arrived with two trunks of city clothing and no more riding experience than an occasional jaunt through Central Park, was fond of telling the tale of his enthusiastic wife leading him on his first horseback tour of the property. At one point Caroline abruptly pulled up her horse, turned to him, pointed with her riding crop, and said, "William, there is a rattlesnake, get down and kill it." Halsted bemusedly went on with his story: "There I was alone in the mountains with this comparatively strange woman, and she wanted me to get off my horse and kill a rattlesnake. She was terribly disgusted when I refused."

His powers of observation and his sly sense of humor intact, Halsted threw himself into the life. He became a good rider, learned to drive a team, as well as the management of a farm that never quite became self-sustaining. Although the cash crops were Caroline's domain, and he rarely interfered, the setting reawakened the Halsted family interest in flower gardening, which was so much a part of his youth at Irvington. Cashiers was a great physical and psychological remove from the city, and from the moment of their honeymoon trip, the old hunting lodge became an institution in their lives.

THREE MONTHS BEFORE their wedding, Halsted had been promoted from head of the dispensary to surgeon-in-chief to the hospital and chief of the dispensary. This was a great show of confidence in his performance, particularly when only a year earlier any appointment at all was in doubt. But a year later, and barely beyond his probationary period, the newly minted surgeon-in-chief went off for more than three months in the country, leaving the surgical service in the hands of his assistant, Finney; Hardy Phippen, the new resident who replaced Brockway; and the new assistant resident. Halsted's summer absences were often stretched to five months: typically, two months were devoted to rest and restoration in the country, for much of the remainder he was totally out of touch with anyone, including his wife. These absences from his duties would become a recurring theme, which more than once brought him to the brink of dismissal.

Dr. and Mrs. Halsted returned to Baltimore in the fall of 1890 and set up housekeeping in a furnished house on Preston Street. Apparently the house was unsatisfactory, and little further mention is made of it. Before settling into a permanent residence, they moved to Madison Avenue in the Bolton Hill section, where they lived for five years. Welch, who continued to live in his two small rooms, was amused by Halsted's pretensions, and wrote to a friend, "Halsted has taken a large house on Madison Avenue, one of the biggest in Baltimore and still feels that he has not enough room to move around."

Apparently he was correct. In 1896, the Halsteds moved into the very large rented house at 1201 Eutaw Place, in the Bolton Hill district as well. Eutaw Place was a grand thoroughfare with an unusually generous, parklike center island, and was among the most fashionable streets of the city. Commanding a gentle curve at the corner of Dolphin Street, the house was a solid, three-story redbrick structure. Bulky limestone balustrades framed the three stone entrance steps, the lowest of which was canted to compensate for the slope of the street. Ornamental iron railings flanked the balustrades and decorated the base of the tall windows that gave onto the street.

The kitchen and dining room occupied the first floor, which was otherwise given over to work space, including Dr. Halsted's surgical library and secretarial space. The second floor housed Halsted's apartment, the centerpiece of which was his beautifully furnished sitting room/work space. Near the center of the room sat his worktable and favorite chair. The large fireplace on the north wall was always ablaze with logs of white oak or hickory, 10 to 18 inches in diameter and aged under cover for two or three years before being shipped to Baltimore from North Carolina. As with most things in his life, Halsted was extremely particular about his fire. Choosing the wood and tending the fire were something of a family tradition, and with pride he would recall his father as "a great student of the open fire and decided ultimately that lignum vitae was the only perfect firewood, burning slowly with small flame and almost without smoke. That time he could buy the rejected pieces of this wood from a manufactory of tenpin ball and it was the most perfect fire I have ever seen. As I cannot command it, I use the next best, white oak or hickory . . ."

Against the wall opposite the fire sat an elegant secretary flanked by bookshelves. Fine Persian rugs and antique furniture completed the setting. In comfortable, old carpet slippers, a dressing gown over his shirt and necktie, Halsted read by the fire, smoked innumerable Pall Mall cigarettes through his ubiquitous white cigarette holders, and frequently worked late into the night. He rarely entertained guests or was visited by his secretaries in his suite, which was largely his private domain. A bedroom and bath completed the apartment. Several small service rooms occupied the rear. Mrs. Halsted occupied the third floor, where her apartment was similarly arranged, though in her case the large room giving onto Eutaw Place was used exclusively as a sitting room. Her bedroom and bath were on the third floor as well.

Windows were open all winter, and only the back half of the house was centrally heated. For the residential area of the house, including the second- and third-floor apartments, the carefully tended, open fires provided heat, which was then distributed through the rooms by the cool, fresh air blowing in through the open windows.

Each took breakfast alone. Halsted prepared coddled eggs and toast on the small gas stove in his private bathroom and ate before the fire in his study. He usually lunched at the hospital, and the couple dined together in the formal dining room on the first floor. For the most part, the hour and a half spent at table was the time reserved for each other. Dinner guests were infrequent. Following dinner, they retired to their respective apartments, Caroline reading or sewing, Halsted at his worktable, reading surgical literature or working on papers. The late 19th century saw the inception of the greatest period of sustained progress in surgical history. Papers were written and published at a furious pace, and it required time and dedication to keep up. For Halsted, this was a necessity and a joy, and until much later in life he was disinterested in any but professional reading.

Unencumbered by city responsibilities, Caroline extended her summer holiday to include the spring and fall as well. On evenings during the months of Caroline's absence, Halsted resumed his pattern of dining at the Maryland Club, while she resumed her life as horsewoman, dog lover, and gardener, soon adding to it the unofficial title of farm manager. The Halsteds renamed the property High Hampton, probably in honor of the ancient Halsted home at High Halsted, in England, and the Hampton family lodge that it had been. Halsted, though every bit the urban patrician, was thoroughly charmed by the country life. He was enthusiastic about his riding lessons and learned to ride comfortably, though never at so accomplished a level as Caroline, and he enjoyed accompanying her through the North Carolina hills, their dogs running alongside. High Hampton was another world, and Halsted was another man when he was in residence.

Returning to Johns Hopkins after that first summer, Halsted resumed work at a breakneck pace, operating almost every day. Surgery began at 8 A.M., and Halsted performed two or three operations each day, assigning the rest to the resident staff or his assistant, Finney, who was already doing double duty as anesthetist on

Halsted's cases. After lunch he conducted formal ward rounds, during which he was trailed by a retinue of residents, interns, and several surgical nurses. He was in the habit of changing dressings on surgical wounds himself, using starched cotton that the nurse first wet and rolled, then trimmed of all loose threads before passing to him for application. It was a rigid routine, followed exactly. Everything adhered to rigid routine. This aspect of Halsted's world was stifling to some, and impossible for others. For those able to find its rhythm, it provided predictable guidelines, and allowed for inordinate freedom of action within the grid of those issues important to the professor. But rigidity did not preclude an open mind, and Halsted was ready to consider better options and change direction whenever clear thinking suggested a better course.

Afternoons, following rounds, were spent primarily in the surgical laboratory. In the four years prior to opening of the medical school, the laboratory work was performed with the assistance of residents and graduate students. Some worked on The Professor's projects, others on problems of their own choosing or "suggested" by him. Few declined, and once involved they were afforded latitude bordering on absolute freedom to work as they pleased. Occasionally they were looked in upon, queried, and helped over hurdles.

CHAPTER SIXTEEN

The Big Four

IN 1888, AUSTIN FLINT, the well-known Bellevue physician, wrote, "What has been accomplished in the last ten years as regards knowledge of the causes, prevention, and treatment of disease far transcends what would have been regarded a quarter of a century ago as the wildest and most impossible speculation."

For the first time, a quantifiable relationship between science and well-being had become obvious. Physicians were able to prevent disease and, in some cases, actually effect cure. In surgery the ability to cure had begun as well, and anesthesia and antisepsis had made it possible to enter any closed space, body cavity, and joint with relative impunity.

Halsted had performed what was very likely the first surgical removal of gallstones on his mother in 1882; the first appendectomy was performed in 1885. Treating all manner of internal catastrophes was no longer beyond the imagination. The greatest strides forward were yet to come, and they would come very soon in an overwhelming cascade of progress. Much of this progress would take place at the new hospital and medical school on a hilltop in the sleepy Chesapeake backwater of Baltimore, Maryland.

By 1890, Halsted had narrowed his focus to a number of issues that would become synonymous with his name. Among them, aseptic surgery and wound healing, the cure of breast cancer, the surgical repair of inguinal hernia, and graduated responsibility residency training would rank among the most important surgical advances in the next half century. These, along with the techniques of intestinal anastomosis, the surgery of the thyroid gland, and the surgical treatment of vascular aneurysm, were topics that would interest him throughout his life.

Halsted exhibited meticulous attention to detail in every aspect of surgery. He insisted on the gentle handling of tissue, and consistently made the point that rough handling of or crushing tissue in an attempt to control bleeding was counterproductive. Devitalized tissue was the perfect medium for infection. He often illustrated the point by opening the abdominal cavity of an animal under sterile conditions, introducing a virulent bacterial culture into the peritoneal cavity, and gently closing the abdomen. With no devitalized tissue to harbor infection, the body's natural defenses would render the bacteria harmless by engulfing and destroying them, and the animal would heal without infection. Conversely, if an animal was inoculated with the same culture and even a small portion of tissue was intentionally devitalized, an overwhelming infection would result, clearly demonstrating the natural defenses of the body and the importance of gentle surgery.

Halsted recognized the need to organize and institutionalize the learning process in order to transform a journeyman surgeon into a scholar. He intended to change the very nature of surgery, and to do that he would train surgeons to train other surgeons. The road would be long and arduous, but the men who endured would be ready to take up positions at the head of other hospitals and universities throughout the country, teaching the gospel and training generation after generation of scientifically grounded surgical educators. The process of becoming a surgical leader would require independent laboratory studies, a complete knowledge of surgical pathology, gradual assumption of surgical responsibility, and teaching one's juniors. All this would take up to eight years, and result in the development of surgeons who would leave their residencies qualified to become surgical leaders at major institutions. Over the years Halsted would train 17 residents, most of whom went on to illustrious careers. He was more interested in training surgical educators and investigators than merely competent surgeons, and it did not take long until he was able to determine which young men met his criteria. His mission was to produce men who were both teachers of the Halsted school of careful, thoughtful, scientific surgery and future contributors to the body of knowledge in surgery.

* * *

IN THE FALL OF 1890, shortly after Halsted returned to Baltimore from his extended wedding trip, Osler saw him in a hospital corridor suffering shaking chills. "This was the first intimation I had that he was still taking morphia," he wrote. As Halsted's physician, colleague, and as one in large measure responsible for his having been given the opportunity to lead the department of surgery, Osler was concerned by what he saw. He confronted Halsted, who confessed that he was, in fact, still taking morphine and could not manage to reduce the dosage below three grains daily, or about 195 milligrams, an enormous amount. The typical dose for severe pain rarely exceeds 40 milligrams daily, usually administered in divided doses of less than 10 milligrams. Halsted was using more than four times the normal therapeutic dose and was apparently undergoing symptoms of narcotic withdrawal. Osler wrote, "On this he could do his work comfortably and maintain his excellent physical vigor (for he was a very muscular fellow). I do not think that anyone suspected him, not even Welch." [1]

---

1 This information was first made public in William Osler, MD, FRCP, FRS, "The Inner History of the Johns Hopkins Hospital," *The Johns Hopkins Medical Journal,* October 1969, vol. 125, no. 4, pp. 184–94. The article included information originally in Osler's hand, with entries impossible for experts to date. The book—locked, sealed with wax, and tied with ribbon—was intended to remain sealed until the centenary

Halsted continued his routine: surgery, ward rounds, laboratory experiments, study of the surgical literature, lunch at the hospital, dinner at home with Caroline, and large daily doses of morphine. In the first years, with the exception of the episode witnessed by Osler, there was no evidence of drug-related disability, but with succeeding years he would sometimes become "ill" and retire from surgery. His summer holidays stretched to five months, and his excuses to the indignant trustees ranged from recurring malarial fever to none at all. It was to become an annual pattern: great productivity, followed by unexplained absences. The length of time during which he was out of contact with Caroline and his colleagues suggest his repeated dalliance with cocaine. Since he confided in no one but Welch, and took great care not to leave written records of his behavior, one cannot reasonably think otherwise. Like Osler, Welch held his tongue.

* * *

BILLINGS AND WELCH had not foreseen the need for a professor of gynecology at Johns Hopkins. The oversight became apparent soon after the hospital opened, and Osler threw his support behind a young phenomenon he had come to know in Philadelphia. Affectionately calling his man the "Kensington Colt," Osler convinced the trustees to offer the position to 31-year-old Howard Kelly. Kelly jumped at the opportunity, gave up his thriving practice and the private hospital he had built outside Philadelphia, and decamped to Baltimore.

Howard Atwood Kelly was the son of a wealthy sugar broker. He was brought up in Philadelphia, attended the University of Pennsylvania, and intended to become a naturalist. After a stint as a cowboy, he

of The Johns Hopkins Hospital, in 1989. Through a series of convoluted decisions the family decided to release the contents in 1969. In addition to the text there are dated notes of questionable significance. Osler goes on to write, probably at some later date, "subsequently he got the amount down to 1 ½ grains, and of late years (1912) has possibly got on without it." This remains unsubstantiated.

returned to Penn for medical school and an internship at the Episcopal Hospital in Kensington. Following the best practices of the day, he traveled to Europe to study gynecology and surgery. Kelly was unusually dexterous and astounded everyone at Hopkins with his surgical skill. Swift and sure, his focus was on clinical gynecology rather than science, and in that role he established new parameters for the specialty.

Halsted and Kelly were polar opposites in every aspect of their personal and professional lives. While Halsted had become a plodding, thoughtful, and rigidly routinized surgeon, Kelly was inspired, balletic, and lightning fast. Halsted observed everything and kept his own counsel; Kelly was garrulous, opinionated, and forgiving. Halsted was a very lapsed Presbyterian, while Kelly was an Evangelical Christian. He prayed before surgery, and he prayed for his patients and colleagues. Paramount among his many spare-time activities was public proselytizing, and he soon became a familiar figure among the fallen women of Baltimore and on street corners where lost souls gathered. He was an abstemious and vocal "anti-saloonist"; an avid outdoorsman; a voracious collector of rare books, portraits, and specimens from nature; a knowledgeable collector of snakes, alive and dead; and perhaps the highest-earning physician in America.

Money was always an important aspect of Kelly's life. Earning it, spending it, and giving it away seemed to bring him equal measures of joy. While still at Kensington, Kelly had founded a private gynecology hospital. He followed the same path in Baltimore, and operated a private clinic concomitantly with the finest teaching service and charity ward yet seen in his field. By 1892, Kelly was ensconced in a huge mansion on Eutaw Place, not far from where Halsted would ultimately live. There he housed his eclectic collections, worked in his library, and with his quiet, German wife raised nine children.

Kelly was a complicated and talented man who could shift from interest to interest and do justice to them all. It was said that watching him operate made other surgeons despair for their own ability.

Exceedingly fast and precise, he demonstrated an innate ability to recognize the proper surgical path and follow it unerringly. He was continually devising and implementing new modalities for the treatment of gynecological disease, ultimately championing the use of radium for the treatment of uterine cancer. Though his colleagues often worried about his increasingly vociferous fundamentalist preaching, their opinions were always softened by his thoughtful gifts, interesting writings, love for his family, and superb work. Over the course of his career, Kelly wrote more than 500 scientific papers. Among 18 books he authored are *Operative Gynecology,* a superbly illustrated surgical manual; *Medical Gynecology,* a comprehensive gynecology text; a number of biographies; books on botany; and *A Scientific Man and the Bible,* a tome justifying the relationship between science and religion.

Along with Welch, Osler, and Halsted, Kelly completed the luminous "big four" that would lead Johns Hopkins to greatness. The interaction among the four, and the time and place in which they found themselves, made the whole of their work greater than the sum of its parts.

CHAPTER SEVENTEEN

Hernia

O F THE AFFLICTIONS AMENABLE to surgical cure, none is as prevalent as inguinal hernia. None has extracted so great a social price, or has dropped so precipitously from the public conscience as inguinal hernia. It has become a curable, nonlethal annoyance, and more the stuff of humorous tales than tragic endings. A cold invading finger, and the eternal "turn your head and cough."

Five percent of children are born with inguinal hernias. Somewhere between 10 and 15 percent of adults develop them, and 500,000 hernia repair operations are performed annually in the United States. Prior to 1889, there was no successful surgical procedure to correct the defect. Findings varied from a small lump in the groin to a huge bulge of intestine expanding the scrotum or vaginal labia. Worse than the incapacity caused by these painful masses was the ever-present specter of a piece of intestine becoming trapped in this abnormal position, having its blood supply compromised by the pressure and the development of a full-blown, gangrenous abdominal catastrophe.

With no cure in sight, something was needed to keep the hernia contained and allow the victim to work. Trusses were just the thing, and an enormous industry evolved. Any gadget, strap, or spring that put pressure on the defect was a welcome thumb in the dike. "Miraculous" and often confounding contraptions came and went, but they offered no cure. Nor did surgery: in 1889 the surgical failure rate was nearly 100 percent.

Clearly, the problem represented a significant economic and physical burden to the individual and to society. Hernias were nothing to be trifled with. Not only are they painful, but they carry the potential to become incarcerated, a situation in which the loop of bowel has insinuated itself into the abdominal wall defect to become trapped. In these desperate circumstances, everything short of surgery was attempted. In 1890, surgery for incarcerated bowel often resulted in fatalities. The first course of non-surgical treatment was called taxis, in which the patient was placed flat, with head flexed and knees drawn up to relax the abdominal muscles, or head down on an inclined bench. Pressure was then applied to the trapped loop of intestine to force it through the constriction and back into the abdomen. But the intestinal loop had often become swollen and compromised, and gentle pressure often proved too forceful, resulting in perforation, peritonitis, and death.

Hernia, by definition, is any circumstance in which part of an internal organ protrudes through a weakness in the containing wall. Usually this refers to intestines protruding through a weakness in the abdominal wall. There are many sites of potential weakness where this may occur. These include the umbilicus, the site of major blood vessels perforating the abdominal wall; any man-made weakness, such as a surgical incision; and far and away the most common of all, the inguinal hernia, in which the ring in the lower abdomen through which the spermatic cord exits is unnaturally expanded to allow the insinuation of bowel, which follows the path of the spermatic cord through the external inguinal ring and into the scrotum. The anatomical variations of inguinal hernia—indirect, direct, and femoral—are different entities sharing common anatomical ingredients within the confined space of the groin. The most prevalent, complicated, and potentially dangerous of these is the indirect hernia, which occurs far more frequently in males.

AS EARLY AS THE Middle Ages, the debilitating symptoms of hernia were of such magnitude that men were willing to endure the brutality and risk of surgery for the chance of relief. Such relief, when it came, was fleeting. More often infection, recurrence, and sometimes death were the result of surgery. Sometimes the testicle and spermatic cord were removed, and a caustic solution or hot iron was applied to the open tissues in the hope that the resulting scar would prevent recurrence. Later, various attempts were made to cure the hernia and save the testicle. Most of these met with failure as well. Then came the idea of opening the groin area, reducing the hernia, and amputating the peritoneal hernia sac into which the bowel had inserted. Soon sutures to tighten the enlarged ring were added to the procedure, with the same dismal result. By the late 19th century surgeons came up with the idea of rolling the redundant hernia sac into a tampon and suturing it into the internal inguinal ring. The success reported for these procedures was never reproducible in the hands of anyone other than the reporting surgeon, making the subjective optimism look more like dishonesty. This led Halsted's New York friend William T. Bull to cite his personal statistic of a 100 percent recurrence rate by the fourth postsurgical year. Bull announced that he would henceforth abandon the term "cure" and resume performing the simplest possible procedure, as its results could be not worse than all the new, more complicated techniques.

Events took a turn for the better on June 13, 1889, when Halsted operated on an eight-year-old boy with a large, congenital right inguinal hernia. This was the first time Halsted would try a radical new technique to reconstruct the hernia defect in the groin. The departure in the technique was the use of the muscle and tough fascial sheath of the oblique muscles of the lower abdomen to reconstruct the inguinal canal floor. Halsted sutured the muscle and fascia to Poupart's ligament, an anatomical inguinal ligament that traverses the iliac bone of the pubis. Strong silk sutures were used to tighten the internal abdominal ring as well. Halsted had gained an intimate knowledge of groin anatomy through innumerable, fastidious dissections. In each case he amputated the hernia sac, created a new internal abdominal ring at the most lateral portion of the wound, and transplanted the spermatic cord superficially. Together the steps comprised what became known as the Halsted hernia repair.

Halsted also inserted several gauze drains beneath the skin and closed it with fine silk sutures inserted into the deep layer, or dermis, of the skin. He had previously shown that the skin was impossible to sterilize. Since these buried sutures did not puncture the surface, they would remain sterile and not introduce infection. Later, sterile silver wire was employed in a continuous buried suture. Silver was believed to possess inherent antiseptic properties, and drains were abandoned. The subcutaneous closure, whether of silk or silver wire, greatly reduced the incidence of dangerous wound infection and wound breakdown in that pre-antibiotic era, and it became part of the Hopkins routine.

Halsted's first cases were reported at a meeting of The Johns Hopkins Hospital Medical Society on November 4, 1889, and subsequently published in *The Johns Hopkins Bulletin* of January 1890. In his historic report delivered to The Johns Hopkins Hospital Medical Society, on October 20, 1890, Halsted referred to his operation as The Radical Cure of Hernia. Among the first 12 patients, there were, as yet, no recurrences.

Edoardo Bassini, a surgeon in Padua, Italy, had been doing a similar operation for some time. He first presented his technique in Genoa, in 1887, in a talk called "A Radical Cure of Inguinal Hernia." This was followed by a 106-page report, published in the Italian, in 1889. The month of publication was not noted, but Bassini had obviously been doing a similar procedure for some time. But he who publishes first owns the operation.

In answer to questions about priority, Halsted wrote to Welch, "Bassini's brochure anticipated my first report by at least a month or two. Whether my first operation was performed before the appearance of Bassini's pamphlet in Italian I cannot say, for the precise date of the pamphlet is not given. In any event I had not heard of Bassini's operation until his German article appeared—possibly about one year after my first operation, neither was I or any American or German, so far as I know, aware of Bassini's first report until the appearance of the second. Bassini unquestionably has the priority. Our operations differed in several respects, but in the essential features were the same."

As early as 1893, Halsted wrote in the *Bulletin,* "Bassini's operation and mine are so nearly identical that I might quote his results in support of my operation."

Halsted wanted nothing to do with jockeying for position in the who-came-first hernia stakes. In the few comments he made on this aspect of the operation, he always acknowledged Bassini.

Over the years, Halsted refined and revised his hernia operation, and carefully correlated each change with results. What became known as the Halsted II operation resembles the original in only the most basic aspects. His residents were so intimately involved with the operation that they became completely comfortable in this anatomically complex region. Patients from all over the country flocked to Hopkins for his care. In the Hopkins system there was only one senior surgeon, William S. Halsted, and very few private patients. Most patients were seen first in the surgical dispensary, where the decision for hospitalization and surgery was made. It was Halsted's service. He performed the operations that interested him and assigned the remainder to an assistant, or the resident. After the initial years spent developing his technique, most of the hernia surgery was passed on to the resident. The system allowed the resident autonomy, and over the years, some residents came to favor other techniques. Rather than insist on strict adherence to the Halsted operation, the department kept careful statistics, which indicated far fewer recurrences when the strict rules of the Halsted operation were employed. Halsted's own cases had a less than 8 percent recurrence rate, and cases done by the residents employing his method were successful as well.

Harvey Cushing, Halsted's fifth resident, a supremely talented surgeon and the man destined to become the father of neurosurgery, achieved distinction in two aspects of the history of hernia surgery. Cushing was independent minded and perhaps resentful of his chief. After a 14-year association, he was one of the great gifts of the Halsted system to the world of surgery. But the trajectory to greatness was painful for Cushing, and his relationship with his chief was complex. Cushing had his own strong ideas and biases, and took issue with Halsted whenever he could substantiate his point of view. Rather than being impressed by the success of Halsted's hernia operation, Cushing made light of the minute details of which it was fashioned and believed that any operation properly performed could cure hernias. Using other techniques, Cushing's recurrence rate of 28 percent proved far higher than the recurrence rate for residents who adhered to the Halsted method, a fact not lost on his mentor.

Others had their own hernia surgery innovations as well. Among them was Howard Kelly, whose superior surgical skill and intelligence made careful consideration of his techniques imperative. Nothing Kelly did in the operating room could be dismissed. Halsted observed Kelly perform his new hernia repair, in which he implanted a marble in the inguinal canal to hold back the hernia sac. Halsted watched closely, and typically, said nothing. Finally, he could no longer avoid comment when Kelly asked him what he thought of the procedure. "Just one question, Kelly, does the marble have to be green or would a pink one do just as well?"

CUSHING DID MAKE a significant and oddly interesting contribution to the treatment of hernia, though it was not, strictly speaking, surgical. Before the development of trained anesthesiologists and sophisticated anesthetic agents, Cushing had become distressed with what he considered "inept anesthetizers." Although Cushing sometimes used chloroform, ether was the anesthetic of choice, and it was difficult to manage. To deliver the vapor, a paper cone containing an ether-soaked sea sponge was held over the patient's nose and mouth by the intern. The first few breaths caused extreme agitation, and attendants were required to hold the patient to the table until the sleep phase was reached. Observation of respirations and pupil size and testing of the eyelid reflexes were the sole indicators of whether the anesthetic level was safe and appropriate. What monitoring equipment existed was, at best, rudimentary. Patients went from agitation to deep anesthesia, and often to too-deep anesthesia. Blood pressure monitoring devices had not yet been invented, and the onset of circulatory collapse could not be anticipated.

Surgery for incarcerated hernia was, and still is, performed on an emergency basis when the trapped loop of intestine cannot be freed by ordinary means. Complicating the situation were the extreme reactions these fragile patients often exhibited to ether and the difficulty in managing them safely. Cushing reasoned that eliminating the general anesthetic in favor of local would serve the patient well.

There was still only one local anesthetic available, and that was cocaine.[1] Knowing nothing of Halsted's history, but recognizing the value of cocaine as a local anesthetic, Cushing took the leap forward that Halsted may have been psychologically unable to consider.

---

1 As safer local anesthetics were developed, they supplanted cocaine. The first was procaine, universally known by the trade name Novocaine. Lidocaine was developed in the 1940s and remains the most popular local anesthetic.

WHEN LARGE AMOUNTS of cocaine solution were injected into the operative site, patients felt a euphoric rush, which soon disappeared, and in its place came shaking, sweating, and palpitations. The solutions were diluted in an attempt to reduce these side effects, and a successful balance between efficacy and toxicity was achieved. Cushing's theory proved correct. Hernia repair was perfectly suited for the use of local anesthesia. Cushing published his experience with the use of cocaine locally in hernia surgery in 1898, and the procedure became standard at Hopkins. On one occasion, Halsted was making ward rounds with the resident and encountered a patient suffering extreme cocaine agitation. Looking at the man, he instructed the resident, Jim Mitchell, "Give him morphia. If you knew how terrible the suffering is with that restlessness after cocaine you would not stint his morphia."

* * *

HALSTED'S WELL-ARTICULATED technique was painstakingly followed with 21 days of hospital-enforced, strict bed rest, which he believed crucial for a successful outcome. To this end, the surgical dressing was covered widely with gauze and plaster of Paris, and reinforced with wooden battens from armpits to knees.

His second hernia patient, George Holdorf, a 20-year-old blacksmith, was banished from the hospital on the seventh postoperative day for "insubordination." Holdorf had left his bed several times and took a cathartic pill without permission. The hernia promptly recurred, and Halsted repeatedly made the point that wound strength is negligible after seven days, and still so compromised at 21 days that he considered enforcing a still longer period of bed rest.

Today's approach to hernia surgery would be unrecognizable to Halsted. Endoscopic techniques, and often the addition of synthetic mesh tissue support, have largely replaced the open, Bassini/Halsted approach. Local anesthetic is routinely employed instead of general, and patients are discharged to home and activity only hours after surgery. The progression of knowledge and technique have made operation and aftercare considerably less daunting for the patient, but the current cure rate for indirect inguinal hernia cannot be much more impressive than the 94.4 percent reported by Halsted more than a century ago.

Halsted often acknowledged the value of Cushing's contribution, but it is very telling that he, the prime mover in both hernia surgery and cocaine anesthesia, did not himself initiate the use of local. Halsted either refused to be openly associated with his nemesis or was psychologically unable to consider it, and perhaps one cannot avoid ascribing the oversight to denial. But cocaine was never far from his thoughts.

* * *

IN ANOTHER INCIDENT, Mitchell was helping Halsted with a thyroid operation. The procedure was still unusual in 1899, and several distinguished surgeons were present to observe Halsted's technique. It was decided to do the operation under local anesthetic, with a dilute solution of cocaine and morphine called Schleich's solution. Halsted injected it sparingly. He opened a large wound in the patient's neck and began applying tiny Halsted clamps to control hemorrhage in what was a notoriously bloody operation. With a flurry of activity around him and numerous clamps hanging from his neck, the patient became agitated and began to struggle. Halsted looked across the table at his assistant.

"Mitchell, I have an awful headache."

With that he withdrew, went into the next room, drank a cup of coffee, and returned to the now quiet patient. He changed his gloves, began to reapply the clamps that had been removed, and calmly set about splitting the neck muscles over the thyroid gland. Again the patient became restless. Again Halsted withdrew.

"My headache is worse. I am going out and rest a while."

After a third attempt to sedate the patient he said, "Now this time you go ahead with the operation. Good-bye."

Only seven thyroid operations had ever been done at The Johns Hopkins Hospital. Halsted had done six, Cushing one, and Mitchell none. Now he faced a complicated operation before an audience of surgical luminaries on the largest thyroid that his chief had ever seen. Somehow, the surgery went well, and the elated Mitchell was entertaining the guests at dinner when a messenger arrived with a package from Halsted. The attached note read, "Dear Mitchell. I telephoned and found you finished the operation and that your patient was all right. Some day you will know what it means to have an assistant in whom you have confidence. I hope you will enjoy this bottle of old Madeira."

Mitchell, who went on to become the leading surgeon in Washington, D.C., very likely had no knowledge of The Professor's enduring drug use.

CHAPTER EIGHTEEN

Establishing the Routine

IN 1890, THERE WERE 100,000 physicians in America, roughly one for every 150 people. Steeped in archaic ideas, they behaved like guild members and aggressively protected their fiefdom and their incomes, but they were rarely able to alter the course of disease or prolong life. Standard practices for medical training were absent, ignorance was rampant, and science didn't have a chance. Bright spots of progress appeared sporadically, but largely, the state of the art was abysmal. All the while, great progress in the laboratory and clinical sciences was being made in Europe. Men like Pasteur, Cohnheim, and Koch had challenged the preconceived notions of the past, and the germ theory was alive and well. Antiseptic surgery, though increasingly practiced in Germany, was still not generally accepted in America, more than two decades after being introduced by Joseph Lister.

The country was ready for change, and the four young men of Hopkins were poised to turn the ignorance on its ear. There was little serendipity involved in these men standing together and finding themselves on the threshold of seismic change. All four, Welch, Osler, Halsted, and Kelly, knew where they had been and where they wished to go. Gilman, Billings, and Welch had been given the general direction and blessed with the wherewithall by Johns Hopkins. The scientific vision was pure and strong and shared. Each of the four came of age when it was necessary to augment an inadequate medical education by studying with the European masters. Each wished to change the situation, and was able to see how that model could be expanded and improved.

In the structure of the new hospital, each would be absolute master of his domain. Similarly, each would head his respective department when the medical school opened. One of the great attractions was the novel idea of departments in the hospital and medical school directed by the same chief. The first six months of operation had been something of a learning experience for all concerned. But they were adaptable, worked as a team, and supported one another, and the hospital was an enormous success.

Halsted was made associate professor in 1890. His operation for cancer of the breast had awakened hopes for a surgical cure, and patients sought help from Hopkins and Halsted. His operation for the cure of inguinal hernia found wide acceptance as well, and despite the unresolved issue of bragging rights between Halsted and Bassini, Johns Hopkins quickly became a center for hernia surgery. From the start, all surgery was performed under what were then the strictest aseptic conditions, and infections became increasingly rare.

* * *

WILLIAM OSLER, the new physician in chief, was not particularly enamored of Baltimore, but it was of little importance since he spent most of his time working. With his resident, Henri LaFleur, and assistant resident, William S. Thayer, he established a routine of hands-on ward rounds and laboratory analysis. Osler saw the value of both German laboratory medicine and British clinical medicine, and his interest in malaria and dysentery kept the house staff at the microscope. All clinical laboratory work, urinalysis, blood examination, and stool examination was performed by the house staff, and this added considerably to their workload. Not only did this work result in established routines and discipline, it was academically rewarding, and the rigorous studies led to expertise and renown for the young physicians.

Initially, Osler was an omnipresent figure on the medical wards, but as routine set in he was no longer fully occupied. Still unmarried, he initially had furnished rooms in the administrative building of the hospital complex, and then kept house off the hospital grounds. With his cousin Georgina serving as his hostess, Osler began an open-door policy that endeared him to the residents and became a hallmark of his presence at Hopkins. He was funny, intelligent, welcoming, and enjoyed a happy evening of drinking and storytelling every bit as much as his young followers. After Georgina married one of the residents, Osler resumed his bachelor life. He was not a clubman in the style of Welch, and did not have the range of outside interests of Kelly. He related well to the residents, and immediately became their older brother. There was none of the standoffishness typical of Halsted, the preaching of Kelly, or the detachment of Welch. Osler was truly the residents' friend, and without doubt, their role model.

Osler was an instinctively great teacher, able to tell the story of disease and the human consequences in a cogent and logical manner. He wrote frequently, but not exclusively, on medicine, and was a prolific producer of prose, poetry, and humor, the latter usually penned by his alter ego, Egerton Y. Davis. Over the years he became increasingly philosophical, and his writing more figurative and dense. But at Johns Hopkins in 1890, he was focused and direct. Among Osler's recurring themes was the diminishing effect of age. During that first winter and spring, he toyed with the idea of writing a comprehensive textbook of medicine. By the following fall he claimed he had sold his "brain to the devil," and signed a contract with the New York publisher D. Appleton and Company for *The Principles and Practice of Medicine.* The $1,500 initial advance proved to be a stimulating omen of things to come. Osler would ultimately achieve a comfortable level of financial independence from decades of sales of his book as revised and updated editions became an annuity.

The book took over his life. The Johns Hopkins Hospital seemed to be taking care of itself, and *Principles and Practice* was a monumental undertaking. Although his huge fund of knowledge provided the skeleton of the work, Osler supplemented what he knew with copious research. Surrounded by handwritten notes and piles of books, he dictated the text to his stenographer. He spent early mornings on the book, a morning hour or two on ward rounds or seeing patients, the afternoon again on the book, and an hour in consultations outside the hospital; then he dined at the Maryland Club and enjoyed a few hours at leisure before his 10 P.M. bedtime.

After his initial flurry of activity, he expended less energy on hospital business. The new hospital was well staffed and not overly busy. LaFleur, Thayer, and the intern cared for the inpatients and the clinic patients, performed all the laboratory work, and ran the day-to-day operation of the service. This was the dawn of academic medicine, and roles were not yet fully defined. There were few hospital beds for private patients, no medical school in sight, and only the house staff was burdened with work.

With an annual salary of $5,000, and some additional income from outside patients, Osler and his fellow chiefs were meant to be free of the business of medicine. Handsomely compensated, they could carry on as they wished. Though Halsted was paid less, he was happy with the new organization of his life, and his operating schedule was soon as demanding as it had been in New York.

Halsted arrived early, changed clothes in his office, and was in the operating room by 8 A.M. The surgical dispensary opened at 10:00, and as surgeon to the dispensary, he tried to attend as soon as his operating schedule allowed. The Roosevelt Hospital Dispensary had become a model of its kind, and making use of his experience there the board of trustees put Halsted in charge of all outpatient services.

The dispensary was the primary source of surgical cases, and the two responsibilities were closely related. As the surgical load increased, Finney assumed increasing responsibility for the dispensary and Halsted spent more of his time in the operating room. Soon he was doing several operations each morning, with Finney administering ether until he was needed in the dispensary. At noon, Halsted retired to lunch with the others.

The nuclear members of the Hopkins staff lunched together regularly. In that fraternal atmosphere someone was always the butt of Osler's pranks. Halsted participated in the freewheeling discussions and parried well with Osler, but he was not the witty raconteur of evenings at the Club. Welch, Osler, Councilman, Kelly, and LaFleur were lunch regulars, joined by a steady stream of visiting dignitaries from around the world who had made the trip to Baltimore to see what the medical revolution at Johns Hopkins was all about. None of the visitors were immune to the infectious goodwill that was palpable everywhere. The Hopkins people were pleased to be where they were, pleased to be in one another's company, and certain they were on the leading edge of medical history.

During that first year, all levels of professional staff lived in close proximity in the hospital administrative wing. Accommodations for the house staff included a well-furnished bedroom and the ultimate luxury of a separate sitting room or study. Senior staff had similar, if larger, apartments. Living together and sharing meals, with waiters, maids, and bootblacks attending to their personal needs, they enjoyed a pleasant environment that fostered a vertically integrated sense of community, to which even Halsted was not immune. Busy as they were at the outset, there was always time for pranks and exercise, and sometimes, women. Baseball and tennis were popular with the staff, and Halsted excelled at both. Those who knew him in later years might find it incongruous to think of the distracted Professor racing the bases or gracefully covering ground on the tennis court. Finney was witness to both the early and late conditions, and as his doubles partner in the early years, benefited from his chief's athletic ability.

After lunch Halsted made ward rounds with Brockway, Finney, the intern, graduate students, and whoever else could be rounded up. It was the resident's duty to make it known that The Professor was en route and see to it that a respectable turnout materialized. Often this included physicians from the Baltimore medical community who were invited to lectures and clinical demonstrations at Hopkins as part of the initiative intended to soften local resentment toward the academic interlopers. Halsted's rounds were long and formal affairs, and not necessarily enjoyed by those in attendance. He spent inordinate amounts of time at the bedside of each patient. Often, an hour of questioning and probing passed without any explanation of his thinking to the assembled staff or the patient. The population of the hospital was overwhelmingly composed of charity patients, with only the occasional private, or paying, patient, and few private rooms to accommodate them. In 1889, surgery for private patients was still performed predominately in their homes, although Halsted was beginning to treat some in the hospital.

During ward rounds, or in the dispensary, he was unfailingly professional and courteous to patients from every stratum of society. His quiet, cold demeanor, and the slavish need to please him exhibited by the house staff, made the chain of command clear. It was rare for a patient to so much as pose a question.

Part of the responsibility of the resident staff was to prepare for Halsted's pointed questions. What are the symptoms? Has the patient's blood count changed? Are there signs of suppuration beneath the bandage? Concise and accurate answers were expected. In the event that the resident was unable to provide the information, he was met with an icy stare and a withering comment. A humiliating "Perhaps you should find a different line of work" drove at least one young doctor away, and surely encouraged others to either fully prepare or absent themselves. Halsted would then turn away and continue his line of thought as if the embarrassing incident had not occurred, and never mention it again. The single transgression that would end a man's career was lying about patient care. When an assistant resident reported a wound to be healing cleanly, having not actually changed the dressing and observed it, Halsted peeled away the bulky gauze bandages to reveal an open and pus-filled wound. In front of the gathered staff, he dismissed the man from his position. If the patients were not intimidated by his presence, and they usually were, the staff certainly was.

Occasionally Halsted's sarcasm or caustic comments provoked an unexpected reaction. On formal surgical rounds, one of the duties of the ward nurse was to prepare bandages for Halsted to apply to the wound. Holding the bandage and attempting to apply it, Halsted became entangled in the untrimmed threads. He was becoming visibly distressed. Raising the now tangled dressing, he said, "In New York, where I was brought up surgically, a nurse would blush to hand a doctor a bandage such as this."

"Ah, but we are more brazen than they," replied the unintimidated nurse.

Halsted said nothing. He reddened from the top of his bald head to his ears and down his neck, removed the loose threads, applied the bandage, and left the ward without another comment.

If he often turned away from confrontation, examples of pure dismissive behavior abound in Halsted legend. So prevalent are they that they must be considered indicative of character. But Halsted had become increasingly aloof, and perhaps out of touch with simple human situations. The same man capable of cutting one off at the knees could be enormously thoughtful and generous. The same man of legendary attention to detail could continually pass the bed of a patient awaiting surgery and repeatedly neglect to schedule the operation.

Often comments that he meant to be amusing either missed the mark or struck accurately, at the expense of others. Among equals or the uninitiated, a joke or prank might be directed at him. At these times he was unable to respond in kind, or accept the remarks in the manner in which they were intended. Osler visiting the operating room and parking his hat, gloves, and walking stick in the sterilizers, provoked an irritated, "Osler, won't you ever grow up?"

The Osler behavior that so endeared him to others caused Halsted to consider him something of a buffoon. William Halsted's humor was predicated on his sense of the absurd, which he happily shared with a very few intimate friends. But all too often it was unpleasantly to the detriment of others, who were not in a position to respond in kind. Not even his peers considered him jolly, but in social circumstances Halsted was amusing and happy to be amused. His blue eyes revealed a smile before his lips turned up, although no one remembers him actually laughing.

At 3:00 in the afternoon, Halsted either conducted a formal clinic in which patients were presented and discussed or he lectured graduate students. Then, at 4:00 or 5:00, he was off to the Pathological and his experimental surgery. From the opening of the hospital on May 7 through the end of the first year, 316 patients were admitted to the surgery ward. Many of these admissions were tuberculosis related, in the form of abscesses, suppurating lymph nodes, and pus-filled joints. Nine patients were admitted for surgery of inguinal hernia and five for carcinoma of the breast. One patient was admitted for appendicitis, though preemptive appendectomy was not performed.

BEGINNING WITH ONLY Brockway, Clark, and Finney, the size of the surgical staff grew to include the resident surgeon, assistant residents, and interns. There were no bad habits to unlearn at Johns Hopkins. The routines established for the house staff were worthy of Voltaire's "best of all possible worlds." The institution was well endowed and could afford the best equipment. The house staff was culled from an admirable pool of applicants, willing to work long hours and remain on call the rest of the time. The position was 24 hours, seven days a week. The chiefs of service were all under the age of 40 when the hospital opened, and they were bright, energetic, and consumed by their profession.

In 1890, Robert Koch, the high priest of the germ theory, made a startling announcement to the world. The man who identified the tubercule bacillus was once again at work trying to conquer the ubiquitous scourge. He believed a substance obtained from tubercle bacillus cultures, which he called tuberculin, would favorably alter the course of the disease, and perhaps cure it. At least it seemed to have cured tuberculosis in guinea pigs in his lab. The world waited expectantly for the result of clinical trials. Through the John Shaw Billings connection, Hopkins acquired tuberculin, and immediately, and with great fanfare, began injecting it into patients with advanced tuberculosis. A momentous day was dawning.

As it turned out, tuberculin did not cure tuberculosis, nor did it positively affect the course of the disease. Much later it was found to be a reliable indicator of exposure to tuberculosis, but as a therapeutic modality it was worthless. The experiment was an abject failure, but Johns Hopkins was in the forefront of medicine. There were no recriminations. The feeling of all concerned was "at Hopkins we try things."

On Monday evenings the weekly Medical Society meetings were held for the general discussion of medical topics, with the first and third Mondays reserved for the presentation of interesting cases and the reading of papers on the work of the staff.

Medical papers were being published everywhere and on every subject, and it was virtually impossible for individuals to keep up with the literature. In Philadelphia, as in Montreal, Osler had organized small groups for the discussion of foreign papers. As a natural extension of the past success, the chiefs organized a Journal Club for themselves and the house staff, which institutionalized the practice of organized discussions of interesting medical papers. Meetings were held on Thursday afternoons in the small medical library of the hospital. This was very likely the first "official" journal club in the nation, with its stated purpose "to enable all members of the staff to keep fully informed as to what is being accomplished by workers in every branch of medical science with the least expenditure of time." It was a good idea, and it spread to every service of every teaching hospital in the country. Specialty specific, journal clubs are as important and popular now as on October 29, 1889, when they began.

In December of 1889, *The Johns Hopkins Hospital Bulletin* was initiated to chronicle medical events at the new institution and scientific papers. So convinced were the participants of the importance of their mission that the *Bulletin* was offered outside the hospital by subscription. The first issue included an introduction to the hospital and its educational philosophy, Johns Hopkins's letter to the trustees and president of the Board of Trustees, Francis King's address on the opening of the nursing school, Hospital Director Henry Hurd on the relationship of the nursing school to the hospital, Halsted on the radical cure of inguinal hernia, Osler on malaria, and Welch on hog cholera. The *Bulletin* also included the proceedings of the Journal Club and The Johns Hopkins Hospital Medical Society. *The Johns Hopkins Hospital Reports* became a vehicle for in-depth exploration of particular medical subjects.

The *Bulletin* was where Halsted reported his first five hernia operations in 1890, and then a total of 82 cases three years later. The *Bulletin,* from the outset, was the propaganda organ of the hospital, albeit with a scientific bent. A great deal of innovative work was being done, and they made it their business to get the word out. The breadth of ambitious medical talent made it possible to fill the pages of the *Bulletin* with stimulating material, and the interest engendered by the papers served the institution well. The Hopkins experiment, as chronicled in the *Bulletin,* made it required reading throughout the world of academic medicine, and its practical value to the practitioner was soon recognized as well.

Welch's time had become increasingly consumed by hospital and university politics, and after a brief spurt of experimental work he produced little more of note. He continued to oversee the work at the Pathological, lecture to graduate students, and perform autopsies, though these last two tasks gradually fell to his assistants.

Kelly was busy from the moment of his arrival in Baltimore. Word of his extraordinary dexterity quickly filtered through the surgical world. Kelly was that unique surgeon able to operate with one eye on the clock and still do the job faster and better than anyone else. He stood in stark contrast to the slow, meticulous, and maddeningly thoughtful Halsted. But Kelly was open-minded about his work and absorbed the "safe surgery" of the Halsted school into his technique. He just did it faster and better, and everyone, Halsted included, respected him for it. Kelly became so busy with operative gynecology and abdominal surgery that he would no longer have time for obstetrics, which would become a separate department under J. Whitridge "Bull" Williams.

Kelly had a host of intellectual and scientific interests, but he was not an experimental surgeon in the manner of Halsted. He was a great technical innovator, a most prolific medical writer and biographer, devoted to his large family, and obsessed with religion.

FOLLOWING THE HEADY and fairly disorganized early months, Osler and Welch were able to free themselves from the constraints of overly busy schedules. Kelly was, by nature, frantically productive, and Halsted was now as busy at surgery as he had been in New York. His personality would be shockingly unrecognizable to those familiar with the Halsted of old, but his energy level and focus were admirable. His dependence on morphine had not yet sapped his strength.

Gradually, all but the drug use would change.

EARLY-MORNING SURGERY soon became 10:00. Halsted would schedule fewer surgeries and hand over increasing portions of these to assistants. Sometimes he did not appear in the operating room for weeks. His attendance at the dispensary would dwindle, and all formal lecturing would grind to a standstill. The experimental laboratory continued to command his attention, but he would rarely spend a full day at the hospital.

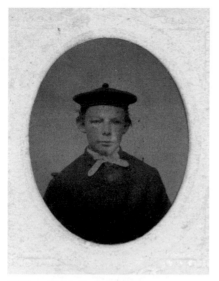

William Halsted, circa 1860.

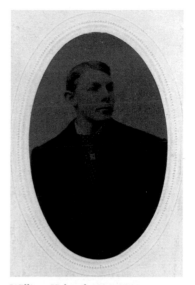

William Halsted, circa 1868.

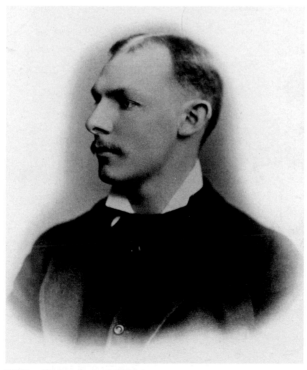

William Halsted, circa 1880.

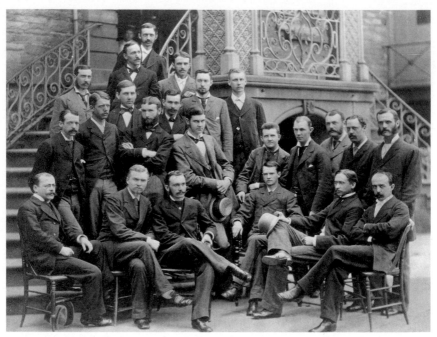

Bellevue interns, 1877. Halsted is fourth from right in second row, under arch.

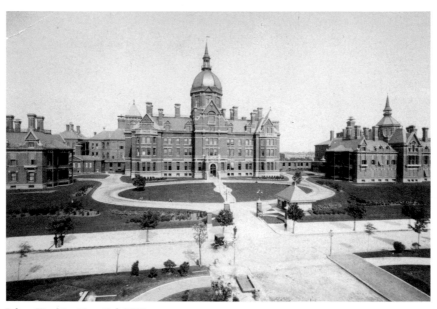

Johns Hopkins Hospital, 1889.

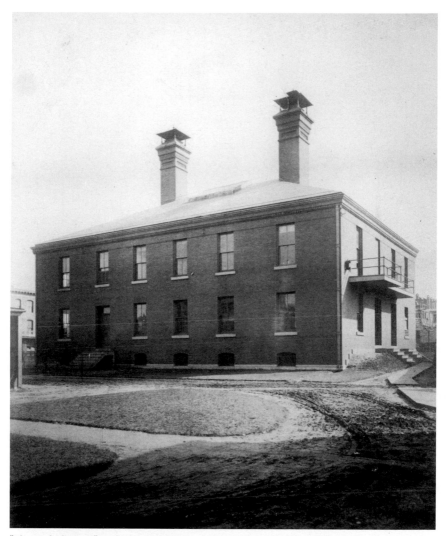

"The Pathological." Pathology building at Johns Hopkins, circa 1890.

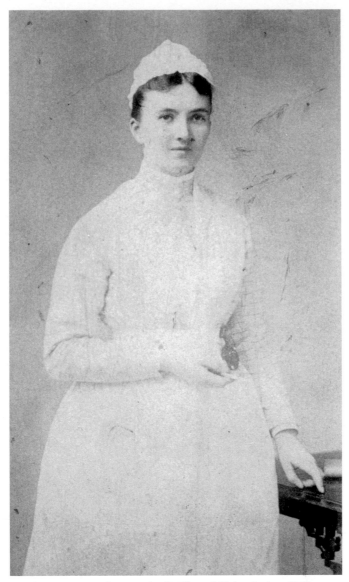

Caroline Hampton, future wife of William S. Halsted, circa 1889.

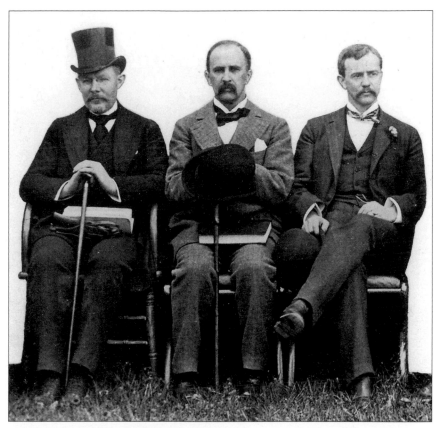

"The three fates." Halsted, Osler, and Kelly, 1897.

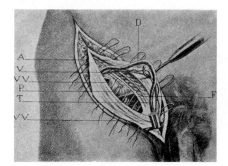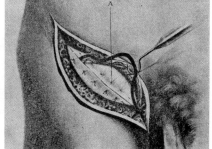

Plates from Halsted's paper "Radical Cure of Inguinal Hernia."

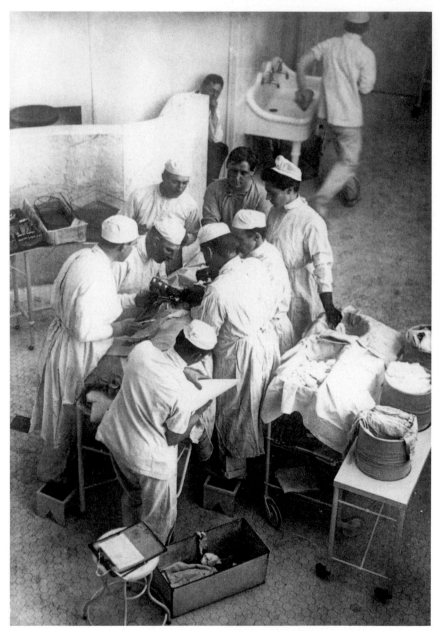

"All-Star Operation," 1904, celebrating the opening of the new operating room. Halsted can be seen at left center bent over patient with mallet in his hand.

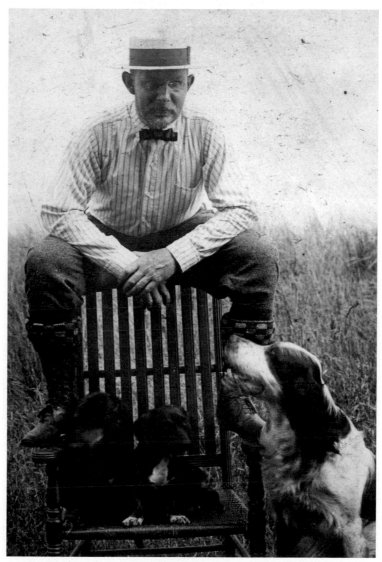

William Halsted, circa 1904, at High Hampton.

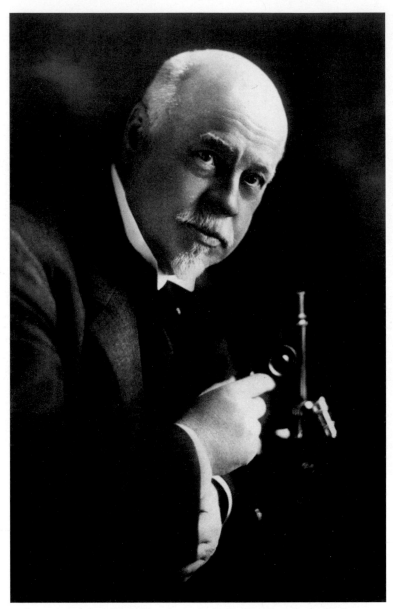
William H. Welch, 1905, the first dean of John Hopkins's medical school.

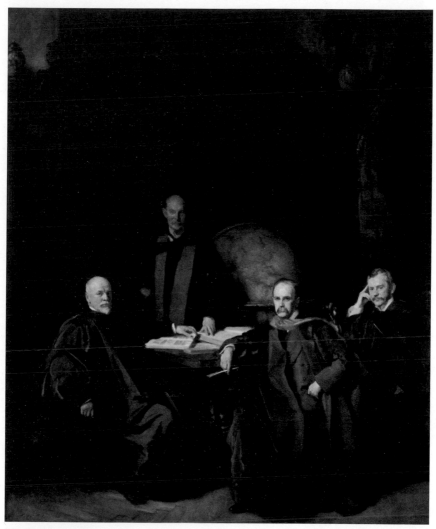

The Four Doctors by John Singer Sargent, 1906.
From left, Welch, Halsted (standing), Osler, and Kelly.

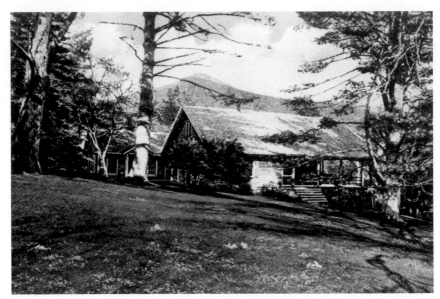

High Hampton, the Halsteds' country home in North Carolina, circa 1920.

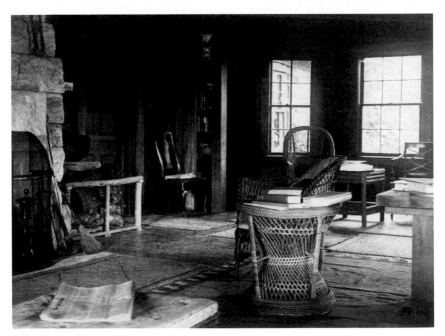

Interior of High Hampton, circa 1920.

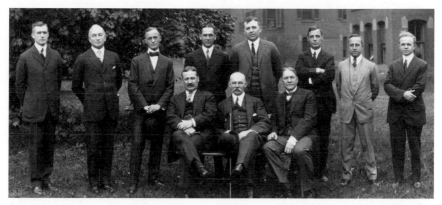

Halsted and his early associates and residents, October 1914. Standing, from left: Roy McClure, Hugh Young, Harvey Cushing, James Mitchell, Richard Follis, Robert Miller, John Churchman, and George Heuer. Seated: John M.T. Finney, Halsted, Joseph Bloodgood.

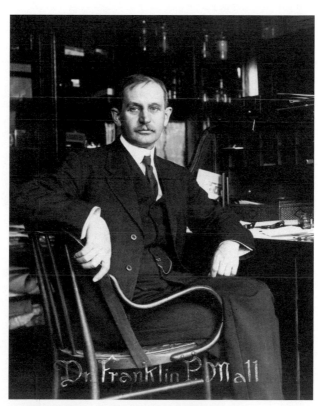

Franklin P. Mall, a famous anatomy professor and one-time laboratory mate of William Halsted, 1911.

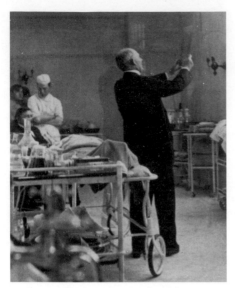

William Halsted studying X-Ray, 1914.

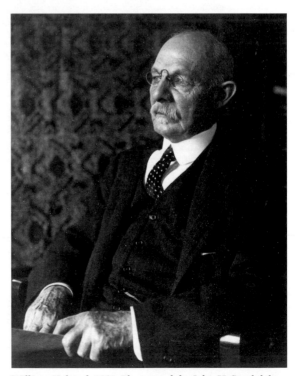

William Halsted, 1922. Photograph by John H. Stockdale.

CHAPTER NINETEEN

Country Squire

FROM THE TIME OF their honeymoon trip in 1890, the Cashiers Valley in the Blue Ridge Mountains became central to the Halsteds' life together. In 1895, Halsted arranged to purchase the Hampton family lodge and the remaining 450 acres from Caroline's aunts. Whether implicit in the transaction or not, "the aunties" became relatively permanent guests, and Caroline's sisters and their children often visited as well. Over the following years Halsted annexed contiguous lands and small farms, until the estate grew once again to more than 2,000 acres.

Halsted's acquisition of the properties usually suited the purposes of both parties, and he was seen as a great benefactor to the hard-scrabble community. But the purchase of an adjoining 50-acre farm in 1897 ended sadly, and resulted in the story of "The White Owl of High Hampton." The tragic tale was often retold in the Cashiers community and memorialized in a painting. As the story goes, Halsted had made an offer to the farmer, Hannibal Heaton, who was amenable to the sale. His wife was not. She became extremely upset and threatened to kill herself if he sold their home. Heaton did not abide her wishes or her threat, and upon returning from completing the transaction found his wife hanging from an oak tree near the house. Legend has it that in the air, circling her head, was a white owl, eerily screeching like a crying woman. Heaton left and never returned to the Cashiers Valley; his wife was buried at the cemetery on the High Hampton property.

Over the years the Halsteds continued to negotiate land purchases through their Charleston attorney, Frank R. Frost. The largest of these was a 640-acre parcel acquired from the heirs of the Preston family at a price of one dollar an acre. Offers made for other nearby land were as low as twenty-five cents an acre.

AS THE LAND ACQUISITIONS restored their control of the valley, the Halsteds began the long process of upgrading the long-neglected buildings. Another cottage was added, along with a guesthouse, both in the unpainted clapboard style of the lodge, which was itself improved in functional ways such as the construction of a pipeline and pump to supply fresh water. The rooms were comfortable and anything but elegant. Furnishings were spare, primarily wicker and wood, and quite unlike the clutter of expensive antiques strewn about the Baltimore house.

The main house and the guest cabins were closely grouped and in the shade of great, old trees. Paths between them were cut and edged, and the immediate grounds were neatly tended. Hiking and riding trails were rough and natural, and often subject to flooding and fallen trees.

The view of the mountains was dramatic. The glittering granite escarpments and waterfalls of Whiteside and Chimney Top mountains, the two highest peaks in the range, were clearly visible, and were as awe-inspiring as any picture postcards. Between the houses and the distant view was a small lake stocked with trout, fast-running streams, and rough-hewn riding trails. Halsted's dahlia garden was located close to the house, and farther away were many acres planted with basic crops such as corn, potatoes, and turnips grown for both human and animal consumption. Yield was plentiful in the rich soil, but the demand so thin that Halsted once wrote, "Our potato crop is so great that we are embarrassed to know what to do with it."

Caroline took an active hand in the farming, often helping with the planting and picking, once bagging 450 bushels of rutabaga with only her young cook to help. A half dozen hands regularly worked the place under longtime farm manager Douglas Bradley, and there was always too much to do. In addition to routine tasks, Caroline oversaw the building of a sawmill to provide finished lumber for their building needs, as well as a water-powered grist mill that turned out excellent stone-ground meal. She supervised the cutting of trails and logging, the care of the farm animals, and personally looked after her constant companions, the family dogs.

For Halsted, High Hampton was a place to read, relax, and indulge in activities he had little time for in the city. Health permitting, he was always available for a hike, a horseback ride, or a drive in the buckboard or buggy. His farming activities were restricted to choosing and cutting dahlias and picking corn. Corn on the cob, freshly picked while the water was set to boil, was a favorite lunchtime treat, and he had perfected a system for determining ripeness that regularly dazzled visitors. Walking among the lines of corn with drying silk, he would roll the ears between his fingers and feel for a telltale crunch that indicated the corn was ready for picking.

Caroline was in charge of projects large and small, and despite its identification with her husband, she was the primary caretaker of Halsted's prized dahlia garden. She arrived at High Hampton in early spring and left in November, the prescribed times for planting new tubers and digging up and separating the old. Each winter Halsted scoured the European seed catalogues and garden literature and ordered the most interesting new dahlia varieties. These would arrive at Cashiers long before he, and Caroline would have the beds prepared and the tubers planted in wide military rows separated by grass paths. The flowers were usually in bloom by Halsted's arrival, and by midsummer they were eye height and bursting with huge heads of brilliant color. Though he had little hand in the care and feeding of his precious garden, Halsted was responsible for choosing the plants for each year's color show. He thoroughly enjoyed the spectacle and in early morning would walk the grass path between the beds, often still in pajamas, robe, and slippers. George Heuer was a guest on a particularly moist morning when the legs of Halsted's pajamas became soaked with dew and clung to his legs. Caroline, already dressed in her usual short, heavy skirt and boots, spotted him from the veranda and called out, "William, how many times have I told you not to go out like that? Look at your slippers, they are soaking wet."

"Yes, Caroline, so they are. I'll take them off." Looking rueful, but obviously teasing, he took them off, and with slippers in hand went on his way. Mrs. Halsted made an inaudible remark, but her body language and shaking head made it clear she considered him hopeless.

In late season, dwarfed by the tall plants, Halsted would bend the stems to him and study the flowers. He would cut fresh stems in the morning dew, carry great bundles to the houses, arrange the flowers, and deliver them to guests and family.

Toward the end of the 19th century, dahlias had become something of a fad for gardeners in both the United States and Europe. The plant, indigenous to Mexico, was known as Dahlia Juarezii. It grew wild, and parts of it were harvested and processed for food. After a single root survived an 1872 shipment to the Netherlands, it was cultivated and cross-bred. The resulting tall, strong stems and beautiful flowers, with a hardy nature and environmental adaptability, became instantly popular. Dahlia clubs soon became a feature on the garden circuit, and Dr. Halsted's garden was widely visited and well respected. Dahlia experts shared their passion, and Halsted took great joy in sending prized new specimens to growers he knew would appreciate them.

Though Caroline, with Bradley and the staff, prepared and planted the beds, they did so according to Halsted's instructions and used the new dahlia varietals he had chosen the preceding winter. Upon arriving, he took charge of the project as if he had been present since inception. He made sure to fill in all weak spots in the show garden with plants from the larger cutting garden, and carried an old wicker "Nantucket" basket filled with wooden name plates to help visitors identify the numerous new specimens.

The growing season for dahlias ended with the first frost. At that time the stalks were cut close to the earth, and the tubers, which had multiplied beneath the surface, were pulled, cleaned of earth, dried, separated, and stored. Most would be given away to make room for the new varieties expected the following spring. Halsted would send gift packages to interested dahlia growers, give others to neighbors, and annually he left a sign at the post office announcing their availability to the community. The local infiltration was so successful that colorful dahlia gardens were everywhere. "One saw in driving within a radius almost reaching Toxaway Lake gorgeous dahlias growing in the little front yards of the poorest cabins."

The mountain people of the area were indeed mostly poor, and poorly educated. Different in every way from the Halsteds, there was an uneasy interaction between them, but the locals clearly held the doctor in very high esteem. Caroline's sister, Lucy Haskell, wrote, "Personally I think that he did not much like the mountaineer—his ignorance, superstition and religion were almost unintelligible to him and he did not enter into the racy shrewdness and humor that is often theirs . . . perhaps they did not show it to him, he was of another world, 'outlander,' a 'furriner.' But for the ill he showed a large sympathy and helpfulness."

Having the doctor among them was useful, and increasingly the mountain folk sought his help and advice. On numerous occasions Halsted arranged for transport of seriously ill neighbors to Baltimore for care at Johns Hopkins at his own expense. Communication between them was usually by letter, and devoted letters of thanks were not unusual. Long lists of symptoms were sent for his attention. These were carefully evaluated, and he helped whenever he could. But the mountain people were a trying breed. Later in life, Halsted arranged for an elderly local woman with a large cancer of the skin of the forehead and eyelid to be treated at Hopkins with the new radium therapy Kelly had instituted and championed. Halsted made the personal effort to see that she was afforded the much sought-after new modality. The woman was living on an undeserved veteran's pension left by her army deserter husband, and later tried to have the pension, to which she wasn't entitled, increased due to her disease. Halsted made clear his distaste for this behavior to friends and colleagues, but he was unfailingly polite in dealing with this woman and others in the community. Although often annoyed by requests for money or medical assistance, he never exhibited the famous sarcasm and biting comments that had established his reputation as a fearsome tyrant at the hospital.

Halsted provided neighbors with a level of help for their medical problems that would otherwise be far beyond their reach. He was called upon to administer to horses, dogs, and cattle, and became increasingly adept at veterinary medicine. Neither of the Halsteds believed in offering charity, and demanded something in kind for their assistance. Often this took the form of goods and services, usually labor and produce.

Halsted, like many physicians, was an amateur astronomer. Consulting with a lens maker in Madison, Wisconsin, he had a large telescope constructed and installed on a platform off the back porch of the lodge. Constantly troubled by difficulty sleeping, he would awaken on clear summer nights and pad off to the telescope platform in pajamas, robe, and carpet slippers to study the heavens until daylight. He acquired charts and maps of the stars and was soon conversant in the constellations and their relationships, which he enjoyed pointing out and identifying to others.

As one might expect, he dressed immaculately in his version of country fashion. Usually this meant a comfortable tweed suit, soft collared shirt, and necktie, sturdy walking shoes, cane, hat, cigarette holder, and Pall Mall cigarette. In warmer weather, shirtsleeves, bow tie, and straw hat might suffice. In a photograph thus outfitted he sits playfully atop the back of a slat-back chair, his country shoes on the wooden arms, trousers tucked into colorful, checkerboard high socks. On the rush seat of the chair are two dark, short-haired dachshunds, and looking up at his master, from the ground, a lovely spaniel. For a man so obstinately photophobic, he seems totally at his ease, perhaps happy, in the photograph. Boater on his head, pince-nez glasses, graying goatee and mustache and smiling face, Halsted looks anything but forbidding.

Caroline, on the other hand, remained consistent in her disinterest in her appearance. Her city clothing was plain, dark-colored, and often homemade. She favored sensible, brogue-type shoes, and her hair was usually tied back in a bun. Though not imposing physically, she was muscular, or at least large-boned, and she reinforced the impression of size and strength with mannish clothing. The country version was largely homemade as well, and decidedly downscale. She wore homespun skirts of shorter-than-ankle length; high, heavy boots; a manly shirt; and a broad-brimmed hat. The locals described Caroline as "salouchy," which meant clean but untidy.

Dogs were a permanent presence in the Halsted household. Nip and Tuck, the favored pair of dachshunds in their lives, among others, were always in residence, usually along with a pair of lively hunting spaniels. The dogs rarely left Caroline's side. Nip and Tuck shared the Halsteds' bed, and one would rarely see her on a buckboard or carriage without a dog or two on her lap, often all four surrounding her. Away from home, Caroline carried Nip and Tuck about in a wicker basket. The dachshunds were lively substitutes for the children the Halsteds had declined to have, and both took great pleasure in their company.

The inevitable deaths of family pets are wrenching events. For the Halsteds, in later life, the loss of the dachshunds, in which they had invested so much love, was totally demoralizing. Halsted wrote his friend William MacCallum of his feelings upon the death of Nip:

> We are very depressed today by the death of Nip. I have just made the autopsy. The cause of death was a valvular disease of the heart, a chronic affair that may have dated from his attack of distemper years ago. He has been ailing for weeks. Mrs. Halsted has nursed him night and day hardly leaving him for a moment. She is quite worn out. I think I wrote you that Silsy died a few weeks ago. So we are without a dog. I have the feeling that Mrs. Halsted will come to town earlier this autumn now that she has no dogs. She will miss their company sadly.

The expression of sadness was genuine, and as heartfelt and emotional as any recorded utterances of his. One must keep in mind that Halsted was a clinical scientist and surgeon, and had, by that time, spent 30 years performing experimental dog surgery followed by autopsy. The fact that he was detached enough to perform the autopsy himself is not unusual among surgeons, and speaks more to his scientific mind-set than to lack of emotion, though Halsted was surely more professionally detached than most.

LIFE AT HIGH HAMPTON consumed time and money year round, and the Halsteds kept scrupulous records of farm expenses on slips of paper, and uncharacteristically not in the form of ledgers, or financial "books." Though largely self-sustaining in the production of hay, potatoes, corn and cornmeal, rutabaga, turnips, poultry, pigs, and beef cattle, little was marketed, and no appreciable income was realized.

Transactions between Halsted and Douglas Bradley, caretaker/manager of High Hampton, were most often handwritten notes on small sheets of paper, rarely utilizing professional letterheads or engraved personal stationery. Occasionally, the notes or small balance sheets were typed by one of two secretaries Halsted employed at home. The nature of the transactions was simply a matter of listing monthly expenses, pay due regular employees and day laborers, money due the Halsteds for bags of milled grain taken, or money advanced to the staff.

The comfortable lodging provided for Bradley, his wife, and children was near the main house, with several windows, fireplaces for heating, and hot and cold running water. There was no mention of an indoor toilet facility. Bradley was paid $40 a month and housing. Most other farm labor was contracted on a daily basis at an average wage of a dollar and a half a day. There were often six or seven field laborers employed. The number decreased during the winter months, unless a specific project such as logging or construction was underway. Planting, growing, and harvesting required more help. A steady stream of communication was kept up from Baltimore to Cashiers during the winter months. Caroline was most intimately aware of the nuances and necessities of the farm, but for what may have been a matter of form and the need to establish authority, orders were often sent by William.

Occasionally, household servants were brought up from Baltimore, but more usually they were imported from Columbia, or elsewhere in the South. Caroline was constantly appalled by the housekeeping and culinary standards of the local people they had attempted to employ, and since she often said of herself, "I am no housekeeper," the quest for acceptable staff was never-ending. At times it became a source of friction, with complaints from Caroline resulting in procrastination from William, who was reluctant to fire household employees. In all, he was often amused, and rarely upset by the situation.

When they were in residence, household staff included a housekeeper, a cook, a laundress, and a house man assigned to care for guests. The in-house staff was black, and frequently treated in the condescending, paternalistic manner prevalent in the 19th- and early-20th-century

South. Generalizations were made about race, and demeaning terms were casually used that are wholly unacceptable today.

"The weather is still cool here. Mrs. Halsted and I are doing the cooking," Halsted wrote. This is a revelation in itself, since neither had any but the most rudimentary kitchen skills. "Our servants have not arrived and it is impossible to find a soul in the valley who can cook."

And later, "Yes, our darkies have arrived at last. You can imagine what a relief it is to Mrs. Halsted and me. I became quite expert in setting the table, washing dishes, etc., and Mrs. Halsted is quite a good cook. I believe that I could now boil potatoes—am still a little unreliable on rice and corn bread."

William Stewart Halsted was an aristocratic and urbane northerner. He was polite and proper to a fault and was not known to swear. In his letters, as in his speech, there was a distance and formality, and the obvious manners of a gentleman. Reading a reference to African-Americans as darkies, no matter how off-putting it seems today, must be seen within the mores of the time. As late as the 1930s, the term "darkies" was routinely used by whites and blacks alike, and was not seen as pejorative. The plaintive 1935 song "That's Why Darkies Were Born" was a national recording sensation, with renditions by both Kate Smith and the great black baritone Paul Robeson. In the same era, in letters to President Franklin D. Roosevelt seeking protection from lynch mobs, Negroes explaining their plight frequently referred to themselves as "darkies"; hence we must not read too much into Halsted's use of the term more than 100 years ago.

Caroline Hampton Halsted's attitude toward blacks was neither virulent nor unexpected. Her South Carolina upbringing, and the loss of the good life formerly associated with slave holding, was probably offset by her uncle Wade Hampton's surprisingly enlightened attitude toward emancipation. There is, however, significant evidence in her letters of a belief in the inferiority of blacks. An example of this can be found in a 1910 letter to Halsted, who was in Paris at the time. Caroline rarely traveled with her husband, having found a European trip made early in their marriage not at all to her liking. William Halsted was devoted to traveling for business and for pleasure, and he spent a large part of most summers in European surgical capitals and at unknown destinations. He did not hesitate to leave, and she was content to be at High Hampton. In the letter, she says:

> The two darkies are having double fits over my last scheme for ridding myself of rats and mice. After some trouble I managed to have got for me two black snakes which are now happily reposing in the attic. They cannot possibly get into the house so I see no reason for their terror. The man announces that the wife has heart disease and if she were to see a snake she might die. She is not afraid of them, but he is. So I have promised to have them removed. They cannot be caught of course but we shall try to catch two others and palm them off. The lower one goes in the race, the bigger fools I suppose they find. I hope you have some of my letters by this time. Not that I have written many, but enough to let you know that I am alive. I am glad that you are enjoying your French lessons. To me your disposal of your summers does seem absurd. Instead of going away from stuffy, dirty cities where you have been living all winter you just go and immure yourself in another buggy place. If you must study French why can you not take it somewhere besides a large city. Still I suppose it is the amusement you want and change, not particularly French. For I do not see what you have learned is of any use to you.

Caroline was nothing if not opinionated. She was a country girl who made no effort to disguise her dislike for city life, and immediately after their marriage she began spending at least half the year at High Hampton. Halsted, too, was absent from Baltimore and Johns Hopkins from May to October, but he spent no more than two months at High Hampton. What he did, and where he went, is the subject of conjecture. He regularly sent letters and postcards from capital cities and small villages, but he was always unaccompanied in his travels, and unless visiting European surgical friends, his whereabouts were loosely established and his routine unknown.

At High Hampton he made every effort to conform to the life Caroline had established. Though anything but a horseman, Halsted had great athletic ability and set about learning everything about horses, riding, and driving, until his skills were estimable. They purchased fine horses and shared long trail rides with the spaniels running before and beside them. Halsted even familiarized himself with enough veterinary practices to care for their ailments. Still, Caroline felt the world of horses was her domain and never quite accepted her husband's increasing competence, just as she never considered herself able or worthy in the flip side of their lives together.

She wrote to Halsted, "I always could have ridden her [a mare in question] I think, but you did not think so. A person who does not ride never can understand how one who can ride does it as naturally as they breathe. You never understood either how crazy I always was to get out and away."

Caroline believed herself entirely self-sufficient, and there is much evidence to support her contention. Though she was at times consumed with managing household servants and field-workers, outdoor physical work was central to her chosen lifestyle. She reveled in being alone at High Hampton in the periods when servants were not present: "The servants left this A.M. and I am happily entirely alone. My dinner has been served and I see no one until the milk comes at 6:30. My personal wants are few and I can always make myself comfortable."

THE HALSTEDS WERE treated with the respect afforded land-rich, moneyed outsiders, but people were not as oblivious to their habits as they seemed. Their comings and goings were noted, and there was a good deal of "general talk" around Cashiers that both Dr. and Mrs. Halsted were addicted to drugs. On one occasion, an agitated Caroline Halsted confronted farm manager Douglas Bradley about a package she had been expecting from Parke-Davis, the manufacturer of morphine. When the package failed to arrive, she sent Bradley to the office of a local doctor. There he picked up a package similar to those received regularly from Parke-Davis or the local physicians.

Morphine was readily available without prescription until the Harrison Narcotics Tax Act of 1914. Chemically, morphine is an alkaloid, and the active ingredient in opium. It is extracted from the poppy plant and structurally very similar to its even more potent cousin, heroin. Morphine was first isolated early in 1804 but was not widely used for the next 50 years. Morphine, like cocaine, found its way into tonics and patent medicines. The passage of the Pure Food and Drug Act in 1906 required the identification of ingredients, but the availability and use of the drugs was not restricted.

Two nearly simultaneous events—the advent of the hypodermic syringe in 1853 and the American Civil War the following decade—were responsible for the first large-scale use and abuse of the drug. Wounded Civil War soldiers found merciful pain relief with morphine, and 400,000 were believed to have brought the habit home from the battlefield with them.

In addition to its primary application as a potent pain reliever, morphine was used to relieve anxiety, nervousness, and sleeplessness, and as an antidote for alcoholism. In the latter instance, the soporific and tranquilizing effects of the drug were seen in sharp contrast to the antisocial behavior associated with alcoholism, and were generally considered more acceptable. Morphine was also tried as a treatment for cocaine and opium addiction, but, as had been the case with Halsted, it proved ineffective. The actual chemical action of morphine is unknown, but specific receptors in the brain associated with the drug have been identified. It is thought to afford relief from pain by preventing neurochemical release. Various studies indicate the involvement of substances such as acetylcholine, serotonin, and catecholamines.

In addition to pain relief, the effects of the drug include sedation, detachment, and a pleasant sense of well-being. Through its action on the medulla, it also suppresses the cough reflex and depresses respiration. Dry mouth, pinpoint pupils and decreased night vision, and constipation are common side effects at therapeutic dose levels.

Physical and psychological addiction to morphine occurs quickly. As tolerance to the drug grows, larger doses are required to achieve the same sense of euphoria, the reward that justifies the quest for the next dose. Barely eight hours pass between doses before the hunger is active again and soon thereafter, withdrawal begins. Starting with chills, nausea, sweating, and restlessness, it builds to the florid complex in 24 to 36 hours with goose bumps and involuntary leg movements, giving rise to the terms "cold turkey" and "kicking the habit." To the addict, nothing is as important as the next dose. Managing the delicate balance becomes an all-consuming priority.

In the late 19th century, women were treated with morphine for depression, dysmenorrhea, and morning sickness, and they soon became habituated. By the early 20th century, the majority of new addicts were women. The term "southern addiction" was often used, which implied a population of middle- and upper-class women with nonspecific complaints who found relief from the ennui of life through use of the drug. Medical personnel with easy access to the drug also succumbed in large numbers, and at the turn of the century it was estimated that more that 10 percent of physicians were addicted. The prevailing philosophy was, "Though a morphine injection could cure little, it could relieve anything."

Morphine is a respiratory depressant. It readily crosses the placental barrier and can result in fetal respiratory distress and neonatal addiction. The number of newborn addictions, birth deformities, and stillbirths that resulted from the rampant use of the drug has not been calculated. As use of the drug became increasingly common, the debilitating aspects of its abuse were recognized and a more protective governmental attitude developed. Prior to legislation restricting its use in 1914, morphine addiction actually carried less social stigma than alcoholism. For a number of years after morphine was designated a controlled substance, it continued to be readily accessible. It was inexpensive and dispensed freely, and doctors maintained supplies on hand and made it available to their addicted patients. Morphine maintenance clinics were opened in many cities, and addiction remained manageable and lawful until 1919, when the United States Supreme Court ruled it illegal to dispense controlled substances to known addicts. When maintaining addicts was no longer legal, a black market in drug traffic blossomed, and narcotic usage soon became synonymous with the darker world of crime and violence. Procuring the next dose consumed and destroyed lives, and it extracted a painful human and economic price from American society.

As a physician, Halsted always had easy, legal access to morphine. He was thoroughly conversant with its effects and side effects and had the ability to accommodate his dosage to his daily routine—or perhaps, his routine to his dosage.

Osler's concern at the time was Halsted's dose management, and not his ability to function. In that regard, morphine was significantly less destructive than alcohol. Halsted's condition, and his struggle to control it, were seen as both tragic and heroic, but not incongruent with a productive life. To Osler and Welch, Halsted was a professional equal with a chronic, but not debilitating, disease. Halsted announced his shame by working to hide all evidence of his problem.

Caroline Halsted fit the profile for "southern addiction" perfectly. She was socially withdrawn, often depressed and tearful, and suffered a decidedly low opinion of herself. Her marriage may have been unfulfilling; she spent large periods of time alone at High Hampton and often took to her suite at Eutaw Place for days on end. In all, she was a perfect candidate for relief from her sadness.

Caroline cannot have been unaware of her husband's morphine use, and witnessing his revival each evening may have seemed just what she herself needed. Halsted's frustration at his inability to extricate himself from addiction makes it highly unlikely that he encouraged her along the same path. Whatever the origin of her initiation, Halsted's drug use and morphine's ready accessibility certainly would have facilitated the process. Shared addiction is not an uncommon phenomenon. Where and when her involvement began are unknown, but the anxiety engendered by the missing Parke-Davis package places Caroline squarely in the picture.

CHAPTER TWENTY

The First Great Medical School

O N APRIL 4, 1892, HALSTED was made full professor of surgery, which elevated him to equal academic status with his peers. Unfortunately, there was still no medical school. Its absence was keenly felt by the chiefs of service, who had been encouraged to expect a pool of young students from which they could cull the most promising as their resident staff.

After the successful opening of the hospital, it had become clear that the medical school endowment, dependent as it was on Baltimore and Ohio stock, was in deep trouble. The value of the stock plummeted, and with it hopes for the medical school. Soon troublesome rumors began to circulate that the hospital itself would attempt to build a medical school unrelated to the university and on the old model, supported by student fees and economic integration of the faculty of practicing physicians. This was exactly what the doctors were trying to avoid. A near insurrection among the medical staff ensued, and a truce was arranged with the board. Part of the compromise was for the hospital staff to give a series of lecture programs for outside physicians, but this proved unpopular and was quickly discontinued, with the fallout from the entire episode being the palpably urgent need to open the medical school. But the whole project was now in doubt, and no one wanted to see the noble experiment drift backward into the sullied past of medical education.

Despite Johns Hopkins's generous endowment, Francis T. King, president of the hospital board, wrote Daniel Coit Gilman, "Where is the man to endow the Medical School?"

As circumstances would have it, no man stood up and assumed the burden, but a group of women, including King's daughter, Elizabeth, did. Four wealthy, educated, and unmarried young women, three of them the daughters of hospital trustees, hatched a scheme to save the medical school. The like-minded four—Mary Elizabeth Garrett, Carey Thomas, Mary Gwinn, and Elizabeth King, all lifelong friends—formed the Women's Fund Committee. Their ostensible goal was to raise an additional $100,000 endowment, which they believed would allow the medical school to open. The trustees estimated the figure at $200,000, but since they believed little would come of the effort, the difference was not made an issue.

The women's fundraising effort was well organized and attracted prominent women in New York, Boston, and Washington, D.C., including the first lady of the United States, Mrs. Benjamin Harrison. Perhaps some contributors were drawn by a desire to further medical education, but more likely the stimulus to contribute came from the committee's demand that women have equal rights to admission to The Johns Hopkins Medical School.

In 1849, Elizabeth Blackwell was graduated from the Geneva College of Medicine and became the first American-trained female physician. The floodgates most certainly did not open, but things changed slightly for the better. Medical schools for women were established, and some of the existing proprietary schools began to admit women. Female physicians could be found in most urban communities, but the elite medical schools and most of the best hospitals still excluded women. Mary Elizabeth Garrett, perhaps the wealthiest member of the committee, was chronically ill and wanted to be treated by female physicians. Other committee members shared this philosophy and believed the best schools should be open to the brightest women to provide the finest female physicians.

The four had been crusaders for other women's causes and had helped found the Bryn Mawr School to provide better college preparatory opportunities for girls, who were excluded from the best schools. Carey Thomas, a member of the committee and an outspoken crusader for equal rights, became dean of Bryn Mawr and favored limiting the enrollment of Jewish girls at the prep school, entirely missing the hypocrisy of her stand. Unmarried, female-centric, and willing to speak their minds, the women used their family positions to enhance the effectiveness of their effort. The trustees agreed to meet with them only because Elizabeth King's father was president of the board. After the meeting, the trustees assured university president Gilman that the women would never raise enough money to become a decision-making factor at the university.

Sentiment in the boardroom was generally against coeducation. Welch agreed, defending his position by saying he would be embarrassed discussing certain subjects in front of women. He later came about a full 180 degrees and was a proud spokesperson for equality for women. Osler came over early and even contributed to the fund drive, but he was far from convinced. Hurd came around, and Kelly was supportive. Halsted was silent.

By the fall, the Women's Fund had raised $100,000. Of this amount, $48,787.50 came from Mary Elizabeth Garrett, the daughter of a former head of the B&O. The funds would be made available to the university if they agreed to coeducation. Now the pressure was on. Rumors were flying that the doctors were unhappy about the prospect of coeducation and were thinking of defecting. Generous offers were being made. Harvard tried to entice Osler and Welch with plans for a new, higher-quality four-year school, including grades for students. Both demurred, but Welch lost his second in command,

William Councilman, who accepted the chair at Harvard in lieu of his mentor. McGill in Montreal tried to repatriate native son William Osler with what was reported to be a king's ransom. He resisted this as well, but a feeling of unrest had replaced the heady atmosphere of the prior years. Something needed to happen, and that something was to make good the unfulfilled promise of a medical school.

Gilman was against accepting the $100,000 and opening the medical school to coeducation. Welch equivocated, but Hurd, Osler, and Kelly strongly urged Gilman to accept. Welch wrote to Mall, who was now in Chicago: "Pres. Gilman and some of the trustees really do not want (sub rosa) the women to succeed, for they do not like the idea of co-sexual medical education. I do not myself hanker after it, but do not see how they can refuse such a large sum of money."

Finally, Gilman reached what he believed was a face-saving compromise. The university would accept the money and allow equal access to women, but the medical school would not commence operation until the full $500,000 necessary to operate had been raised. The women continued their work, and in December 1892, Mary Elizabeth Garrett personally contributed another $306,977, bringing the grand total to $500,000. But she was not about to hand over the money and leave. With her position solidified, Mary Garrett became the conscience of The Johns Hopkins School of Medicine.

She now insisted that all students must have earned a bachelor's degree, as other graduate schools at Johns Hopkins already required. To this she added a working knowledge of French and German, and the premedical requirements of biology, chemistry, and physics. The medical degree would require a four-year course of study. These demands had not materialized from thin air, nor had they been invented by Miss Garrett. They were largely the requirements that had been spelled out by Welch at the behest of Billings and the trustees, in the earliest stages of planning. They were not appreciably different from still earlier suggestions made by Billings to Gilman in 1878. On both occasions Gilman praised their high-mindedness but dismissed the requirements as unrealistic. Pointing to the lax requirements at even the finest medical schools, and the additional year required when others programs were only three years, he doubted they would attract enough students to fill a class.

The trustees were totally undone. Fathers applied pressure to daughters, meetings were held in small groups, and everyone outside the women's committee tried to convince Mary Garrett to soften her terms. Instead of softening them, she added a few more. The most important was that women would not be admitted as separate but equal with men, but on the same terms, guaranteeing the "same" medical education to women. Garrett also stipulated that no more than $50,000 of her gift be used for the Women's Fund Memorial Building. Negotiations had become so acrimonious that Garrett named a committee of six women who would operate in perpetuity to ensure that if the terms of her gift were violated, the funds would be returned to her estate. As it turned out, she had reason to retain the lever of financial power. As the new anatomy building neared completion, relieving pressure on the already expanded Pathological, Garrett insisted the Women's Fund name be inscribed on the outside. Gilman wanted an inscribed tablet inside the building, and Welch, as the first dean of the school, stepped in to remind Gilman that this was not a fight they would win.

Now the great experiment could begin in earnest. Welch, as dean, set about recruiting both the most accomplished men to teach the preclinical sciences and members of the first class of medical students at The Johns Hopkins School of Medicine.

Gilman convinced William H. Howell, a distinguished physiologist, to leave his post at Harvard and return to Hopkins. Howell would be replacing his old professor H. Newell Martin in the post. Martin had become an increasingly debilitated alcoholic and had been convinced to resign. Next on the list was Franklin P. Mall, the anatomist. Mall had left Hopkins for Clark University, and then moved to the University of

Chicago as professor of anatomy. There he spearheaded plans for integrated departments of basic science and experimental research into disease. Halsted was confident that Mall would return to the fold no matter how rich the carrot at the end of the other stick. Mall had been talking about building a $4 million anatomy institute at Chicago, while the income available to him from the Women's Fund was barely $20,000 a year. Still, Mall telegraphed, "Shall cast my lot with Johns Hopkins," and they were off to the races. The next recruit was John J. Abel, a pharmacologist and chemist then at the University of Michigan. All would soon distinguish themselves and Johns Hopkins.

In the fall of 1893, 18 students registered for the first-year class at The Johns Hopkins School of Medicine. The 15 men and three women were about to participate in a very trying experiment. There was no formalized curriculum in place, and the clinical and laboratory faculty greatly outnumbered the student body. Lectures were largely replaced by laboratory work; experiments were devised and carried out to reach conclusions students would otherwise be taught. Scientific papers in the original languages were required reading instead of textbook distillations. Students found themselves with free time, and very little direction. Mall welcomed the first-year students to the anatomy lab, and after a long wait for dissecting material, presented them with a cadaver and a scalpel, and left. He provided no text, lectures, or instructions. The students were being treated as scholars, and they didn't seem to like it.

Welch later wrote, "As it turned out, the embarrassments and difficulties we feared in the novel venture of co-education in medicine never materialized."

Osler, on considering the high standards for admission to the new medical school, commented, "Welch, we are lucky to get in as professors, for I am sure that neither you nor I could get in as students."

CHAPTER TWENTY-ONE

Teaching without Teaching

THE SECOND-YEAR CLASS WAS 40 strong, including eight women. What they shared with the inaugural class was dissatisfaction with the instruction they were receiving, or weren't receiving. From the first day there was a running battle with Mall, who not only had not procured cadavers for dissection, but didn't know how to properly embalm and store them when supply became plentiful. What sharp contrast this was from the P&S anatomy instructor, William S. Halsted, who was ever present in the dissecting room and provided excellent examples of proper dissections for the students to study. Mall offered no instruction. He expected medical students had no need for spoon-feeding of so basic a subject; that's what books were for. Nor did he bother with formal lectures. He was, however, available to the few who were interested in experimental projects. The medical students didn't simply dislike Mall, they detested him. He, in turn, wasn't going to be bothered with students unwilling to educate themselves. When a student complained about having nothing to do, Mall handed him a broom. He simply refused to teach "shoemaker anatomy for the pill doctors." He did pay enough attention to one of the female first-year students to marry her. However, marriage disqualified students, and the new Mrs. Mall dropped out.

The students complained to the dean. Welch tried to mediate, but the students soon found that he, too, was among the missing when it came to teaching. Simon Flexner, who had come to him as a graduate student in 1890, was his assistant when the medical school opened. Welch had regularly scheduled lectures for the class, which he rarely attended, sending Flexner, who was a fine researcher but a less than dynamic speaker, in his stead. Welch and Mall shared the philosophy that American medical students were taught too much, and not allowed to learn. The students thought they were simply lazy. Their colleagues, particularly Osler, believed both Mall and Welch were lazy and derelict in their duties to the medical students.

John J. Abel, the third laboratory scientist whose fame was meant to attract the best student population, was another teaching dud. Having spent seven years in Europe after earning his PhD at Michigan, he returned home with an MD degree but very little desire to practice medicine. In the laboratory he was among the first to isolate epinephrine, did important research on insulin, and was respected as a biochemist and physiologist. But as well-meaning as he was, Abel was a boring lecturer, not at all interested in teaching, and impossibly inept at laboratory demonstrations.

The biggest problem, however, was Halsted. In the fall of 1895, the students were beginning their exposure to clinical subjects. As the moment marking the transition from student of basic science to fledgling physician, it was much anticipated and meant a great deal to the already disgruntled students. Halsted had been scheduled to lecture on wound healing the previous spring, but the course never materialized. The Professor was nowhere to be found; having left Baltimore for the mountains of North Carolina and parts unknown, he began the extended absences that became the hallmark of his erratic behavior. Not only had he not planned the formal lecture series and the introduction to surgery, which sorely disappointed the now third-year students, but he was frequently absent from the hospital as well. Hospital superintendent Henry Hurd repeatedly confronted him, and Halsted repeatedly assured him of his future compliance. Finally, exasperated, Hurd reported the problem to the board of trustees, who declared that attendance regulations must be "rigidly observed."

Morphine and, possibly, cocaine were at least indirectly responsible for these episodes of erratic behavior and absences. At the time, Halsted's daily dose was three grains of morphine, enormous by any standard and, naturally, difficult to manage. He was a changed man in so many ways that it didn't take a great leap of imagination to assume drug implications. His slower, more intense pace may have been in some respects an intellectual epiphany brought about by the tranquilizing effect of morphine. Since only Osler and Welch were aware of his drug use, students, colleagues, and the trustees had to judge the man by his actions. And his actions were very confusing.

The work being produced by Halsted was a resplendent feather in the Hopkins cap, and the staff and trustees were justifiably proud of the international fame that followed it. In 1890, he had reported on his new hernia operation, and in 1892, he published the results of 82 cases. Hernia surgery was now an elective reality. In 1894, Halsted reported on 50 cases of his radical operation for breast cancer, again devising an operation considered the gold standard by the American Surgical Association, an honor whose rewards would accrue to The Johns Hopkins Hospital. The trustees of the hospital were in an uncomfortable position. They were facing a problem they would rather ignore, and they never took action.

Absenteeism was not the only issue. Halsted had no relationship with the medical students and made no effort to develop one. Not only did he often skip his weekly lectures, but the subjects upon which he lectured were so far over the heads of the students that they felt excluded. The same applied to his clinic and ward rounds. The students were required to attend, but it was as though they were invisible. Questions, when The Professor asked them, were often unrelated to the patient in front of them, or were aimed at the senior resident who was expected to be in command of the literature. Often, Halsted would discover a symptom or curious finding, quietly contemplate it, examine the patient with no time constraints, and with no explanation, move on. Worst of all, his radar would sound at the slightest blip of untruth or lack of knowledge. The medical students tried to hold their tongues and duck questions. But somehow The Professor found the ones with great holes in their knowledge and exposed them publicly, which did not add to his popularity. Finney said, "To the good student, he was a great stimulus, to the poor one, a constant terror."

Formal ward rounds were interminable. The students commonly referred to them as "shifting dullness," a parody on the flat percussive note caused by a collection of fluid in the abdomen that had shifted with the patient's position.

MacCallum believed Halsted taught by example. Others were less kind. But medical students could learn little of the master's methods if they didn't first learn the basics. A method that was good for the residents was not necessarily good for students. Halsted had been the ultimate quizmaster in New York, plying students with facts, teaching them to think, and drilling, drilling, drilling, and proud that his students routinely finished at the top of the class. Was this an entirely different approach, or simply neglect? If this change in methodology was intentional—and there were those, like MacCallum, who believed it so—then it was congruent with the style evolving in the hands of Mall, Abel, and Welch. Whatever the case, the students may not have been taught in the traditional sense, but they did learn. And disgruntled or not, they became the envy of their peers.

CHAPTER TWENTY-TWO

Residents

A S SURELY AS THE PROFESSOR ignored the medical students, the interns and junior residents often felt excluded as well. They were at the bedside and in the laboratory to do a job. Instruction was provided by their seniors, technique was learned by doing, and the rest was learned by observing The Professor's every move.

On hospital rounds Joe Bloodgood ordered his junior, Jim Mitchell, to make a complete blood count on a sick patient every half hour. Mitchell protested that it was impossible for a man to do that and clean his instruments between counts.

Halsted asked Bloodgood, "Have you ever made a blood count?"

Bloodgood acknowledged that he had not.

"Neither have I," said the Professor, followed by a long silence that the recipient felt more stingingly than a reprimand.[1]

---

1 The complete blood count reflects changes in the response to infection by an increased number of white cells, or leukocytes. Changes in the red cell count and hemoglobin would reflect blood loss but would be unlikely to change on a half-hourly basis. These tests are now performed by automated equipment. Drawing and transporting the blood takes far longer than the test. In 1893, it was a tedious and time-consuming process. Blood was drawn by the doctor, dilutions done, slides prepared, and the slides read under the microscope.

It was the rare junior that caught his eye, and those who did found their future assured. For those who ascended to the residency, the course could be difficult as well. Some, like Bloodgood and Mitchell, saw the best in The Professor and refused to respond to the rest. Other early residents, like Hardy Phippen, were not constitutionally able to do so. Phippen was already trained as a surgeon when he followed Brockway into the residency. Finney had liked him when they worked together at the Massachusetts General Hospital. But Phippen left the Hopkins service abruptly, claiming he could not get along with Halsted. Superintendent Henry Hurd was distressed by both the resignation without adequate notice and the resident's complaint that his self-respect would not allow him to continue in his position. Halsted did not discuss the matter.

For all his posturing and complaining, Hurd was the ultimate advocate for the house staff. He was known to become apoplectic over less serious infractions than losing a resident and marched, red-faced, to the trustees to complain of the disruption caused by loss of a resident, and Halsted's behavior.

Positions on the surgical house staff were challenging. Not only were the hours painfully long and the work hard, but it was not a democracy, and there was no room for argument. Halsted was soft-spoken and courteous, but he was also cold, demanding, and painfully honest, at least with regard to other people. Most were able to see the forest for the trees and found him the perfect role model; others found him insufferable. But nearly to a man they persevered, and were better for it.

JOSEPH COLT BLOODGOOD arrived at The Johns Hopkins Hospital as a surgery intern. He had graduated in medicine from the University of Pennsylvania the previous year and had very little surgical experience. The first thing Halsted told him was to read everything that Joseph Lister had published. Lister's antiseptic techniques were about to morph into Halsted's aseptic techniques, and it was important for the young man to be thoroughly versed. Bloodgood recalled:

> When I went to the little library in the Johns Hopkins Hospital I had no difficulty in finding the correct places in all of Lister's articles published in the *Lancet* and in the *British Medical Journal.* Each article was indicated by a torn piece of blue paper which Dr. Halsted always employed in his correspondence. Thirty years later, when we sat in Halsted's library during his funeral services and I looked about on the books on the shelves around the four walls, I could see protruding from the top of almost every volume little pieces of blue paper. I advise any young surgeon who reads this article to do as I was advised by Halsted: read everything Lister wrote. To this I would add: Learn by heart everything that Halsted has written in his surgical papers.

Halsted must have seen something special in Bloodgood, for after only six months he sent him off for a year of study in Europe. Upon his return he was made resident surgeon. Bloodgood would distinguish himself in many ways, but he is best remembered as the chronicler of Halsted's surgery, and the first true surgical pathologist. In the former role he compiled the statistics for Halsted's signature operations for hernia and breast cancer. In the latter, he took up what The Professor believed to be a critical step in surgical care. Halsted was known to study pathological anatomy on the surgery table during surgery. He would find the mass, touch it, roll it between his fingers, squeeze it to see if the core was solid, and in the early glove-wearing days, he would remove his gloves for a better sense of feel, move the mass between his fingers again, feel the lymph nodes, and contemplate. All the while, progress of the operation had stopped. He would remove the breast, pectoral muscles, and lymph nodes, and carry the specimen off to a room in Welch's laboratory to study it every bit as carefully as he operated.

Bloodgood returned from Europe with a new microtome for cutting frozen sections, and new staining techniques that allowed nearly instant analysis of a specimen. Halsted saw the frozen sections as a way to corroborate his diagnosis after surgery, not during surgery.

Bloodgood observed, "He made few mistakes in his gross pathological diagnosis at the operation. During the first seven years of my close association with Halsted, we never used the frozen section to help us in the operating room. The frozen section, however, allowed us to see the sections more quickly after the operation to satisfy our curiosity."

Welch's lab in the Pathological was a brisk five-minute walk away, and there was not yet blind faith in microscopic diagnosis. Many of those reading the sections were far less experienced than the surgeon making the gross diagnosis. Welch himself said that in these cases "the experienced surgeons were always right."

The true advantage afforded by frozen sections is to guide the surgeon's decisions during the procedure. Is it cancer? Is it benign? What is the nature of the tissue in the mass? Should we go on? Halsted was so confident of his preoperative and intraoperative judgment that he considered this an unnecessary crutch, and it would be years until surgeons at The Johns Hopkins Hospital relied on frozen sections for guidance in the operating room. Frozen sections remain imperfect, but for a century they have provided useful information upon which to base surgical decisions. Given the circumstances—the relatively recent development of the frozen section, the imperfect staining technique, and the physical distance between operating room and pathology lab—it was neither hubris nor shortsightedness that kept Halsted from realizing the full potential of the new technique.

JIM MITCHELL SHOWED up in 1893, a small, solidly built, clean-shaven, fresh-faced young man, looking for work. He was a native of Baltimore, and not exactly a stranger to Johns Hopkins. The Mitchells lived near President Gilman on Cathedral Street, and the families were friendly. Mitchell graduated from Johns Hopkins, and in the absence of a medical school at Hopkins had just completed his second year at the University of Maryland Medical School. That spring, he corralled Finney, whom he had known for years as well, and got a summer job helping out in the dispensary. Soon after beginning work, Finney made the following proposal: "Jim, I have a good job for you which may be a great thing. Dr. Halsted is away and before leaving told me that, if his operating room head nurse should leave during his absence, he wanted a man in charge . . . If you make good when Dr. Halsted returns, you will be all right. If not, you can go back to the University of Maryland in the fall."

Halsted had been at war with the administration over O.R. nurses since the departure of his wife, Caroline Hampton Halsted. Isabel Hampton, the superintendent of nurses, appointed replacements without consulting him, and in the spring of 1893 the situation had come to a head. The most recent appointment had been unacceptable to Halsted, and he rejected her. Isabel Hampton said something to the effect of "this person or no one." Rather than fight the administration again, Halsted ducked it and left for the country with the issue unresolved. The escalating problem landed in Finney's lap. He had already learned not to make suggestions to his boss, and the best tactic seemed to be to make decisions and allow Halsted to think they were his own. The idea of installing Mitchell was Finney's, and he received no support from the superintendent of nurses, who objected to a man taking the position, and particularly without her permission.

Superintendent Hurd thought that no good would come from the confrontation and wanted to hide from the issue as well, saying, "We had better let things drift for the present until a satisfactory solution of the impasse is presented."

There was a sort of loving give-and-take between Hurd and the house staff, and when Mitchell was ultimately given his job in the operating room Hurd protested, claiming the residents wanted him to take up the slack so they could go off and play baseball in the afternoon, leaving Mitchell in charge of the hospital. Finney responded that would not happen because "we want Jim for the team." Of course, that set Hurd off, just as Finney knew it would, and everyone enjoyed the show.

LATER, THE RELENTING Hurd installed Mitchell in housing on the top floor of the administration building along with Mall, Barker from Medicine, and Flexner from pathology. Obstinately, Hurd refused to provide furniture for the rooms. The residents playfully festooned the apartment with party decorations and spit balls, and Mitchell made do with a bed from the ward and some crates for tables.

Finney and Bloodgood tutored Mitchell in making dressings and passing instruments. He became familiar with the routine, learned to sew, and was functioning as operating nurse by the time Halsted returned. Mitchell did everything he could to make a good impression. He would meet Halsted at the front door in the morning, "Take his hat, coat and gloves, follow him on his rounds, and assist him as nurse in all his operations in the hospital and in private operations outside."

Though the effort may have been appreciated, Halsted said nothing. Mitchell had been well briefed by Finney and took the silence as a good sign. Shortly after Halsted's return to Baltimore from his summer hiatus, he and Mall inspected Mitchell's almost bare rooms on the residence floor of the administration building. Halsted made no comment, but immediately arranged for a complete set of mahogany furniture to be delivered to the apartment. Mitchell considered this a good sign as well.

Halsted was in the habit of spending the time between operations in his dressing room, reading and chain-smoking cigarettes. It was still several years prior to the introduction of the prerolled and packaged Pall Mall cigarettes that Halsted would come to favor. He used Cosmopolite papers and Bob White tobacco, and would smoke one cigarette while rolling the next, then light one from the other. One morning, having forgotten his tobacco, Halsted searched through Mitchell's pockets and found his. Dissatisfied with the young man's choices, he proceeded to lecture him on the virtues of the preferred brands. Thereafter, Mitchell saw to it that Halsted's table was stocked with Cosmopolite papers and Bob White tobacco.

From the outset, Mitchell, as a second-year medical student at another university, spent more time with the chief of surgery than anyone on the Johns Hopkins staff. The nature of surgery in the early 1890s was such that more affluent individuals still insisted on being treated in their homes. That meant that the operating room would have to come to them. With the adoption of aseptic technique, the traveling staff had to transport increasing amounts of equipment. Often three or four assistants would leave their hospital responsibilities behind and join Halsted on the journey. They packed large glass dishes for soaking the hands and arms in mercuric chloride, and others for the carbolic acid instrument soaks, in two large steamer trunks along with sterile linens, instruments, and bandages. On one such trip, a particularly long affair, while the group waited to change trains after an overnight ride, Halsted led them to a nearby field where he somehow produced sandwiches and a coffeemaker and served breakfast. On these occasions, Halsted, Mitchell, and the residents would spend entire days in one another's company, something that The Professor rarely allowed in Baltimore, the consequence of which was that they came to see a fuller range of his behavior, and sometimes caught a glimpse of his thinking, as his reserve slipped away.

Since elective surgery was still in its infancy, these operative trips were mostly in response to emergency situations. It was not uncommon for express trains to make special stops to afford the surgeon better proximity to the patient's home. On one occasion, Halsted, who had been complaining about the attitude of the new, young nurses, engaged an older nurse to accompany the team. The nurse interrupted

several times during a difficult operation and in an entirely uncharacteristic rebuke, Halsted raised his voice and ordered, "You shut up
and get out of here."

It was a rarely seen display of temper, and nothing more was said
following her exit. The remainder of the operation was spent in silence.
The next day he approached Finney.

"I'm not as much stuck on that old woman as I was. She talks
too much."

In the operating room, on the wards, or traveling to operate in
patients' homes, Mitchell became accustomed to Halsted's intense
concentration, his unbending demands for excellence, and the attention he lavished on even the most trivial detail of his surroundings.
When Mitchell produced a photograph of Halsted, Kelly, and Osler,
which had been dubbed "The Fates," Halsted, already known to be
pathologically camera shy, looked at the photograph and recoiled.
Mitchell wondered what faux pas he had committed, and was
surprised when his annoyed boss remarked, "Mercy! My hat never
looked like that."

Mitchell explained that the picture of the three men had been
cropped from a larger group photo, and the cropping accounted for
the irregular appearance of the silk top hat he so carefully tended.
The explanation satisfied Halsted and relieved Mitchell, who wanted
to avoid the wrath of his employer at all costs. Increasingly he seemed
to be courting it. One morning after returning from holiday, Halsted
was called away during a surgery, leaving Bloodgood to close the
abdomen. Bloodgood, too, was called out, and the junior resident, a
notoriously lazy individual, turned to Mitchell and said, "Here, you
damn nurse, sew up this belly," and left.

No sooner had Mitchell begun to work than Halsted returned. He
watched for a few minutes and quietly asked, "Mitchell, do you close
all the abdomens now?"

"No, sir, not all of them."

Halsted left again, and Mitchell thought his job was lost. Instead, from then on Halsted would not allow anyone else to make his dressings. The operating room joke was that Mitchell could anticipate what his boss wanted by the wrinkles on the back of his neck.

The relationship between employer and employee was quietly satisfactory. Mitchell was fully aware that he'd been thrown into the DNA of surgical evolution, and expected to return to medical school at the University of Maryland far the better for it. It was the fall of 1893, and The Johns Hopkins Medical School was about to welcome its first class. With no preamble, Halsted said, "Mr. Mitchell, I have taken the liberty of entering you in our first year class and have arranged with Dr. Mall, Dr. Howell, and Dr. Abel that you may attend classes when you wish, so you can go on with your work in the operating room."

Apparently his efforts had been appreciated. Mitchell was overwhelmed, and gratefully accepted the appointment. Nothing more was said, and Mitchell did double duty for the next two years. Finally, physically exhausted and having lost a great deal of weight, he was ordered by Osler to give up the nursing work. He did service again as an undergraduate intern; then, after graduation in 1897, Mitchell became first assistant to Harvey Cushing, who had come from Massachusetts General Hospital to begin his tenure as resident. Cushing would virtually invent neurosurgery and become the brightest star in the pantheon of Halsted trainees. Three years later Cushing was about to begin an extended European tour, and Halsted announced with no time to spare, "Mitchell, Cushing is leaving tomorrow and I have taken the liberty of naming you as his successor. What do you say?"

Mitchell tried to express his gratitude, and was waved away.

"Don't say anything. Just get to work."

The pattern was becoming clear to those close to The Professor. If one was insecure enough to require reassurance and compliments, one was certain to be sorely disappointed. By the same token, abject disapproval would be reserved for those in mortal disfavor and would be delivered unemotionally, in a quiet and withering tone, with an expressionless face and unyielding ice blue eyes. In one case Halsted told a resident, in all seriousness, that he should specialize in operating on piles (hemorrhoids), as it would not be too taxing for his abilities. Offended and dismissed, the young surgeon fed on the insult and built an admirable surgical career, at least in part stimulated by his determination to show The Professor that he had been wrongly judged.

Halsted was often aloof, but it would be erroneous to assume that he did not register everything significant to him. In the pursuit of excellence, he drew no boundaries between the precise manner in which a suture should be placed and the precise place on a skin from which shoes should be crafted. His intense concern with subjects in which he was interested left little time for consideration of issues that didn't interest him. Assistants marveled that a man who would spend an intense hour palpating the skin and lymph nodes about a cancerous breast prior to surgery could be the same man who was often unaware of the identity of his junior staff. Asking Mitchell, a senior student, to join his staff after graduation, he was surprised to be told that Mitchell was already on the staff. Another member of the first class, Tom Brown, was apparently from a prominent family. Halsted asked Mitchell to point him out.

"He comes of good stock and I want to know him."

Later he asked Mitchell if he thought Brown would like to join the staff, only to be told he had been on the staff for months. At other times he would simply forget to schedule surgery on patients who spent long days and more awaiting their turn. He could be reminded of his forgetfulness only at the risk of his wrath.

At surgery Halsted demanded help but did not welcome suggestions. Multiple assistants attended every operation and were expected to anticipate his every move without a word being said. Cushing and Mitchell were proud of their ability to identify and cross-clamp every tiny vessel in the potentially bloody mastectomy surgery before it could be cut. Dozens of clamps hung from the specimen waiting to be tied or released, and everyone worked quietly. Everything was done with precise technique, and no task was too unimportant for personal attention. Halsted personally assumed the tedious task of winding silk suture material around glass bobbins before sterilization. Everything was to be just so. Tissue was brought together in a tension-free manner with small sutures of fine silk that had been threaded on sterile straight needles and stuck through sterile towels in precise formation. Skin sutures were carefully buried beneath the surface to minimize the possibility of seeding infection from the skin. Later, buried silver wire was used for the task. Bacteriological studies had shown that gold and silver had properties that inhibited bacterial growth, and after abandoning gold for its expense, silver wire closure became the method of choice until the advent of truly aseptic technique with the adoption of sterile gloves, caps, and masks.

Halsted came to believe the only true barrier against infection was sterile gloves. Infection was often the difference between success and failure, and for the first time it became clear that the manner in which surgery was performed was important. Gentle tissue handling diminished devitalized tissue, and hence did not produce a good medium for bacterial growth. Dead space—a gap between the sides of a wound—was to be avoided for similar reasons, though Halsted did believe allowing a clean blood clot to form in the wound would promote healing. The anesthetists, who were initially residents, interns, or the ubiquitous Finney, were told to give less ether, not more. The order shocked Bloodgood, who had been taught precisely the opposite in Philadelphia. Halsted devised an ether cone, which would allow a greater admixture of air for the patient to breathe. Blood loss was sharply reduced, aseptic technique ruled, anesthetic dose was reduced, and in abdominal operations sterile gauze soaked in sterile saline solution was used to protect the intestines from trauma and drying. Patients were kept warm after surgery, the foot of the bed was raised slightly, and replacement fluids were given by rectum to prevent postoperative shock. Day after day, and year after year, it became abundantly clear that thinking and technique counted. Safe surgery was good surgery.

CHAPTER TWENTY-THREE

Changes

A DECADE AT JOHNS HOPKINS had passed fruitfully for Halsted. Dealing daily with unyielding personal demons, as well as the growing pains of a revolutionary organization, he had reinvented himself as the leader of the scientific surgery movement and conceived a surgical philosophy that would be adopted worldwide. He had devised and popularized two gold-standard operations, put surgeons' hands in sterile gloves, and begun a training system that would prove itself by providing three generations of the most influential surgeons in America

But by 1896, The Professor had changed appreciably. Pushing his starting time back to 10 A.M. may have been the first signal of a waning ardor for the daily grind of surgery. He was doing fewer operations, rarely completing them, and quite regularly handing them off to his assistants. "You know what I want done," he would say, leaving the room. He frequently carried the specimens to the lab, where he dissected and pondered them himself. In later years, as Bloodgood established the surgical pathology service, he would oversee the tagging and sectioning of areas of interest to him. Experimental work in the dog lab consumed more of his time as he became increasingly involved in the newly evolving issues related to the thyroid gland, and the techniques of what would become vascular surgery.

For the first year Halsted operated every day, followed every hospital patient, and was regularly present in the dispensary. Gradually, according to plan, the resident assumed responsibility for more of the surgery and aftercare. As Halsted's comfort level with the resident rose, his oversight diminished. Soon the resident assumed primary teaching responsibilities for his juniors, and a functioning system was in place. Gradually, The Professor became a visitor to his wards and a less frequent operator. By the end of the first decade, he had established a routine in which he would visit the ward and politely ask the resident whether he would mind if "I examined this patient." Similarly, he would choose a patient whose problem interested him and ask permission to do the surgery. This, of course, was nothing more than a polite sham, but it became the manner in which he laid claim to his interests and allowed the rest to pass to the resident.

He frequently arrived late for surgery, casually offering excuses varying from lame to the bizarre. These were duly noted but never challenged. Some were too comical to imagine, including the morning he claimed to have lost track of time while he and Mrs. Halsted were killing rats in their cellar. Often, he said he had been working late into the night preparing a paper or studying the literature on a surgical problem and was too tired to operate, deliver a scheduled lecture, or conduct a clinic. In these events he issued a last-minute note or telephone call to the resident, asking him to serve in his stead. Standing instructions were issued to start surgery without him, should he be late. Few outside the administration were bothered by his absences. The resident was pleased with the opportunity to perform more surgery, and the medical students learned early in their tenure that Professor Halsted was not the answer to their prayers.

After pioneering abdominal surgery techniques, he rarely performed them, preferring to study the problem and pass the actual surgery to Finney and the residents. Breast and hernia surgery held fast as the "routine" procedures in which Halsted maintained a working interest, but they had become the magnet attracting patients to Hopkins, and the volume was shared. For his entire tenure, he was the only senior surgeon at The Johns Hopkins Hospital and the only professor of surgery. Not even the long-serving Finney had the privilege of caring for his private patients at the hospital. All patients on the surgical service, private or not, were Halsted patients, to whom he would dispense care as he wished. Customarily this took the form of assigning operations to the resident surgeon or Finney, while reserving those of interest for himself. This, too, would change.

In retrospect, much of the tardiness and the absences must have been due to the effects of the large doses of morphine. Surely some of the "poor health" that caused him to retire from surgery in mid-case was too much, or too little, morphine. On many occasions Halsted was sweaty, weak, and dizzy, which he routinely blamed on palpitations from excessive smoking. The claim was sympathetically accepted by those unaware of his history, and to some extent this might have been true, but the more likely trigger was morphine, as it had been in 1891 when Osler had observed his symptoms and learned the truth.

In April of 1891, Halsted had written the trustees requesting an extension of his summer leave to a full six months to cope with what he presumed to be malaria. The malaria letter to the trustees was one of the few concrete instances in which he plainly lied. It may be valueless parsing to harshly contrast a claim of "malaria" to "ill health" or "a racing heart," but the malaria excuse strikes a particularly outlandish note. The malaria-causing parasite had been identified by then, and Councilman and LaFleur had made the Hopkins laboratories central to the investigation of the disease. After a tragic misdiagnosis, Osler had issued a dictum that the diagnosis of malaria was never to be presumed without the verified presence of the parasite in the red blood cells. All this was well known, and one wonders how Halsted expected to get away with his claim without a blood test. Perhaps he knew he would never be challenged. What he was doing for those six months is unknown.

He managed the decade well enough, remaining enormously productive, if not energetic in the manner of the first few years. More of his time was spent studying at home, but he would appear daily at the hospital, albeit often briefly. The experimental surgery laboratory at the Pathological again became the focus of his energies as he became increasingly involved in issues related to the thyroid gland, and the techniques of what would evolve into vascular surgery. As his operations for hernia and breast cancer became more widely adopted he could rest upon the impressive statistics being compiled by Bloodgood, but he rarely operated. It is unlikely that his colleagues among the "Big Four" registered the change, since Welch and Osler had slipped into much more comfortable routines, and Kelly was far too frenetic to notice.

* * *

THE HALSTEDS FINALLY rented the grand house at 1201 Eutaw Place. Howard Kelly and his family lived just down the street in an enormous house at 1406, but the two couples did not socialize. In the countrified atmosphere of the Bolton Hill district, one could feel pleasantly isolated from the grit of downtown and the harbor. The short journey to the hospital across town immediately dispelled that isolation for all but the blind and anosmic. Central Baltimore was still an unsanitary backwater without municipal sewers. Bathwater and manure flowed freely across the cobbles and drainage swales. The central water system was efficient but unprotected from contamination, resulting in regular and costly outbreaks of typhoid. Osler and Welch publicly executed a campaign to correct these public health offenses, which they observed daily en route to the citadel of modern medicine and laboratory science. Amidst the dirt and debris, the old Baltimore custom of early-morning scrubbing of the stone steps in front of the homes seemed a quaint anachronism.

In the early years, Halsted made the journey to the hospital on the hill in East Baltimore by meandering bobtail horse cart or omnibus. Later, he drove an old horse cart of his own, after acquiring driving skills as a country horseman. After a few years of driving himself he graduated to an elegant liveried carriage, which he used until the advent of electric streetcars and motorized taxis. His advancing age, and perhaps a rejection of the flashy roadsters in which the young doctors sped about town, resulted in Halsted's general disinterest in the automobile, which his contemporaries had quickly embraced—particularly the well-compensated Kelly, who was driven around in the largest and finest of motorized steel chariots, with several spares in the carriage house attached to his home.

The large house on Eutaw Place made possible the separate living arrangements that suited them, and Halsted had room enough to establish a working office and formal library on the first floor. There he had access to medical texts and papers from his extensive personal collection, and worked with his secretaries on correspondence and Johns Hopkins business. Books and papers on his current interests were pulled and stacked in his second-floor study, where what he considered the real work took place. This arrangement freed him from interruptions but further isolated him from the hospital and his residents. If his attention was urgently required, they could reach him by telephone or send a messenger, but one rarely made the mistake of too casual an interruption.

Most evenings were spent at home. After dinner Halsted would retire to the second-floor study, exchange his suit coat for a comfortable silk dressing gown worn over his shirt and necktie, exchange his shoes for old carpet slippers, and read and write into the night. Caroline, who was a voracious reader, would retire to her sitting room on the third floor to sew and read. Her tastes in literature favored what Halsted termed "trash." His reading was primarily the medical literature, but in later years he expanded his horizons, often seeking consultations on books from bibliophile friends before setting off for his annual holiday.

Their lives remained essentially separate until the next evening, when they would reconvene at 7 P.M. to dine and chat until 8:30. If Halsted chose to spend the day at home they would lunch together. Mealtime conversation covered a wide spectrum, from science and medicine to farming, etymology, and evolution. Caroline often expressed appreciation for her husband's forbearance and interest in her, and felt herself to be his intellectual inferior. "He was very patient with my ignorance but did gratify me by saying that he thought I had a scientific mind. He did not add what its limitations were but I fully appreciate how much I have lost . . . by not being more educated."

In their unconventional manner, the Halsteds were devoted to each other. Caroline felt her purpose was to make life pleasant for her husband and facilitate his ability to do his work. However, some of her letters to him when she was away at High Hampton seem laced with irony, if not anger. In most cases the anger was directed at her husband's fastidious nature:

> I wanted to write you a full account of my adventures yesterday but a headache stopped me. I started at 3:30 in a drizzle. It poured a deluge and my only worry was your buggy. I knew you would rather have me stuck on the road a week than have one thread injured . . . I do not think your wagon is injured. I covered everything . . .

But there is little evidence of overt friction between them. Caroline regularly suffered migraine headaches and not infrequently took to her bed for days. She was by her own admission often feeling forlorn and depressed. In the same 1896 letter from High Hampton, she wrote, "I don't suppose that anyone will know what a struggle it has been to me getting through this summer. I have seemed apparently well but I think that I have forced my physical recovery at the expense of a heavy toll on my nervous system. I can't sleep and I feel like crying most of the time."

There were few regular guests at the house on Eutaw Place, and the legend of the reclusive nature of the couple continued to build with years of absence from the hospital social scene. Although Halsted did attend medical banquets and dinners for visiting dignitaries, he was invariably unaccompanied. On the select occasions when visiting surgeons were entertained at his home, Mrs. Halsted did not appear. Most of his socializing took place at the Maryland Club. His friends were usually in attendance, and he could count on good company. In the first years the group was made up of Welch, Halsted, Mall, and two longtime club members, Major Richard M. Venable, an attorney, and Francis H. Hambleton, an engineer. Central to the gatherings was William Welch. Osler, who had been a club member since arriving in Baltimore, was part of the unlikely group of chatterers and pranksters but rarely joined in after his marriage in 1892. More often he entertained house staff and students at his home on Franklin Street.

For a time Major Venable lived at the Maryland Club, and later he frequently hosted the group at his home. An able lawyer and Latin scholar, he was a notorious local character. The *Baltimore Sun* wrote of his membership on the City Council, "Although the Major's constant breaking of the rules by perpetuating jokes upon his fellow councilmen interfered at times with the dignity of the branch, he assisted in accomplishing needed civic improvements."

Dr. William Lockwood and Dr. Frank Donaldson joined the group a short time later, but Venable and Welch were the central figures who provided both the intellectual and mischievous leadership.

While climbing the stairs of the Maryland Club, Welch complained of pain and pounding in his chest. Concerned, Halsted pressed an ear to Welch's chest and was met by a jolting protean rhythm. This, it turned out, was caused by an inflatable rubber bulb connected to another in his pocket, which Welch squeezed at irregular intervals.

Another time, Welch placed an inflatable bladder under Halsted's plate and watched with feigned disinterest as The Professor studied the intermittently jiggling dish.

Most of their practical jokes were either sophomoric or at the expense of making others uncomfortable. Welch once invited his assistant, Simon Flexner, lately arrived from Louisville, to join him at Venable's home for dinner. Venable's reaction upon seeing the young man was, "I suppose you want him to stay for dinner."

"Yes," said Welch.

"I suppose it's all right. I suppose there's enough to eat." Then Venable told the maid, "I suppose there's going to be enough soup for one extra. If not, don't give any to Flexner."

He continued the routine throughout dinner, though there was quite obviously more than enough to go around. After dinner, when the stories began, the young man was temporarily relieved, only to find himself repeatedly the object of the loudest laughs.

Halsted was at ease with the group, and there was genuine fondness among its members. Most importantly, they provided an amusing and safe outlet, and the relationships were predictable and formal enough to preclude intrusion or intimacy. The interaction among the men included a good deal of intellectual teasing and scholarly one-upmanship. It is unclear whether Welch's and Venable's pranks annoyed Halsted as much as did Osler's, but his own idea of humor tended more toward the sharp and sarcastic.

For all the portrayal of The Professor as out of touch and absent-minded, the detachment provided a functional cover from which he could choose the situations in which he wished to interact and ignore the others. But that did not mean he was unaware of them. He was, if anything at all, a most acute observer, and the fact that he rarely shared these keen observations was a useful tool he honed sharply over the years. He would question a new acquaintance with great interest, listen attentively to the response, and say very little. Disarming and effective, he was able to draw people out and judge their knowledge, and value quickly. Boastfulness, inaccuracy, and dishonesty were instant disqualifiers.

Many of his casual observations were amusing commentary on the world according to William Stewart Halsted, and resound more fully when juxtaposed.

He remarked to the pediatrician Edwards Park, "At medical meetings the best looking men are the internists: the worst looking men are the dermatologists, and the surgeons come in somewhere between."

To Edwin Baetjer, the Hopkins radiologist, with whom he was strolling down the corridor as Joe Bloodgood passed, he turned, followed Bloodgood with his eyes, and finally said, "There goes Bloodgood. He can draw more general conclusions from a single instance than anybody I ever knew."

Bloodgood was a mediocre surgeon and an excellent surgical pathologist. He conducted his private practice of surgery elsewhere but was always in attendance at Hopkins, where he operated very occasionally. He was very well liked and often the butt of Halsted's humor. Once, in the early days, Osler asked Halsted and Bloodgood to see a patient with what Osler called a "squint of the cock," referring to a chordee, a condition in which the erect penis is bent.

"Doctor Bloodgood, how would you treat him?" asked Halsted.

"Oh, by massage, Doctor Halsted."

Halsted turned to him with a smile. "Oh, Bloodgood, you don't mean that, do you?"

FINNEY TELLS OF A telephone call from an associate regarding a patient with acute abdominal pain, for which neither he nor Halsted could find a cause. The patient was a particularly unattractive young woman who worked as a practical nurse. Prior to coming to the hospital she had been drinking tansey tea and taking cathartics. Tansey tea was believed to stimulate menstrual flow and abortion. Finney diagnosed a ruptured tubal pregnancy. The associate demurred, thinking about the patient's appearance.

"Wait until you see her. It can't be that."

At operation the patient was found to have a ruptured tubal pregnancy, and a belly full of blood. When Halsted was told that Finney had made the diagnosis over the phone, his first comment was, "Did Finney do that? Make a diagnosis right off over the telephone without seeing the patient?" Then he added, "Well, come to think it over, after all it isn't as astonishing as it might appear. Of course, you and I, Pancoast [the assistant], wouldn't be expected to know the significance of tansey tea and cathartics, but Finney, with his knowledge of the world, he would know."

He later added, "It is better to make no diagnosis than the correct diagnosis without a reason."

* * *

A FEW PEOPLE WERE fairly regular visitors at 1201 Eutaw Place. Among them were Caroline's old friend Sally Carter, her aunts, and in later years, the wife of Halsted's former resident, Samuel Crowe. Crowe, the son of a physician, had first encountered Halsted at the end of his first year as a medical student. He and two friends were on holiday in the North Carolina mountains in a covered wagon, pulled by two enormous Percheron horses, when one of their hired horses became immobile and seemed to freeze. At a loss for what to do, they began asking around the nearby town for a veterinarian. Crowe let it be known to the suspicious locals that he was a medical student from Johns Hopkins, which of course were the magic words. He was directed to High Hampton, some two miles away, where he would find the "doc," who had the only barn in the area large enough to house the huge horse.

Halsted had gradually become expert in treating farm animals and pets, as well as his ailing neighbors, and was all too frequently called upon to do so. Crowe found his way to High Hampton, and to his surprise, was welcomed by a maid in full uniform. Dazzled by the fine views, elegant plantings, and wide lawn, he waited uncomfortably for The Professor, who soon materialized from his hike in spotless white flannels, a silk shirt, patent leather pumps, and his walking stick.

Halsted had his buggy rigged and the young man led him to the ailing horse. Crowe had expected the stable man, not the doctor, to make the journey, and was even more impressed when Halsted stood in the mud for 20 minutes, quietly examining the horse. He diagnosed the problem as muscular rheumatism, and the horse was coaxed back to the big barn at High Hampton, where it spent a week wrapped from head to hoof in oilcloth and was rubbed down regularly by the professor of surgery at The Johns Hopkins School of Medicine.

Crowe was treated as an honored guest while the horse was recovering and got to know both Halsteds quite well. Halsted warmed to his guest and over the next few days spoke movingly of the beauty and demands of medicine. Young Crowe was dumbstruck and inspired by the entire experience.

The occasional resident visited the Halsted home, usually for special occasions, and few were invited more than once. There were exceptions, and in later years some spent a great deal of time at Eutaw Place and High Hampton. Few hosts were more concerned with the comfort of their guests than Halsted. But some of his closest friends and hospital associates never entered his home and rarely encountered Mrs. Halsted, if at all. William MacCallum, Halsted's friend, collaborator, and biographer, was a frequent visitor to the private quarters but met Caroline for the first time just several months before her death.

On the rare occasions when the Halsteds entertained, Caroline ceded the entire process to her husband. It was he who scoured the vast Lexington Market for delicacies and chose the menu. He chose the china, planned the placement and the flowers, and saw to it that every wrinkle and fold was carefully ironed out of the tablecloth after it had been spread on the table. The dinners were elegantly planned and presented multicourse affairs. Fine wines were served with every course, and Halsted would politely sip with his guests, perhaps drinking a total of a single glass of wine over the course of an evening. Otherwise, he rarely drank at all.

Despite his propensity toward solitary evenings at home, Halsted did attend some hospital functions and professional dinners, though he preferred small gatherings with his friends. After years of such sparing attendance, his presence at any gathering was dutifully noted, remembered, and reported upon, largely because these occasions were among the few social contacts many individuals had with the distant, aristocratic man who was otherwise unapproachable. Reports of these sightings were usually underscored by anecdotes of his sly sense of humor and unexpected comments.

Halsted's passion for antique furniture, fine old Persian carpets, paintings, and all manner of decorative artifacts flourished at 1201 Eutaw Place. The first three floors of the large house were soon filled with his purchases, but the issue was less about furnishing than collecting, and the result had the effect of a disorganized storage facility. Cushing described it as "a great magnificent old stone house full of rare old furniture, clocks, pictures and what not in topsy turvy condition, cold as a stone and most unlivable."

One of his associates in the acquisition of these antique treasures was a burly Baltimore physician named Crim. Their shared love and knowledge of antiques appeared to be the sole basis for the friendship. Dr. Crim had among his patients many of the now impoverished old Baltimore aristocracy, with whom he would barter services for antique furniture. Crim was personally unclean and medically inept, and an unlikely individual for Halsted to embrace.

Observing knee surgery on a patient he had referred to Halsted, Crim watched as the heroic preoperative preparations for sterility were carried out. The surgeons scrubbed, dipped, dipped again, and gloved. The patient had gone through overnight applications of antiseptic solutions, was painted with antiseptic on the table, and draped with sterile white towels. When asked exactly where the symptoms had begun, Crim laid his dirty, unwashed, and ungloved hand on the carefully prepared knee and promptly contaminated the sterile field. Crim was banished from the room, and the entire preparatory procedure had to be redone.

Despite this sort of medically ignorant transgression, Crim managed to retain his relationship with Halsted. How he was perceived as a physician is another matter entirely, but socially Crim was well known and well connected. He was famous primarily for his collections and conducted an auction at which some of Halsted's finer pieces had been purchased. Halsted was active enough in the world of antique furniture to find it worthwhile to retain an old German carpenter on his household staff to repair and maintain his acquisitions. Some of the furniture made its way to High Hampton, though the environment there was decidedly more spartan. In general, collecting was a city passion, and his dahlias, and sometimes his telescope, the country passions.

The only source of heat in the living quarters on the north side of the Eutaw Place house were the open hardwood fires, which were often inadequate compensation for the open windows. The service wing on the south side of the house was heated by a modern furnace. Among the books, and clocks, and fine furniture in the big, cold house were any number of dogs. It seemed that dachshunds and spaniels were everywhere. Halsted was fond of the dogs, but they were Mrs. Halsted's constant companions, particularly the dachshunds.

When Halsted was in residence, a secretary, and sometimes two or three, worked alongside him in the first-floor library. Household staff scurried through the back of the house, and during the winter season Caroline Halsted, who sometimes spent entire days alone in her third-floor aerie, tended to the dogs. For exercise and excitement she often drove their large-wheeled, high-seated "dogcart" through nearby Druid Hill Park, with the dachshunds seated beside her and the spaniels running alongside. The lightweight cart was well balanced and had the seat situated over the two large wheels. It was fast and maneuverable, and she drove aggressively. On one occasion the cart overturned, and Caroline suffered bruised ribs and a broken femur. Halsted had been away at the time and Finney cared for her at home. After cabling him to return home, Finney met Halsted's train the following day and told him that Mrs. Halsted had suffered an accident. Sizing up the situation, he asked, "Is she dead?" with the clinical detachment that was his trademark.

By that time it was clear that her condition was stable, Finney reassured his chief, and hinted at how difficult his patient had been. Caroline had insisted on engaging an old attendant, who would tolerate being bossed around, instead of a qualified nurse. She recovered grumpily but uneventfully.

Finney had the opportunity to treat her once again, this time for acute appendicitis. He operated early, using the new "McBurney incision,"[1] and her course was uncomplicated. As usual, Caroline refused to follow instructions. She invoked her nursing training regularly, and very soon after surgery began to complain about lying around in bed. Finney knew what was coming and anticipated her.

---

1 In the late 19th century, several surgeons recognized the value of early diagnosis of appendicitis and surgical removal prior to rupture. Removal after rupture was generally associated with a nearly 25 percent mortality rate, so the standard procedure was to wait for rupture and abscess, then drain the abscess and hope for the best. An early innovator was Charles McBurney, at The Roosevelt Hospital in New York City, who identified the tender point at which maximal pain from appendicitis is localized. He was also among the first to remove an acute, nonruptured appendix, and devised an incision in which the oblique muscles in the right lower quadrant of the abdomen were spread apart and not cut. This allowed access to the appendix. When the wound was closed the fibers of the two muscles, which were oriented in opposite directions above each other, reformed the abdominal wall without the weakness prevalent in muscle-splitting or muscle-cutting incisions. McBurney's point and the McBurney incision have been in the medical lexicon for more than a century, though the diagnosis is often confirmed by scan, and the incision has become of historical significance with the advent of laparoscopic appendectomy.

"Why don't you sit up in this armchair?"

And he carried her to the chair just as Halsted entered the room.

"Finney, you get your patients up sooner after operation than I do."

"Yes sir, some patients," Finney admitted to The Professor, who was slyly smiling, no doubt happy to see the burden transferred to his assistant.

CHAPTER TWENTY-FOUR

Into the 20th Century

THINGS WERE GOING ALONG better than anyone could have predicted in the Department of Surgery at The Johns Hopkins Hospital. Halsted had done several hundred hernia repairs and dozens of operations for breast cancer, and was beginning to experiment with new techniques for surgery of the thyroid gland. The entire surgical staff was wearing sterile rubber gloves at surgery. White surgical shirts and trousers were universal, and aseptic techniques were rigidly, or almost rigidly, adhered to. Most surgeons now wore hats, but masks hadn't yet appeared, and when Halsted really needed to get a feel of something, he would still remove his gloves. No one made much of it because he was the chief, and, more important, postsurgical infections had become increasingly rare.

Halsted had virtually banned the use of catgut sutures. Fine silk was used for internal sutures and ties around blood vessels, and wounds were closed with silver wire. Halsted found fine silk the least irritating, least disturbing material for internal use. It would become the rule. The outcome was excellent so long as the surgeon was skillful, delicate, and cognizant of the inadvisability of crushing tissue beneath the ties. In the hands of average, careless surgeons, he believed gut sutures were less problematic. So, although he insisted on the use of fine silk sutures by his staff, he was well aware of the habits of the surgical world at large and acknowledged the existence of second-class surgeons. Wounds were no longer routinely drained to provide an exit route for infection. Sutures were not brought out through the skin, a change that prevented stitch abscesses. New types of dressings were being tried, and laboratory studies of wound healing, intestinal anastomosis, and thyroid and arterial surgery were moving forward. Joseph Bloodgood was inventing surgical pathology, though he may not have known it at the time, and he was preparing to organize and compile The Professor's surgical experience.

In 1897, the first medical school class was preparing to graduate, and applications for future places were outstripping availability. When one of the three female students in the first class had married Franklin Mall, the scourge of the medical student, and dropped out, Osler quipped that at that rate there would be no women remaining to graduate. Otherwise, resistance to coeducation had dissipated, and varying numbers of women entered succeeding classes. However, an undercurrent of displeasure with women in medicine persisted. Most thought women did not have the physical ability to tolerate the grind. There were comments about the loss of femininity and sexuality necessary for them to succeed, and even Osler was said to have commented on the three classes of humanity: men, women, and women physicians.

The chiefs were pleased to have their first homegrown class of young doctors from which to choose their interns and residents, and things were finally going along according to the original plan. The same professors of clinical medicine had been responsible for teaching the rudiments of scientific medicine to the students. And students who had shown an aptitude for independent thought and research were being rewarded with positions under their mentors.

The dog surgery course finally got off the ground late in 1895, and it was a resounding success. Halsted had made good on his promise. He had structured an experience that accurately mimicked human surgery, and the students were not only consumed by the opportunity, but aware of being part of an important transition in medical education. The vision and the syllabus were his, and he taught the course whenever he could, and then whenever he felt like it, and then not at all.

Perhaps the greatest disappointment for the third-year students was the absence of surgical teaching beyond the dog lab. Lectures were frequently canceled, and when they took place, were too esoteric to be worthwhile. Halsted still didn't get it. His interests were in unsolved surgical problems, in difficult diagnosis, and the correlation between disease and surgical pathology, all far beyond the scope of undergraduate surgery. The students were interested in learning the day-to-day clinical practice of surgery. The residents understood this and attempted to fill in the gaps.

Friday surgical clinics were a great success. These took place in the amphitheater. Halsted held the floor; patients were presented and discussed. The medical students in the rows of benches did their best to keep out of sight. After Halsted's presentation, he asked questions on a wide range of topics. In a discussion that wandered to the muscles of the neck, William Rienhoff recalled The Professor asking the students gathered around him, "What made the larynx go up and down when one swallowed?"

After a significant silence, Halsted answered his own question. "The inferior constrictor of the pharynx," a muscle located in the back of the throat.

Rienhoff didn't accept the answer. The next day he went to the anatomy building and dissected a human neck. His dissection demonstrated that the muscle responsible for laryngeal movement was, in fact, the stylohyoid. With trepidation, Rienhoff reported his findings. It was this sort of curiosity that Halsted sought, and Rienhoff remained a favorite thereafter, ultimately earning the position of resident.

Despite the disorganization and disappointments, the popularity of the school grew. The Johns Hopkins School of Medicine stood alone in the country, and was being recognized for the phenomenon that it was. By 1896, the entering class was more than 40-strong. Women were filling more of the places, and the quality of the female students was generally excellent. Even skeptics like Welch were speaking out for coeducation.

Not all the bright, young students fit the mold, or were able to thrive within the system. Gertrude Stein entered with the class of 1901. Having studied experimental psychology with William James at Radcliffe, Stein returned to her family in Baltimore and enrolled at The Johns Hopkins School of Medicine. From the start, she was anything but popular with fellow students. The butt of pranks and unflattering sobriquets, she was thought generally unpleasant in manner and mannish in appearance—two accurately portrayed traits, which she incorporated into her persona.

Stein developed close relationships with feminist voices in the community, including Dr. Claribel Cone and her sister, Etta, who were wealthy art collectors. Claribel was doing postgraduate work at the medical school, and she and Stein built an enduring friendship. Stein openly espoused her lesbian philosophy and lived outside the mainstream of student life. She did well through the two preclinical years and idolized professors the other students despised, particularly Mall and Halsted.

In the clinical years Stein failed miserably, and by consensus she was denied her degree. For a period she remained at Hopkins studying neuroanatomy with Mall, but that, too, ended in failure. With no aptitude for medicine, Gertrude Stein moved to Paris and gained fame as a writer. Stein coined the term "The Lost Generation," for the young, intellectual expatriates struggling to find themselves in postwar Paris, including her friends Ernest Hemingway, F. Scott Fitzgerald, and Sherwood Anderson. She befriended Picasso and Matisse; claimed that Cézanne's painting *Madame Cézanne*, beneath which she sat while writing *Three Lives*, was the inspiration for her book, and went on to amass a brilliant collection of Impressionist art. For that collection alone, she will always be remembered. Stein's influence on the literature of the day was significant, if debated. Much of her writing was obtuse, and though few believed her work to be as great as did she, much of it has survived.

AS THE CENTURY drew to a close, The Johns Hopkins Hospital was filling its beds and changing the way medicine was practiced. Everyone was working well, no one was working excessively hard, and each of the Big Four was rapidly becoming a caricature of himself. Welch was wearing too many hats and spending too little time in each. His lectures were mostly given by assistants, who were not nearly so dynamic and embracing as speakers. The joke was that his courses were "too much Flexner and not enough Welch." His laboratory work and scientific paper production had dwindled to near nothing. He spent some time as dean of the medical school, some time as pathologist in chief, and lots of time at the dining table.

Halsted was fond of writing letters, but he was notoriously slow in responding to his mail. Knowing this, he often began the return letter with a disclaimer and apology for the piece having slipped to the bottom of the stack. Welch, on the other hand, was completely hopeless. In 1896, he had founded the *Journal of Experimental Medicine,* which he also edited. Prominent scientists gladly contributed their work, only to lose touch with their manuscripts and hear nothing from Welch. Requests for return of the manuscripts went unheeded, and Henry Hurd was asked to intervene. Hurd began to periodically slip into Welch's study when he was away for his weekends, rummage through the stacks of unopened manuscripts, and return them to their worried authors.

Welch's library was furnished with eight chairs and a desk, all piled high with unopened mail. The disorder was staggering, but Welch, it seemed, had a system: "On that armchair there I have the letters that have come during the past week; I hope to read these in the near future. On that chair I have the letters that have come within the last month. On the other chairs are letters and magazines anywhere from six months to a year old which I hope to get to sometime."

He had reserved one small corner of his desk for writing. The bulk of the surface was reserved for storage. When the desk became too littered he would spread a newspaper over the letters and papers, and start again. Hugh Young recalled seeing four such layers on the desk. Young offered a Dictaphone and stenographer to help restore order. When the first cylinder was returned for transcription, the only message on it was a salutation, followed by, "Young, I can't use this machine. Send your boy around to get it."

WILLIAM OSLER REVELED in the success of *The Principles and Practice.* He drew the finest residents around him and was absolutely beloved by the medical students, who endured the first grueling years of basic sciences awaiting their exposure to the great man. Osler could regularly be seen walking the halls with an arm on the shoulder of a student or intern. He was the only senior faculty member who regularly socialized with the students, even inviting groups of them to his home on Saturday evenings for dinner or dessert. He was on close terms with the residents, not only those in his department, and beloved by all. And he was a congenital jokester. His pranks were generally enjoyed, other than by Halsted. He continued to compose verse, often on hospital issues, and was, in the eyes of all, particularly his juniors, the beating heart of the institution.

Kelly was operating constantly. Hunter Robb, who had been Kelly's assistant, and preceded Bloodgood as the first man to wear surgical gloves for surgery, had become resident. "Bull" Williams, who led obstetrics, was a difficult and biased man. He was intensely disliked by the female medical students, who found his offhand, sexist remarks offensive. Kelly was too busy to take up the cause, but it was his nature to defend honor and decency, even when he wasn't asked to do so.

Kelly's fees were extremely high, and his popularity enormous. He had already written the two-volume text *Operative Gynecology* and was thought to be the best surgeon in the country.

Halsted's fame was nearly equal to that of his peers, about which he was honestly unimpressed, and the surgical service was busy. His private practice had grown with his fame, but he was operating less and relying more on his assistants. Fewer private patients were treated in their homes, and increasingly the resident performed the surgery when the patient was hospitalized.

The charity wards provided the overwhelming percentage of surgical patients. Initially, the wards were racially integrated, in the spirit of the founder. The board of trustees—founder Johns Hopkins's fellow Quakers—generally favored integration, and Francis King, the president of the board, personally saw to it that the hospital opened with racially integrated wards. In short order, protests and unrest festered among staff members and the patient population, both black and white. The experiment in integration was abandoned shortly after it was begun, and segregated wards were created.

All charity patients were treated by Halsted with the same gentlemanly intensity and detachment as were his private patients, but gradually, this aspect of his life became less central. There always seemed to be something that demanded his attention—a project in the lab, a paper he was working on, a problem at home, or simply his feeling out of sorts. As Halsted withdrew from the operating room, the burden fell increasingly on Finney, Bloodgood, and Mitchell. The occasions upon which he verbalized his thanks to those picking up the slack were few. It had become an unspoken part of the job.

* * *

THE ENORMITY OF the success of the Hopkins experiment could only have been the result of the unique celestial alignment that brought together Welch, Osler, Halsted, and Kelly. Other institutions were working to move medicine forward, and many began to adopt elements of the Hopkins style. Laboratories were integrated into the great hospitals, aseptic surgery was slowly accepted, and postgraduate training became available. The better medical schools instituted more stringent admission requirements and some moved to a four-year curriculum, but abandoning the old ways was a slow process. Hopkins soon stood alone far ahead of the pack, and it would take the organized outrage of the Carnegie Commission to fully turn the page. By the time that would come to pass in 1910, there was Johns Hopkins, and there was everyplace else.

But a big shake-up was headed for the Department of Surgery. It came in the form of an assistant resident, the son of a wealthy Cleveland doctor, by way of Harvard and the Massachusetts General Hospital, and in the person of Harvey Cushing. A slight, dark-haired young man, Cushing was aristocratically handsome, with a beaklike nose and strong jaw, and was as tightly wound a "type A" overachiever as one could imagine. With boundless energy, enormous technical skill, scientific curiosity, and great intelligence, all packaged together with soaring ambition and no small amount of hubris, he moved into the world of Johns Hopkins. Not surprisingly, Cushing would be the first of the Halsted residents to stamp his own mark on the surgical world.

CHAPTER TWENTY-FIVE

Harvey Cushing

I N 1910, MAJOR GENERAL Leonard Wood was about as distinguished a military man as could be found in the United States. Among his other accomplishments he commanded Theodore Roosevelt's Rough Riders, was military governor of Cuba and later military governor of the Philippines, and on top of it all he was a physician interested in public health. His energetic exploits had made him a household name, and he was next in line to become army chief of staff. As his fame and military importance were growing, so too was a large, nearly half-pound, tumor in his brain.

Harvey Cushing had been at Johns Hopkins for 14 years. He had performed hundreds of craniotomies, usually to release pressure on the brain and relieve symptoms. He had removed brain tumors as well, but with very limited success. Still, he was the most experienced man in a field of general surgeons with an interest in neurological surgery. No one specialized in neurosurgery, because little was known about surgery of the brain, and the results of meddling were consistently bad. Prior to Cushing taking up the task, postoperative infection killed the patients that the operation hadn't. Finding one's way into and out of the brain was difficult enough; achieving tangible improvement for the patient was nothing short of a miracle.

Wood's left-sided weakness and seizures had become too severe to ignore. After years of procrastinating, he found himself on Cushing's operating table. Cushing followed his routine and personally shaved the general's head, just as he would the head of an indigent ward patient. He had already proven that the skull and brain were insensitive to pain and planned to do the surgery under local anesthetic, using a dilute cocaine solution to numb the scalp. Patients could lie comfortably awake for hours, chatting away, as the surgeon dug into the recesses of their brains. After preparing the scalp with antiseptic, Cushing draped the area with sterile towels, in much the same manner he had been taught by Halsted to do in general surgery. Then Cushing changed his mind, and Wood was anesthetized with chloroform. He cut through the skin of the scalp to the richly vascular loose connective beneath it. He applied pressure to the scalp beyond the incision, thereby controlling bleeding, and applied fine Halsted clamps to the blood vessels. When the field was dry, he incised the deepest layers of connective tissue, the galea and periosteum, and exposed the bone of the skull. The next, brutal, step was to drill holes through the skull with a hand-powered trephine. A wire blade, called a gigli saw, was threaded from hole to hole and the saw pulled back and forth until the skull between the holes was opened. This then could be lifted out like the lid of a jack-o'-lantern, or left partially hinged to the scalp. It was a bloody and time-consuming procedure.

Cushing looked beneath the flap and encountered a very large, superficial mass. Calculating the difficulties already incurred in simply trying to control bleeding, he opted to withdraw, close the skull flap, and begin again another day.

Several days later, this time with the patient under local anesthesia, Cushing lifted the skull cap and faced the pulsating mass. Cushing thought the better of having Wood awake for the struggle, and he was given chloroform once again. It was an enormous and daunting tumor. Cushing began digging. The tumor appeared to be a meningioma, originating from the fibrous layers covering the brain. It had pushed into the soft substance of the cerebral cortex, causing symptoms by its space-occupying mass, but was not actually invading the brain. After hours of painstaking dissection separating the benign meningioma from the normal brain surrounding it, Cushing believed he had removed the entire tumor, or as much as could be seen. The challenging task of controlling bleeding was time-consuming as well, but that, too, went Cushing's way. The operation was completed by reversing the steps made to enter. The dura was sutured closed, the skull cap replaced, and the galea and scalp sutured in place.

General Wood recovered quickly and fully, and Harvey Cushing became a national hero.

AFTER INITIALLY PLANNING to study medicine with Osler, Cushing switched gears and spent a year as a surgical intern at Massachusetts General Hospital. By all measure the ablest and most ambitious intern in the group, the obvious thing for him to do was to head for Baltimore and study the new surgery with Halsted. After an unsuccessful attempt to secure a position at Hopkins, Cushing was preparing to leave for a year of European study when an assistant residency became available. In September 1896, Cushing arrived in Baltimore ready to work.

Harvey Cushing wasn't the usual self-effacing junior resident reporting for duty. This one arrived with his wardrobe, his books, and the first X-ray machine ever seen at The Johns Hopkins Hospital. In Wurtzburg, Germany, Wilhelm Roentgen had recently passed a high-voltage electric current through a vacuum tube and noted an odd form of light that was not absorbed by a screen, but instead was projected across the room. On November 8, 1895, Roentgen used the apparatus to produce an image of his wife Bertha's hand. It clearly showed her bones as well as the wedding band on her ring finger — the first X-ray picture. The implications were enormous, and Cushing leapt into the fray. He, and others, at the Massachusetts General Hospital experimented a bit, then purchased a tube and a hand-cranked static electricity generating device, and began taking X-rays of fractured bones. Cushing provided most of the money to purchase the device and after some wrangling took it with him to Baltimore.

The first X-ray ever taken at The Johns Hopkins Hospital was a dramatic image of a bullet lodged in a woman's spine. Taking the X-ray was a tedious 45-minute affair, particularly for Joe Mitchell, who had to crank the generating apparatus while Cushing adjusted and readjusted the exposure. Cushing had arrived in a blaze of glory, bringing with him the newest and most obviously useful medical device. He continued to do all the X-ray work for the hospital until he became resident the following year.

Massachusetts General Hospital was very large and very busy, and Cushing was both surprised by the comparatively slow pace of Johns Hopkins and disappointed by the boring, backward city that Baltimore was at the time. In Boston the volume of surgical work had been great. Speed and technique were of the essence, and the idea of surgeons wearing rubber gloves was laughable. There was "No encouragement to follow-up a bad result, whether to its home or to the dead house."

This was the difference between the Halsted system and all the others. For Halsted every case, every patient, and every manifestation of disease had to be carefully studied before surgery, meticulously executed at surgery, and examined for lessons learned after surgery. Results were analyzed and methods continually changed, in the constant search for better solutions.

Cushing had no prior experience with laboratory tests, bacteriology, or surgical pathology. His learning curve was labor intensive, but he recognized the value of the work and was soon publishing papers on various laboratory-based topics. He wrote:

The talk was of pathology and bacteriology, of which I knew so little that much of my time the first few months was passed alone at night in the room devoted to surgical pathology . . . looking at specimens with a German text book at hand . . . . It was most disconcerting to me, after the hurly-burly of Massachusetts General Hospital, to have my new Chief come into Ward G; ask if he might be allowed to examine a particular patient; to have him spend an hour fiddling over a patient with cancer of the breast . . . if he were sufficiently interested he might ask that he be permitted to do the operation; and if he came and did operate, so soon as the breast was removed leaving the huge closure and skin graft to Bloodgood, he would depart with the tissues.

Cushing was the most impressive and possibly the most able and ambitious of the 17 Halsted residents. He was the first to utilize local anesthesia in hernia repair, the first to operate on the pituitary gland, the first to routinely open the skull to decompress the brain, the innovator of numerous neurological techniques, and the developer of prototypes for exactly how neurological operations should be performed. Simply put, he invented neurosurgery. All this transpired while Cushing worked as Halsted's assistant in the department of surgery. Cushing was an able and enthusiastic teacher, and in the laboratory he directed a team of assistants on research projects, increasingly involving the pituitary gland. In his spare time he performed the bulk of Halsted's surgery.

Halsted's legacy was built on two equally potent, unimpeachably world-altering platforms. The first was the establishment of the school of scientific, safe, and anatomically correct surgery; the second, a working environment that shaped the education of generations of surgeons and propelled American surgery to its preeminent position in the world. The former brought about an undeniable surgical revolution, proven by consistently superior results; the latter was a more complicated and personal equation, and Harvey Cushing was the perfect case in point.

Cushing came to Hopkins with curiosity, intelligence, and intensity. There he found the proper environment for his talents to prosper. He was neither groomed nor nurtured, but was allowed to take from the environment everything he needed to excel. He was the first to carry the Halsted tradition to greater heights, and he became far better known than The Professor himself. Cushing was the product of the scientifically enriched surgical environment created by Halsted. He fully utilized the Halsted springboard to realize his ambition of greatness, but he was the least vocal of disciples in praise of his chief.

Shortly after being named resident in 1897, Cushing became ill with abdominal pain, which he initially blamed on bad food. William MacCallum, a fourth-year medical student who had uncovered the physical properties of the parasite that caused malaria, was assigned by Cushing to repeatedly perform a count of the leukocytes in his blood. The white count, elevated at the outset, rapidly rose to a level indicative of active, acute infection. The professors were called in. Both Osler and Halsted adopted a wait-and-see posture, though it remains unclear what they were waiting for. The JHH experience with appendicitis was growing, and early intervention, before rupture, had finally become the rule.

IN 90 CASES OF appendicitis treated since the hospital had opened, the mortality rate was about 25 percent. Cushing didn't want to be among them, and he pushed for the surgery. Halsted, Finney, and Bloodgood were all in on the operation the following day. Cushing was anesthetized with chloroform, and by his own account, "all six hands were inside of me at once—and big hands at that." Nonetheless, the surgery was uneventful. The early postoperative course was smooth, but just when it seemed his problems were over, a wound infection developed. It was the first in a summer-long record of 200 consecutive cases without wound infection. Though Cushing recovered fully, he complained about the silver wires buried in his abdominal wall whenever anyone would listen.

When Cushing fully assumed the responsibilities of resident, he became more acutely aware of Halsted's absence. He wrote home, "The chief rarely operates. Today I did all of his private cases . . . ." Gradually, Cushing became disenchanted with his chief. He respected Halsted for all he had accomplished, but was outspoken about finding him both difficult and odd. At times he seemed to be compiling a dossier on what he considered Halsted's dereliction of duty; at others he was happy for the opportunity to assume responsibility and garner experience.

This, in fact, became the conundrum of the Halsted method of teaching. Had negligence and dodging of duty facilitated the graduated assumption of responsibility by the resident, or was all this according to plan? Cushing thought the worse of it in the early going, and the better of it in retrospect. Most residents shared the latter opinion. There can be little doubt that it was not a black-and-white issue. With increasing frequency, Halsted missed lectures, failed to appear at surgery, and did not follow up on research projects. There is no precise information on the extent of his drug use at the time, but things were getting worse.

HALSTED AND CUSHING had more in common than the single-minded pursuit of their goals. Both were Yale men; both had been athletes at college, and neither could brag about having spent any time in the Yale library. Halsted was impressed by Cushing during his first year at Johns Hopkins and chose him above senior men as resident. Cushing was ambidextrous and was a skillful operator from the start. This he credited to his earlier training in Boston, where so much emphasis was placed on technique. When lecturing, he would write on the chalkboard with both hands simultaneously. He was a competent representational artist and illustrated his charts with drawings of each operation. The drawings became part of the Cushing legend, and a useful device adopted by many surgeons to come.

Cushing worked tirelessly and was as demanding of assistant residents, nurses, and ancillary staff. On one occasion he so humiliated a junior resident that the man cornered him in the changing room, locked the door behind them, and threatened to give him the beating of his life unless he apologized. Cushing backed off but didn't change.

A perfectionist, he was rigid in his rules both inside the operating room and out, sometimes obsessively so. Samuel Crowe recounts that Cushing insisted his patients be fed soft-boiled eggs, bacon, and toast with bitter orange marmalade for breakfast, pureed spinach for lunch, and a list that went on and on. Hearing that Crowe forgot to order pureed spinach for a patient, Cushing flew into a rage, again nearly precipitating a physical clash.

But Cushing was just as hard on himself. When he lost a patient his first inclination was to blame himself, and in those early days he often complained to his wife that everyone he touched died. As he began to explore the uncharted world of brain surgery, failures far exceeded successes, and the self-flagellation became so intense that it almost smothered his enthusiasm. By 1899, he had already thrown himself into the deep water, achieving great success in an operation to control the debilitating pain of trigeminal neuralgia. Commonly known as tic douloureux, it is a life-altering affliction involving the sensory component of the fifth cranial nerve. Patients were known to kill themselves rather than endure the pain, and all prior efforts had failed for anatomical or technical reasons. Cushing was trained to become expert in the anatomy. He was technically proficient and he had great surgical courage, a combination that would lead him from success to success.

AFTER COMPLETING HIS residency in May 1900, Cushing set off for his first European tour. He observed the state of European neurosurgery, made a number of cultural side trips, and generally enjoyed the experience. He had already written numerous papers and was well known, and received job offers from hospitals in Boston, Philadelphia, and New York, eager to install a famous, young Halsted-trained surgeon. The most comfortable possibility was going home to Cleveland, where his father practiced, and set up as a surgeon. But everything considered, the future of medicine still resided at Johns Hopkins.

It was difficult to negotiate with Halsted. He either ignored the situation or refused to make a decision, but he wanted Cushing to return. Part of the inducement to draw him back to Hopkins was allowing him to take over the operative surgery course for third-year students, which occupied Friday afternoons, and the lectures on surgical anatomy two afternoons a week. Mornings were reserved for learning everything he could of neurology. He attended at the dispensary daily and did whatever operative neurology cases he could find on Friday mornings. For the first few years he saw private general surgery patients each afternoon from 2:00 to 3:00, in a small office in his home at 3 West Franklin Street. Throughout, he continued his work in the research lab.

Cushing restructured the operative surgery course, giving students roles in the care of the "patient" that mimicked human medical practice: family doctor, surgeon, assistants, and anesthetist. They dressed for surgery, observed proper aseptic technique, cared for the canine patient with a charted "history," and kept anesthetic and surgical records. One of the rules of the laboratory was, "An autopsy shall be performed in all cases of death occurring in the laboratory. These autopsies shall be conducted with the same respect and formality in the pathological department of the hospital and the findings shall be recorded in the laboratory record."

All this brought with it the feelings of joy and despair attendant upon any surgeon in the care of patients.

Halsted appreciated the improvement in the course he had created. Under Cushing it became the highlight of the student experience in surgery, and the envy of other medical schools. Halsted later wrote Welch, "I embrace this opportunity to express my indebtedness to

Harvey Cushing, for thirteen years my brilliant assistant, for his zeal in elaborating these courses and placing them on such a substantial basis that they are now regarded as one of the dominant features of the surgical curriculum for the third year medical students at the Johns Hopkins University and are being adopted by other medical schools of this country."

CUSHING SHARED THE rented house on West Franklin with two other young Hopkins doctors. Their neighbors at Number One were none other than the William Oslers. The relationship between Cushing and Osler had been excellent from the start, and it grew closer and more familial with the years. Osler welcomed the young men to the neighborhood with wine and cigars. An open-door policy, or at least an exchange of keys, was established, which was quickly dubbed the "latch key club." Cushing and the others often spent the late evening in the Osler library, working or socializing. The relationship became closer still when Cushing and his new bride, Kate, took over the house. Cushing, always a bibliophile, regretted the absence of a fine library and loved spending time among Osler's wide variety of well-bound editions. The Oslers adopted Kate as well, and the arrangement seemed to suit both families perfectly.

Osler was the glue between the volatile Cushing and the enigmatic Halsted. The 33-year-old Cushing was intemperate, at best, and the string of people he casually insulted gradually enveloped him and threatened to strangle his career. Rumors of his bad behavior spread beyond the Hopkins medical community. After one incident Osler called Cushing out for deprecating remarks he made about colleagues, which had found their way back from New York. Osler finished with the advice, "Keep your mouth."

Cushing also confessed to his wife, Kate, of being rude to Halsted: "Sorry, but I couldn't help it. Some day I will tell him I don't like him and pack up my duds and go home and bury my head in your lap."

A destructive pattern of behavior had developed. If Cushing did somehow learn to hold his tongue, much of the credit belonged to Osler. Beyond his father, there were few people who could influence Harvey Cushing. Years later he would win the 1926 Pulitzer Prize for his book *The Life of Sir William Osler.*

LITTLE OF WHAT irritated Cushing about Halsted was untrue. He was often absent from surgery, he did miss lectures, he did not communicate with medical students, and he was away from the hospital for almost half the year, and worked at home or in the experimental lab for a good deal of the time that he was present. He was, unintentionally or otherwise, oblivious to the feelings and the needs of those working for him, critical in a quiet and diminishing manner, and certainly niggardly with his compliments.

Cushing's negative attitude toward Halsted was evident during his residency, but The Professor's delinquencies had provided more opportunity and experience for him, and he was mollified by his own profit. Later his anger jelled around the difficulties in extracting a clear delineation of his position should he choose to return to Hopkins after the European tour. After a stimulating year "opening the box," as he referred to brain surgery, he had every intention of making a career of neurosurgery. Halsted had written him and offered such a position in the department of surgery. Later, Halsted suffered recriminations, thought there wouldn't be enough work, and made other suggestions unacceptable to Cushing, among them adding orthopedic surgery to his responsibilities. Tempers flared, or at least Cushing's did. Halsted said nothing. He backtracked and procrastinated, and was unable to make a decision. Finally, with some urging from others, the deal was struck and Cushing won all his points, but lost respect for The Professor.

For his part, Halsted recognized the unique talents before him and allowed them to blossom. He believed himself to be both encouraging and appreciative, and was apparently unaware of the animosity the young neurosurgeon harbored toward him. As early as 1899, Halsted wrote him, "If you should break down I would be in my grave in a month." There is no evidence of Halsted believing their relationship was anything but mutually beneficial and friendly, and later Cushing may have been the only former resident that Halsted treated like an equal.

It was Halsted who suggested Cushing pursue the exploration of pituitary function, which later resulted in his greatest scientific breakthrough, and it was he who allowed him the latitude to develop neurosurgery. As death and disappointment followed Cushing's every step forward, Halsted was said to have quipped that he didn't know whether to say "poor Cushing's patients, or Cushing's poor patients," but he was always supportive and never interfered.

Opening the skull was a daunting enterprise. It was approached infrequently, and the demise of the patient was the most frequent outcome. Intraoperative death was usually related to bleeding, and postoperative death the result of swelling of the brain and infection. X-rays could not differentiate brain tumors from the surrounding soft tissue, and tumors were therefore difficult to localize. Neurological examination and past experience could indicate the general location of a lesion, but finding it within the substance of the brain was fraught with disaster. One could not dissect indiscriminately through the substance of the brain without expecting to pay a dear price in neurological deficit.

The pressure of expanding tumors causes swelling and fluid accumulation, and pushes the brain against the skull. This results in seizures and a whole range of neurological deficits. Cushing reasoned that even if he couldn't localize the tumor and remove it, he could drain fluid and blood, and offer temporary relief until the tumor increased in size. It would be palliative at worst. He applied the lessons learned from Halsted; rigid asepsis and scrupulous hemostasis were the rule.[1] The towels draping the head should be as free of bloodstains and spatter at the conclusion of the operation as they had been at the start. Time-consuming and precise, the preparations made further exploration feasible, in a controlled environment.

The infection rate in Cushing's cases plummeted. His subtemporal skull flap provided both adequate decompression and a strong muscular layer to keep the brain from herniating through the trapdoor in the skull when the cover was not replaced. A year after devising the approach, he had performed more than two dozen successful decompressions. Cushing took his show on the road, and was harsh with surgeons who advocated surgery only when the tumor could be localized. With better technique and a more aggressive attitude toward palliation, his reputation grew, and along with it the courage for wider exploration and tumor removal. But he was still groping in the dark.

The popular course in operative surgery was held in cramped and inadequate quarters on the ground floor of the old anatomical building. Cushing, MacCallum, and a group of students successfully petitioned the trustees for a larger space. The resulting effort was called the Hunterian Laboratory of Experimental Medicine, after the pioneering British anatomist and surgeon John Hunter. Built in 1905 at a cost of $15,000, the new building housed laboratories for surgery

---

1 Cushing had brought a blood pressure cuff and measuring device home from Europe. In addition to monitoring pressure during surgery, he pioneered placing the cuff around the scalp, below the area of incision, to control blood flow from the vascular scalp. When this proved cumbersome, he developed a technique in which he and the assistant applied pressure to their side of the proposed incision before cutting the skin and galea. This would control bleeding until clamps could be applied and blood vessels tied. After drilling holes in the skull and connecting them with the gigli saw, he lifted the bone flap and stemmed the bleeding from the skull by applying bone wax, a technique devised by Horsley, in England. Cushing was obsessed with expanding the use of his blood pressure monitoring apparatus called the Riva-Rocci cuff, and Michael Bliss wrote of an obscure footnote in which he "... decided to apply the cuff to his own neck, he and a colleague observing the results as he strangled himself to the brink of faintness and nausea."

and pathology. Cushing favored naming it for the 19th-century French physiologist François Magendie, a particularly insensitive choice. Magendie made great contributions to the knowledge of neuroanatomy, which accounted for Cushing's interest, but he was a well-known vivisectionist, who caused great outrage in the United Kingdom with his thoughtless dissections of live animals. In a particularly revolting demonstration, he nailed an unanesthetized greyhound to a board and demonstrated the nerves of its face by dissecting it live. The direct result of this was the English laws banning cruelty to animals.

"The antivivisection group in Baltimore were very active at the time and Magendie's name was anathema to them, so at the suggestion of Dr. Welch we thought we should use John Hunter's name instead," Cushing wrote. "It was not a bad solution, for it mystified a good many people who thought the term had something to do with a pointer or a setter, and after all we did have something to do with them for we began to have a good deal of veterinary work."

Averting the public relations disaster was wise. Wiser still was the service rendered to the community. With their wide knowledge of animal diseases and their unheard-of facilities for care, Halsted and his staff treated many local pet dogs, saved many canine lives, and won over the community.

The Hunterian was the site of great experimental activity. Halsted was working on surgery of the thyroid gland, arterial aneurisms, and his eternal search for the best method for end-to-end intestinal anastomoses. Cushing had begun work on the pituitary, soon to be known as the "master gland."

Cushing began writing and speaking about diagnosing brain tumors by examining the retina. Increased pressure from tumors put pressure on the retinal nerve, resulting in an easily visualized sign called a "choked disc." His fame spread, and brain tumor patients came to Johns Hopkins for surgery by Cushing in the same way that breast cancer and hernia patients sought out Halsted. Revolutionary work and frequent publications got the word out, and in 1909 and 1910, Cushing operated on more than 100 suspected brain tumor patients. In the *Bulletin* he reported an apparent cure of 30 of the last 100 patients, with a "complete absence of the old-time post operative complications. A meningitis or fungus cerebri [infection] is almost inexcusable today."

Tumor cases were carefully followed, and Cushing, ever creative, had all patients write him on their birthday. If they didn't write, he contacted them or their families. In this manner a great deal of information was amassed on the natural history of brain tumors, which helped direct efforts in the future. He was thoroughly devoted to his patients, and they to him. Though his energy, enthusiasm, and difficult temperament were pillars of his personality, he was socially charming, and always so with his patients. He was willing to go where others had declined to venture, and his patients and their families accepted the risks and felt his concern for them.

Cushing passed on his teaching responsibilities to others. He performed increasing numbers of long, tedious operations and had begun his work on the pituitary in earnest. He had his own assistants and staff, and an average census of 40 patients in the hospital, including many private patients. A legion of medical students and assistants worked with him on the wards and in the Hunterian Laboratory, and he had risen to associate professor at the medical school.

BY THE TURN OF the century there was a general awareness of the importance of the strange, ductless glands like the thyroid and the parathyroid. Halsted was at the forefront of examining the function and malfunction of both. The adrenal glands, ovaries, testes, thymus, and pancreas are also ductless glands, a category that came to be called endocrine glands. These glands somehow delivered regulating substances to the body, not through a connection or duct, but directly into the bloodstream. Whether these glands were interconnected was unclear. What was clear was that animals without thyroid glands could not survive. Animals without parathyroid glands perished as well. The pituitary gland is a small, bilobed, pea-sized structure sitting at the bottom of the brain in a bony saddle called the sella turcica. The position of the gland made it uniquely accessible to surgery, and Cushing assigned three medical students—Lewis Redford, Samuel Crowe, and John Homans—to remove the pituitaries of a series of dogs.

After 100 procedures it became clear that the dogs would die without the gland—often slowly, but they would die. The next step was to see whether the two lobes, the anterior and posterior, had separate functions. Most of the dogs that lost most or all of the anterior lobe died. In one of the surviving dogs, Cushing noted a loss of energy, lack of growth, asexuality, and a fatty slothfulness reminiscent of the symptoms of Frohlich's syndrome, an enigmatic state linked to atrophy of the optic nerve, which happened to be in direct proximity to the pituitary. Cushing surmised that if lack of pituitary secretion, or hypopituitarism, was responsible for the condition, perhaps tumors of the pituitary could cause hyperpituitarism. The symptoms of hyperpituitarism were well known, and termed acromegaly. They included gigantism, thickened bones, large hands, protruding jaw, and vascular defects.

Cushing became consumed by questions of pituitary function, constantly mindful of the close relationship between the pituitary and the sella turcica in which it rested. Enlargement of the gland eroded or deformed the bony sella turcica and therefore was visible on X-ray. Clear cases of pituitary abnormalities began to surface, X-rays aided in the diagnosis, and Cushing began to perform surgeries. He had easy access to the pituitary under the upper lip, through the nose, and into the brain. Peering in with a miner's headlight, he easily removed cysts and tumors of the pituitary gland, although with inconsistent outcomes. Cushing rushed to publication with his hastily assembled *The Pituitary Body and Its Disorders,* but there was far more to the master gland than he understood. Still, Cushing had opened the box for brain surgery, and opened the door to the understanding of the master gland.

Cushing's single-minded pursuit of information brought him to study an acromegalic giant named John Turner. Cushing had cared for Turner, but when he died in Washington the family refused an autopsy. Undeterred, Cushing dispatched Crowe to the undertaking parlor with a bag of instruments, and at 3 A.M., unable to single-handedly remove the giant from his coffin, he operated in the burial bier, removed Turner's pituitary, and brought it back to Hopkins.

THE TWO-STORY HUNTERIAN Laboratory of Experimental Medicine was the scene of more triumphs than Cushing's alone. It was there that MacCallum discovered the relationship between the parathyroid glands and calcium metabolism, and where he proved that removal of the islets of Langerhans of the pancreas caused diabetes, setting the stage for the isolation of insulin. It was also where Walter Dandy would do the monumental work in pneumo-ventriculography that resulted in a method of visualizing the interior of the brain, and making Cushing apoplectic.

Cushing was on the national stage after treating General Wood. Things were going remarkably well for him, but he was ready to move on. Osler, his father figure, had left Baltimore five years before to assume the Regius professorship at Oxford, leaving a personal void that remained unfilled. Cushing had a young family around him, but his life was his work. He was 42, ambitious, and felt continually thwarted, and he was eager to bring glory to himself and his new specialty in his own department, rather than remaining at the whim of an eccentric professor. In 1912, he left Hopkins to become chief of surgery at the new Peter Bent Brigham Hospital, and professor of surgery at Harvard.

CHAPTER TWENTY-SIX

All Quiet on the Home Front

B Y THE CLOSE OF the 19th century, Halsted had eased into the life that he would lead for the next 22 years. Sustained by his work, enabled by a devoted, if strange, wife, isolated by a demanding addiction, and ignoring or handing off responsibilities, he showed no evidence of unhappiness with his situation. If Halsted was not oblivious to the discomfort of others caused by his behavior, he certainly gave no outward sign of acknowledgment. His enigmatic distraction was by now Hopkins legend, and those who knew him best simply shrugged their shoulders and took it in stride. In the heat of the wrestling over Cushing's fate, Osler was asked if he had any idea what Halsted was thinking. His response was, "No, nor has anyone else."

Halsted maintained an outward calm even as he ceded the de facto operation of the department to a succession of residents. Each year the census on Ward G, the primary surgical ward, increased. Patients didn't enter the hospital, have surgery, and leave. This was particularly true for the charity patients. Hospital stays were protracted affairs, often lasting months. At a time when the elaborate dressing on a hernia wound remained in place for three weeks, with the patient immobile, in bed, one can only extrapolate the lengthy hospitalizations required when recovery was complicated.

Even into the early 20th century, surgery was still being performed in people's homes. On one occasion Halsted took his traveling surgical troupe to Providence, Rhode Island, where he was "detained for 4 and 1/2 days." The patient and his family were difficult, and Halsted, having had enough of it, departed, leaving Cushing to care for the patient. Cushing was upset by the demands of wealthy patients in general, and this one in particular, and let Halsted know about it. Halsted was effusive in his apologies, adding, "Dr. Cushing please submit your bill, I will add it to mine." Included in his fee for services was an additional $200 for assistants, easily five times what was customary for two residents and two nurses, and exactly the figure Cushing had demanded.

Halsted did not maintain separate offices for private patients, nor did he openly promote his private practice. Fee-for-service patients were seen in their homes, their hotel rooms, or at the hospital. He demanded numerous assistants in the operating room, and when he traveled, he rarely did so alone. He charged handsomely for his services and for those of his staff. Typical fees were up to $75 per hour for time spent outside of Baltimore. His surgical fees slid readily up and down the scale, according to the patient's ability to pay. He was often tempted to alter the bill based on the patient's behavior but rarely did so, as the financial deal was typically struck prior to surgery. His notes on fees billed and paid offer a rare look at his world through his eyes, as well as at his cutting sense of humor.

An operation for intestinal obstruction performed in a farmhouse in Maryland was described as "Terrific operation, also highly dramatic; electric lights gave out; lamp nearly exploded, and set the house on fire; patient stopped breathing; artificial respiration; inexperienced assistants; ether gave out because etherizer had so asphyxiated the patient, he got neither air nor anesthesia; life of patient saved thus far; 5 hundred dollars by agreement, should be $5000."

Another bill, for a complicated amputation performed in stages, was for $13,825, quite a sum—the 2009 equivalent of about $250,000.

After examining a three-year-old girl with swollen glands, he noted: "A terrible kid, consult $50 at least, one hour's torture by child." Sometimes he even noted when the bill was paid: "Paid within 12 hours." Or when he was paid in the operating room: "This doesn't happen too often." "Very wealthy, outrageously small bill." "Very much of a gentleman, more like a New Englander."

Halsted's initial salary of $2,000 was raised to $3,000 when he was appointed surgeon in chief and professor, one-third of which was paid by the university. With his salary, the funds he received from his father, and the income from his private practice, Halsted was certainly well off, but never considered himself rich. His spending habits were neither outrageous nor ostentatious, but they were free and unusual, and he did make the grand gesture now and again. When Mitchell engaged and trained a stenographer for him, Halsted then hired her as his private secretary on a one-year contract. The woman soon asked Mitchell if he could help her find a new position, as Dr. Halsted no longer needed her. Mitchell easily placed her with Henry Hurd, with whom she got on famously for years. When Mitchell finally asked Halsted why he had discharged the woman, the indignant reply was, "Mitchell, she would use perfume and I told her I objected to it, that it was distasteful to me, and what did she do but change the brand: so I gave her a year's salary and let her go."

His outside income afforded a level of comfort that his salary alone could not provide. In 1900, beefsteak sold for 10 cents a pound, a roast beef dinner and all the trimmings for 25 cents. With his income, Halsted was able to subsidize salaries in his laboratory; employ a full staff of household employees, including several at High Hampton; employ several private secretaries and a liveried coachman; and travel the world with impunity. He generously aided community projects in Cashiers, and even subsidized the small Episcopal church on the grounds of High Hampton, although he did not attend.

A bespoke tailor made his conservative, dark suits and country tweeds. He favored black silk socks and highly polished, square-toed shoes, which were made for him by the half dozen pair by a Parisian bootmaker. Each pair was fashioned from a particular portion of the skins personally selected by Halsted, and upon delivery he would scrutinize them closely and discard the shoes he found beneath his standards. His gloves and hats always appeared fresh and new. English travel bags, leather goods, and brushes were perfectly cared for, and his handkerchiefs were of such fine linen that it seemed a shame to use them.

Halsted's shirts were all of the finest cotton and linen, and made to his measurements at Charvet, the famed French shirtmaker at 28 Place Vendome, in Paris. Charvet shirts were an extravagance shared with generations of famous men, including Oscar Wilde, Gustave Eiffel, and Henri Matisse. By 1920, the cost of each bespoke shirt had risen to nearly $9, driving Medill McCormick, the United States senator from Illinois, to tell the *New York Times* how outraged he was by the manner in which Americans were being taken advantage of by the French.

In Halsted's dressing room at Eutaw Place was a large wardrobe with many shelves piled neatly with stacks of perfectly laundered shirts. Claiming that he was unable to find anyone in this country who could adequately launder a dress shirt, he would have his shirts shipped back to Paris to be washed and ironed. When he traveled to Europe in the spring or summer, he would pack the soiled shirts and deliver them himself. Later in life, believing he had found "a little place in Baltimore where they laundered shirts sufficiently well," he gave up the long-distance laundry.

His suits usually included a matching waistcoat, and they draped well over his top-heavy, long-armed frame. Even with his odd walk and his arms bowed at his sides, the fine lines of his suits were obvious. The cravats Halsted favored in the earlier years were replaced with conservative modern neckties, and striped shirts and bow ties were a favored country combination, worn with either flannels or tweeds. He wore a perfectly cared-for traditional silk top hat around town until his later years, when he adopted the more modern, black derby. That, too, always appeared new and spotlessly clean.

Among the Hopkins men were any number of fashion plates, and very high on the list was William Osler. Osler was a bit flashier than Halsted in his dress, as in his demeanor. He wore brightly colored cravats, frock coats, and striped trousers and always had a rose in his lapel. The choices in his dress and the little extra touches were more lighthearted and quick-stepped than those of the somber Halsted. Finney recalled walking in the hospital corridor with Halsted, when they met Osler, who was unattended by his usual retinue. "Very soon here came Billy Thayer, hurrying to catch up with 'The Chief.' He too was faultlessly attired. Following him and not far behind came Barker, as I recall, also in frock coat and top hat. As each one hurried by, Dr. Halsted, after exchanging greetings, cast an envious glance out of the corner of his eye after him. Last of all came Sladen, in a great hurry. He was the epitome of sartorial elegance. This was a little too much. After Sladen had passed, Dr. Halsted stopped, turned around, and cast an admiring glance down the hall after the retreating medical men, remarked, 'Fine dressers, these medical men, aren't they?'"

His obsessions did not end with perfectly cut suits. The white oak and hickory logs he favored for the open fires in his rooms were equally important, and Caroline frequently scoured the suburban suppliers when the woodpile was running low. He was equally serious about his coffee, and every bean counted. Individual coffee beans were chosen to match in color and size, brewed black and thick, in the Turkish fashion, and said to have a lasting effect. Halsted's coffee was blamed for the sleepless nights of those who had been honored with dinner invitations, and he did not trust others to prepare it.

Halsted was also an inveterate letter writer, sometimes exchanging letters with his sister Bertie in French. It was believed he had help with this affectation, as he was not fluent in the language. But he was fluent in German, and corresponded regularly with a host of German surgeons. He wrote often to Caroline, and she to him, when she was away at High Hampton, or he on his medical travels and journeys to parts unknown. Her letters, brimming with facts of day-to-day living, also offer a window into her frustration with his character. One wonders if the veil of formality was dropped in his letters, but sadly, all that remains is a one-way correspondence. Immediately upon Caroline's death, her sister Lucy Hampton Haskell destroyed all of Halsted's letters to his wife, without reading them, she claimed, believing they were private and should not survive the recipient.

Through the late 19th century Halsted wrote with duck quill pen and ink. Lewis Waterman perfected and patented the design for the fountain pen in 1884, and when Halsted fell in love with the writing gadget, he fell hard. For years he bought large quantities of fountain pens, far more than he would ever have any use for, and stored them in his desk.

His care and preoccupation with material objects and style should not be confused with venality, for Halsted was anything but venal. It was more about an obsession with excellence. He rarely mentioned money and never mentioned the cost of his extravagances. Of course, one can be happily oblivious to finances when money is simply there.

So it was for a good part of his life: not quite wealthy, but never wanting, and never caring. If there was enough to do whatever one wished in the manner one wished to do it, what was the problem? Halsted was not only unconcerned with finances, he was believed by those close to him to be shockingly inept in business matters. The lack of interest might well have been a simple matter of choice in the absence of necessity. Edwin Baetjer, Halsted's lawyer, commented, "The gulf which separated his higher intellectual capacities from the ability to understand or deal with the business or ordinary affairs of life, was unfathomable."

In a 1914 letter to the wife of surgeon Herbert Evans, Caroline Halsted wrote:

When I was married, Dr. Halsted had $3,000 a year and some debts. After he began to practice it seemed that money came so easily that I could not understand why he should do almost everything but positively decline cases so as to devote more time to the hospital. He became more devoted to his work and finally took up spending a good part of his salary on the hospital. The trustees did not enough for the salaries of certain employees considered necessary and to keep them Dr. H added enough to induce them to stay. One year I know his whole salary went back to the hospital. The young men grew up, got married and soon had motors [automobiles]. I candidly say that I did at times feel sour when I was waiting on a corner for a car to see the young people passing in their autos. We decided that we did not care for a family which of course saved considerable. We entertain very little for Dr. Halsted likes to have his evenings undisturbed for work.

I am gradually making the place [High Hampton] more self supporting. As I am there six months or more every year and my needs are small. I buy coffee and flour and pay for my cooking and washing and house work the enormous sum of $3.75 a week. My clothes are home made and cost little. So in the end I am glad the decision was for science and not money.

By this time private practice had been abolished among the chiefs of service at Hopkins. They were meant to be working full time for a fixed salary. For Halsted, it represented far less of a change in his routine than it did for others, as he was not operating frequently, saw few private patients, and was spending most of his time on his research and writing.

Caroline also referred to her loneliness as "one who paddled their own canoe . . . For I go off alone, stay on the farm and travel home alone. I might go on to say that I live alone on the third floor. All the rest of the house is given up to stenographers and books."

There appeared to be no substantive changes in the nature of the relationship between the Halsteds as the years passed. The decision not to have children was made early in the marriage. After frequently hosting young nieces and nephews at High Hampton, they congratulated each other on having made a proper choice. The unconventional match seemed to thrive under living conditions characterized by separation and isolation.

The arrangement apparently suited them. Both husband and wife had entered into the contract with unusual expectations. Halsted surprised himself with his interest in Caroline. For her part, she made plain the appreciable changes that marriage would make in her life circumstances. If Caroline appeared mannish and unattractive in dark clothes and work shoes, it was a package that did not seem to disturb her new husband. Of his feelings, little can be said other than that he took delight in her southern manner and ancestry, breeding having been a favorite theme over the years. Caroline worked happily at providing an undemanding environment in which her husband could follow his intellectual star, and only after some years of marriage were there signs of discontent or feelings of neglect. Still, Caroline Halsted voluntarily spent six months of each year away from her husband.

Whether it was a marriage with infrequent sex, or any sex at all, is a matter for conjecture. Halsted's sexuality is a muddy pond. There are no stories of adolescent infatuation; there is no known previous involvement with women, and no evidence of the desire for any sort of relationship until nearly age 40. Nor is there any evidence of homosexual relationships. His Yale friend and roommate, the Reverend Bushnell, commented, "While he liked girls he did not go in for social things." Cushing believed both Halsted and Welch to be homosexual, and hinted at a relationship between them, but there is no evidence beyond innuendo. Sexual inversion, the operative term for homosexuality at the time, would not have been tolerated at Johns Hopkins during the Halsted era. And just as his drug addiction, at the time a far less damning trait, was hidden, one would not expect Halsted to openly admit homosexuality, or perhaps even admit his unrealized desires to himself. His close relationship with Mall, and the letter in which he predicted Mall's surprise that he was engaged to marry a woman, can be read as misanthropic humor, which is likely given the waspish jibing that passed between them.

CHAPTER TWENTY-SEVEN

After Cushing

A S A RULE, HALSTED made infrequent appearances on the ward; hence, the level of organization of the service varied with the energy and ability of the resident surgeon. All the residents were competent; some were great, but that greatness was measured in different ways. To be chosen as resident was a singular honor, and the competition for the post was intense. Halsted often passed over senior men to appoint a particularly talented junior, as he had with Cushing.

Halsted picked interns from among the students he knew, and since he spent a great deal of his time in the laboratory, that was a good place to catch The Professor's eye. The favored students were those who asked insightful questions at the bedside or in the formal clinic.

Whenever possible, his choices for resident were made from among those who had shown an aptitude for the laboratory. Surgical stars did not shine as brightly in the eyes of The Professor as did inquiring minds, and he was not at all reticent about deciding what career path a man was suited to follow. Some trainees were made to detour from general surgery while waiting to become resident, and establish themselves in the evolving world of surgical specialties. Others had decided on their future only to have The Professor abruptly change their plan. This was sometimes done by fiat and at other times accomplished by gentle suggestion, which implied a fall from grace if disregarded.

Some, like William F. Rienhoff, Halsted's last resident, had an easier time predicting their future. Halsted had learned from Mac-Callum that Rienhoff, as a medical student, was interested in working in the experimental surgery laboratory. Rienhoff recalled:

> He had every intention of keeping me on later if I worked hard and carefully and of having me follow into the residency. It interested me very much that he had planned things so very far ahead. I was convinced that if I attended to my business, my chances of being trained into the residency were good. He relieved my mind of any apprehension about getting on and put me in a position where I could spend all my time in working and need not worry about the next year. I know that he had similar conversations with two others of his residents. It is true, of course, that the men he did not care to keep on, had no interview with him on the subject as he would not permit it. He made up his mind in these three instances at the very beginning of our hospital careers and from then on, these men were given advantages in assisting and time to work in the laboratory that other men did not receive.

Choices were made by a committee of one, and although instances abound of men assuming new positions without his knowledge, Halsted's tacit approval of the individual had already been demonstrated. Distracted and unorthodox as Halsted was, his choices for resident were unfailingly excellent.

The operating room diminished as the primary focus of his interest as he moved on to another phase of his career, and Halsted summed up the state of affairs in his own words: "Surgery would be delightful if you did not have to operate."

* * *

NOW, 20 YEARS AFTER founding the department of surgery at The Johns Hopkins Hospital, Halsted changed yet again. He had become intensely interested in the thyroid gland and was experimenting with vascular surgery, while performing clinical surgery only once or twice a week. The combination of his reduced surgical burden and the departure of Harvey Cushing for Boston drove him to reenter the world of teaching. He resumed leading the course in experimental surgery, and he was present more regularly at the Friday teaching clinic. His interaction with the residents increased as his dependence on a single man abated, but mostly, his mind was on his research.

The resident following Cushing was James Farnandis Mitchell. Mitchell was a superb general surgeon, but he was not Cushing. There was a gap to fill, and with Cushing gone, it was the time for others to shine.

* * *

HUGH HAMPTON YOUNG was the Virginia-born son of a Confederate general. His grandmother was a cousin of Wade Hampton II, Caroline Hampton Halsted's grandfather. Young was an unusually bright student, and in a single four-year period at the University of Virginia he earned bachelor's, master's, and medical degrees. After medical school, Young moved to Baltimore and found work under Osler as a graduate student in the dispensary. Somewhere along the way he developed an overriding interest in bacteriology, and always carried around a pocket full of culture tubes. It was not unusual to see Hugh Young poking around the hospital and culturing everything in sight. On one occasion he cultured a patient's lower lid abscess and identified the first case of anthrax seen at the hospital.

In 1895, he decided to seek training in surgery and wrote Halsted to apply for internship. When he next met Halsted, Young introduced himself.

"I wrote you applying for a position on the surgical staff."

Halsted nodded stiffly. "Oh, yes, Young, I got your letter, but there isn't any place for you." Halsted had nothing more to say.

Disappointed, Young found summer work in bacteriology. In September, a surgery intern at Hopkins telephoned to ask him to be his substitute during his vacation. The intern returned from vacation, but in October two intern places opened. Young and two others, a total of three, hoped to secure the two spots. All three continued to work under Finney's supervision. When Halsted returned from his summer holiday he said nothing about filling the positions. Young decided to simply stay on until they kicked him out, and the others followed suit. After a few weeks one of the three became ill with typhoid fever and withdrew to convalesce, and the problem solved itself. Halsted was unaware of the issue and expressed no surprise whatsoever at seeing Young on his staff, accepting him as though the hiring had been his idea.

The next year Young worked on Ward E, where the urology patients were assigned. One of the patients he was caring for was incapacitated by the need to urinate every 15 minutes, and no one knew how to deal with his problem. Young's examination revealed the man's bladder had shrunk to the capacity of a tablespoon. It seemed reasonable to believe that he could dilate the bladder by forcing fluid into it. Young rigged a 15-foot-high pole with a fountain syringe on top. He fixed the tube against the tip of the man's penis and forced fluid up the urethra and into the bladder—first a tablespoonful, then as the bladder dilated, an ounce, and then two. Gradually, the man's bladder capacity increased to normal, and the frequent urge to urinate disappeared.

The procedure was used thereafter whenever a similar problem presented itself, but always with the overriding fear that fluids forced into the bladder might back up into the ureters and the kidneys, risking serious infection. Young studied the question by pumping tinted fluid through the urethra into the bladder of fresh cadaver. When the bladder was blown up like a balloon with a full quart of tinted liquid, Welch and the other observers backed off, expecting the dam to burst. But it didn't. Young cut into the ureters and found no backflow of the colored fluid. The fluid remained sequestered in the bladder. The experiments were presented to much acclaim at the Johns Hopkins Medical Society. Halsted said nothing, and Young continued on as an assistant resident.

The following October, Young turned a corner in a hospital corridor and ran head on into Halsted, nearly bowling him over. Catching The Professor before he hit the floor, Young began to apologize profusely.

"Don't apologize, Young, I was looking for you to tell you we want you to take charge of the Department of Genito-Urinary Surgery."

Young demurred, but didn't have the courage to outright refuse. He had finished his time on the G-U ward and was looking forward to general surgery, and besides, he didn't know anything about the subject.

"Welch and I said you didn't know anything about it, but we believe you can learn."

Young yielded to The Professor's pressure, and he did manage to learn quite well.

One of the new methods for studying the internal "plumbing" of the genitourinary system was the cystoscope. The device was basically a thin tube inserted into the urethra through the penis, which had been numbed with cocaine. The surgeon would look around the bladder through the long, thin metal device with illumination provided by a tiny lightbulb. This illumination was an advance over the pre-Edison models, which were lit by a glowing platinum loop, which would burn the bladder if not properly cooled with ice water. Young further improved the instrument by adding a prism at the tip, which afforded more panoramic visualization.

Then, as now, prostate cancer was the plague of men of late middle-age. Young recognized its nature as a slow-growing tumor and saw the value of catching it early. Just as he had previously run around culturing everything, he now began doing rectal examinations on all his male patients, ushering in the era of early diagnosis of prostate cancer and greatly increasing the chance of cure with surgery. He improved on the bloody suprapubic prostatectomy and introduced a new method called the perineal prostatectomy, performed through an incision beneath the scrotum and above the anus. He popularized the new operation and gained fame for performing 125 perineal prostatectomies without a fatality. This arcane record led a New York urologist to quip, "The prostate makes most men old, but it made Hugh Young."

In addition to being a world-class tinkerer, Young was a very good surgeon. He was bold and confident, and a fine leader and teacher, but when Halsted hovered behind him in the operating room, it all disappeared. He was known to break out in a sweat and fumble in Halsted's presence, and afterward throw his sweat-soaked scrubs on the dressing room floor, kick them across the room, and curse himself, asking, "Why can't I get over this feeling of inferiority when The Professor is around?"

Few men other than Finney, Cushing, and Richard Follis appeared fully comfortable in his presence, and even then, their apparent comfort might not have been what it seemed. Halsted was well aware of the unsettling effect he had. He rarely did more than quietly ask the surgeons what they were up to. He never commented, never corrected, and rarely brought the subject up later. Only the most grievous error brought unsolicited comment, and the worst punishment of all, banishment from the operating room. For the senior staff, nothing was missed by Halsted, and they knew it. But occasionally, a nod or a sly smile gave him away. If he enjoyed the discomfort he caused, and he probably did, Halsted was nothing but helpful and supportive when the operator was truly in trouble. Even with staff members whose technique disappointed him, The Professor castigated himself for not becoming aware of their shortcomings earlier, but did not confront them or try to change what had already become ingrained.

TAKING THE LEAD from Halsted, who believed that many of the answers to surgical mysteries were found in the study of laboratory specimens, Young performed microscopic examinations on all prostate samples he removed. As the first surgeon to do so, he greatly expanded the understanding of the disease. In older men, benign enlargement of the prostate is responsible for difficulties in passing urine. The usual cause is enlargement of the central bar of the prostate, which compresses the urethra, blocking urine flow. Young modified a cystoscope through which was passed another instrument with a biting tip. Several bites with its jaws removed enough of the obstruction to allow normal urination. This relatively minor procedure replaced an extensive, invasive, and very bloody one, in which an incision was made over the pubic bone and into the bladder, and a section of the prostate excised.

This simple advance quickly changed the lives of many thousands of men. Among the earliest patients to benefit from the new procedure was James Buchanan Brady. The legendary "Diamond Jim" underwent the operation and had a rough postoperative course, but he could urinate. Brady became a great patron of Young's and endowed the first urological institute in the country, which bears his name at The Johns Hopkins Hospital.

Under normal circumstances, urine is a sterile fluid. The complex urinary tract begins with the kidneys, where urine is manufactured. The ureters carry the urine from the kidneys to the bladder, and from the bladder it reaches the exterior via the urethra. The entire system should be sterile, but it is subject to retrograde infection from the outside. Once seeded, these infections are difficult to eradicate. Fifty years before the antibiotic era, Young was searching for an antiseptic solution to maintain sterility and treat infections of the bladder and urethra. In 1919, after years of experimenting with numerous chemicals in the labs at the Brady Urological Institute, Young and his staff settled upon a relatively nontoxic compound of mercury, which they named Mercurochrome. The new, red-brown antiseptic became instantly popular and was soon used universally to treat scrapes and cuts. Children knew it as "monkey blood" because of its color, and for decades no household was without it. Young was convinced of its miraculous powers and used it in virtually all his procedures, believing it could cure everything from septicemia to bladder and kidney infections.

As a victim of chronic bronchitis, Young coerced his colleague Sam Crowe into injecting Mercurochrome between his vocal cords and into his trachea and bronchi. Crowe performed the procedure quickly and expertly, and remembers, "An immediate series of explosive coughs sprayed me, the ceiling, and the surrounding walls with the bright red drug."

But the mess wasn't the worst of it. Apparently, enough Mercurochrome was absorbed for Young to develop signs of kidney failure, which only slowly resolved. This extremely dangerous episode didn't stop his experimentation with the drug, and some time later he managed to have his resident administer an intravenous injection of Mercurochrome to prevent an abscessed tooth from requiring extraction. There is no record of how this ill-conceived adventure turned out.

Mercurochrome is still a popular antiseptic everywhere but in the United States. Because of the alleged potential for mercury toxicity, and its unproven effectiveness, the FDA has banned interstate commerce in Mercurochrome, and the substance has disappeared.

Young's residents went on to found urology departments at universities around the country, among them Harvard, Yale, Cornell, and the University of Pennsylvania. Advances came quickly, and based on his experience with the Journal Club at Hopkins, Young recognized the need for the exchange of information. He founded the *Journal of Urology,* a project he personally funded for years. A man of wide-ranging mechanical inspirations, his creations varied from Mercurochrome to a mechanical soap dispenser to seaplane landing gear.

Hugh Hampton Young never achieved his goal of resident in surgery. Instead he became the father of urology.

* * *

JUST AS HALSTED identified the moment and the man for urology, he seized upon Frederick Henry Baetjer to be the first official acti-nographer[1] at The Johns Hopkins Hospital. After an internship in medicine under Osler, Baetjer was appointed assistant resident in surgery. He had worked on the hand-cranked X-ray machine with Cushing since medical school, and when Cushing finished his residency the work seemed to fall to Baetjer. He signed on to the job full time in 1902 for the lofty salary of $900 a year, for which he developed the specialty of radiology, lost most of his fingers and an eye, and developed lymphatic cancer.

Baetjer was a rotund and happy individual with enormous scientific curiosity. Carefully following his findings on the roentgenograms into the operating room, he was able to dramatically demonstrate the diagnostic possibilities of the new technique. Just as Cushing had done at the beginning, Baetjer focused the X-ray beam on his hands and often held the patient in place while exposing the plate. At the time, the long-term effects of radiation were unknown. As late as the 1940s, fluoroscope machines in shoe stores produced a moving X-ray image to demonstrate the fit of the bones of the feet in the new shoes. The miraculous toy delighted children until the dangers of radiation became known. Baetjer learned the lesson earlier.

The field was still in its infancy. There were no protective lead aprons and gloves, and the radiologist was not separated from his subject by an impermeable shield. X-ray tissue damage is cumulative and takes years to express itself. Among the first signs of trouble are thinning of the skin as a fibrosis of the blood vessels sets in. Once set

---

1 Actinography was the term used for the measurement of X-ray exposure. An actinographer is one who creates the images of X-radiation, and is known as a radiologist today.

in motion the process cannot be reversed, and yesterday's exposure continues to manifest itself today.

On June 3, 1908, the *New York Times* said:

> Dr. Frederick Baetjer, widely known as an authority on roentgen rays, today underwent a surgical operation for the removal of his right eye. His friends thought that the trouble might have been aggravated by his continuous experiments with the rays, but the oculists say it was the result of an accident during his college days.
>
> Some time ago Dr. Baetjer was attacked with a particular partial shriveling of the arm and hand from which he recovered. It was attributed to the effect of the X-rays.
>
> Dr. Baetjer is a member of the Johns Hopkins Hospital staff.

The *Times* story was probably incorrect, and later accounts believe the cause of the lost eye was radiation. Baetjer underwent more than 100 operations and ultimately lost part, or all, of eight fingers, but his spirit was never broken. The lifelong bachelor was much loved and a great favorite of everyone at Hopkins. His relationship with Halsted was always good, and The Professor both appreciated him and enjoyed making jokes at his expense. Typically, when Baetjer was demonstrating a finding, he held up an X-ray film and started his talk with, "This is an image of the skull."

To which Halsted responded, "Really, Baetjer, I had that thought myself."

After learning the price of exposure, Baetjer abandoned the mechanical side of radiology and concentrated on reading films and clinical correlation.

CHAPTER TWENTY-EIGHT

New Horizons

THE THYROID GLAND SITS like a butterfly on the neck, just below the larynx. The two lobes straddle the trachea and are joined together by an isthmus called the body. The gland is fairly superficial, readily visible when enlarged, and covered by layers of flat, vertically oriented muscles. With a normal weight of barely 30 grams, the thyroid is a powerful regulator of human activity.

Through the last quarter of the 19th century very little was known of the gland's function. It was a surgically accessible, ductless endocrine gland and was associated with Graves' disease, a dangerous condition characterized by a goiter (enlarged thyroid), bulging eyes, weakness, swelling of the shins, and rapid pulse. Removing the gland reversed the symptoms of the disease but rarely saved the patient, so the surgery was infrequently performed.

Prior to coming to Baltimore, Halsted had assisted his mentor, Henry Sands, on a single thyroidectomy at Roosevelt Hospital in New York. The gland, particularly when swollen, is invested with a very rich blood supply, and in the hurried surgery of the day, hemorrhage was a constant problem, so the patient was seated in a chair with a rubber bag tied around his neck to catch the blood flow. The surgery was ugly and dangerous, but Graves' disease, or Basedow's disease, as it is called in Europe, was not uncommon and could be deadly.

Other forms of goiter were not associated with the symptoms of Graves' disease but could cause asphyxiation by the pressure of the expanding neck mass on the trachea. Surgical intervention came as a result of attempts to cure Graves' disease. Simple goiter, it turned out, was related to iodine deficiency and was cured by dietary supplements.

Halsted had been exposed to research on the thyroid in Europe. Although he had little or no experience with thyroid surgery, he was curious about a number of its elements. If the thyroid gland was necessary for life, how much had to be removed to cure the disease, and how much must be left for the patient to survive? How did it function, what did the thyroid produce, and why did patients with the entire gland removed suffer both the weakness and fatigue of hypothyroidism, along with spasms, twitching, and seizures?

Years earlier, in 1887, with the questions clear in his mind, Halsted had gone looking for answers. He started at his laboratory at the Pathological and worked his way to the operating room. Setting up his research model in anesthetized dogs, Halsted began the arduous process of removing sequentially larger portions of the gland, ultimately sacrificing the animals and studying the remaining gland. The results of these first experiments were baffling. The remaining portion of the thyroid gland rapidly increased in size. When the new growth was studied under the microscope it had no similarity to the cellular appearance of the thyroid gland. The cells had become taller and fuller. And colloid, believed to be the thyroid secretion, first accumulated along with the growth of the cells, then abated.

The microscopic changes looked exactly like Graves' disease, and yet the dogs had no symptoms. Confusing.

The confusion continued for the next 20 years. Meanwhile, Halsted developed a surgical technique for dealing with the formidable enlarged gland of Graves' disease. He treated the tissue gently, tied off the small arteries and engorged veins with fine silk, and divided them without blood loss. The large superior and inferior thyroid arteries were then identified and dealt with, maintaining the bloodless field.

In most cases, removing all of one lobe and most of the other cured the symptoms of Graves' disease. The remaining gland enlarged enough to sustain life without causing hypothyroidism—sluggishness, weight gain, thinning hair, and mental degradation known as myxedema. Still, the balance between how much needed to be removed and how much had to be left remained unclear. And there was more. Often when the superior and inferior thyroid arteries were tied off, both patients and experimental animals developed severe twitching and seizures called tetany, which often resulted in death. Halsted recognized that these were the symptoms of compromised calcium metabolism brought about by removal of the parathyroid glands, four tiny structures associated with the thyroid. But even when he tried to spare the parathyroids, the symptoms often arose.

Since the patient faced death without treatment, Halsted tried everything. Fresh bovine parathyroid was recovered from slaughterhouses and fed to patients. It temporarily relieved the symptoms, but the patients found the volume and presentation of the organs quite disgusting. Halsted tried parathyroid transplants with questionable results. Later an injectable parathyroid extract became available, which seemed effective, and finally the use of calcium salts managed to prevent tetany. The patients improved, but the underlying issue persisted. How does one cure hyperthyroidism and not cause tetany?

In 1907, Halsted asked MacCallum to study the parathyroid glands at autopsy. After 67 consecutive dissections, MacCallum reported the two pairs of tiny glands were most often found in the posterior lateral surface of each thyroid lobe. Significantly, the lower parathyroid gland was always closely associated with the inferior thyroid artery. It was not quite the revelation Halsted had hoped for, so he had a medical student, Herbert M. Evans, study the specific blood supply to each parathyroid. The goal was to find the place where the large arteries to the thyroid could be divided while still sparing the blood supply to the parathyroids. Evans found that each parathyroid had a small, dedicated artery emanating from the inferior and superior thyroid arteries respectively. That was what Halsted needed to know. Now he could formulate a plan.

The safest strategy would be transecting the large arteries after the dedicated tributaries had been given off. This required delicate dissection within the substance of the thyroid gland itself, a very trying technique, but one for which Halsted was perfectly prepared. Dealing with the distended web of veins and fine arteries was tedious work. Innumerable fine, pointed Halsted clamps were applied, the veins were tied and transected, the arteries to the parathyroids identified and preserved within a surrounding nubbin of thyroid tissue, and then the larger arteries were taken. Special care had to be taken to protect the recurrent laryngeal nerve, which was dangerously close to the inferior thyroid artery. Surgeons had learned by bitter experience that injury to the nerve could paralyze the vocal cords and desperately affect breathing and voice.

Six hundred and fifty cases later, Halsted reported on the overwhelming success of his technique. He taught other surgeons how to approach the gland surgically, but he could not fully unravel its mysteries. In 1920, he published *The Operative Story of Goitre,* which, from the surgeon's point of view, was all there was to know about the subject. But the essence of thyroid physiology remained elusive. The veil of frustration would not be lifted until the nature of the feedback mechanism between the hypothalamus in the brain, which produced hormones to stimulate the pituitary, and the pituitary, which produced thyroid-stimulating hormone, was fully understood. And this would not come to pass within Halsted's lifetime. Meanwhile, The Professor had other things on his mind.

※ ※ ※

LEVIN WATERS WAS a fair-skinned Negro laborer. At age 52, he was strongly built and had white, closely cropped hair and a full beard. Waters had been in robust good health prior to his April 1892 admission to The Johns Hopkins Hospital. At first, he had noticed a small, nut-sized mass under his left clavicle. The mass grew rapidly, and soon he could "feel it beat like his heart." There was also a slight numbness in his left arm and hand. On examining Waters, Halsted noted an enormous tumor that now enveloped the clavicle and reached to the left shoulder. It was a pulsating arterial aneurysm, measuring some 42 centimeters in circumference.

The aneurism was located in the left subclavian artery, which is the first branch off the aorta. The left subclavian gives branches to supply blood to the head and neck, before continuing on as the main artery of the arm, where it is called the axillary artery. An aneurysm is a weakening and bulging of an arterial wall. The danger it presents is that the constant pounding of pulse pressure will rupture the thin arterial balloon, risking death by hemorrhage. This was the situation in which Halsted found Waters.

Twice previously in recorded surgical history attempts had been made at excising an aneurysm in this location. Both resulted in death for the patient. With some trepidation, Halsted made a long incision from the sternal notch over the aneurism,[1] and down the arm. Skin flaps were laid open and the aneurysm was carefully isolated. Heavy silk ties were placed on the vessel before and after the dilation. The aneurysm was excised and the wound closed. Where skin had been excised as well, a dressing of natural latex, gutta-percha, was applied.

---

1 The sternal notch, or jugular notch, is in the midline at the top of the sternum (breast bone) bordered by the heads of the right and left clavicles.

Shortly after surgery Waters felt a slight tingling in his fingers, and then full sensation returned. The wound healed without incident, and Waters left the hospital and returned to work.

The first successful excision of an aneurysm of a major vessel had proven two things: that good surgical technique is increasingly the key to success as more intricate surgeries are attempted; and of specific importance to vascular surgery, that smaller communicating vessels in the area, called collateral vessels, can fill the gap, bypass the interruption in flow, and supply the dependent tissues.

The audience at the meeting of the Johns Hopkins Medical Society was spellbound as Halsted presented the dramatic and groundbreaking case, especially when Waters appeared. He was barely a month postsurgery, completely cured, and rehabilitated. Halsted went on to describe the surgical tour de force. But then, in his usual modest fashion, he left the room before Welch could begin the discussion. Welch praised the surgeon in the highest terms and spoke volubly of his immense value to The Johns Hopkins Hospital. The audience concurred, and the field of vascular surgery was off and running.

Halsted had described the operation as "a tedious one" since it took more than three hours to perform. Any surgeon reading this statement realizes that it belies the conventional wisdom that Halsted was a slow, plodding surgeon. In the world of modern surgery, a complicated vascular procedure can easily take the most adept surgeons more than an unremarkable three hours. But following so closely behind the era of five-minute amputations, it must have seemed a lifetime. Halsted routinely spent more than an hour and a half repairing an inguinal hernia. Other surgeons did their hernia procedures significantly faster, often in 15 minutes. But Halsted's operation succeeded, while all the others failed. In all but the most extreme examples, surgical time is a relative measure.

Once the commitment was made to absolute asepsis and gentle tissue handling, to tying off every blood vessel with silk so fine it would snap if knotted tightly enough to crush tissue, and to close a wound carefully, layer by layer in anatomically correct position, then surgery took more time to perform. Not too much time, simply more time than was taken in the sloppy, careless, and usually disastrous techniques of old.

Halsted had not been miraculously transformed to a new identity after having been among the best of the slash-and-dash surgeons. He had evolved into a surgeon who understood that aseptic technique, absolute knowledge of the anatomy, and gentle respect for that anatomy would change the world of surgery forever.

Categorizing William S. Halsted as an operating surgeon remains difficult. Few are qualified to pass judgment, and those schooled enough to do so must, by definition, be surgeons themselves. Unless one attempts to perform the feat oneself, the ability to separate flash from excellence becomes confusingly subjective. Looking back on their long professional association, Joseph Bloodgood wrote, "During the operation Halsted was a surgeon, a pathologist, and a thinker. He always had in mind improvements in the operative procedure and carefully studied every bit of tissue exposed by the knife."

In the end, judgment lies in how well the patient is served. Using this yardstick, Halsted was indeed among the greatest surgeons of his day. Impressions of his surgical ability were blurred by the intensity of purpose with which he performed and the new vocabulary of surgery that he devised. Although not as naturally gifted as Kelly, he was an unquestionably facile and adept operator. And, as was so often said, he was a surgeon of the head, not the hand, meaning a thoughtful surgeon rather than a dazzling technician. Being a surgeon of the hand was what he least aspired to, finding routine performance boring and thoroughly unsatisfying. Over the years Halsted established a pattern of mastering a surgical problem, then moving on. He was fascinated by the many technical issues of intestinal surgery but performed few such operations, and only five operations on the stomach, over his entire career at Hopkins. Many of the emotional moments of his professional life were associated with gallbladder surgery, but his interest in performing the procedure dwindled to devising gadgets to deal with sticky problems associated with exploring the common bile duct.

His work in that specific arena revolved around the difficulty of controlling bile loss after opening the common duct for removal of gallstones. Stones often occlude the common duct and impede passage of bile from the gallbladder, where it is stored and concentrated, into the intestine, where it is necessary for digestion. This results in the backup of bile in the gallbladder and biliary tree, painful colic caused by contraction of the duct against the stone, and often inflammation and infection. Hence the common bile duct has to be opened to extricate the stone.

Immediately after opening the common duct, bile does not yet flow freely to the intestine even though the obstruction has been relieved, so some artificial mechanism is necessary to drain the excess to the outside. Bile is rich in digestive enzymes and electrolytes, and its chronic loss is quite debilitating. Leakage of bile into the abdominal cavity is irritating and inflammatory, and long-term external drainage through the skin depletes essential elements. Halsted designed a device that looked like a small rubber hammer, which, when inserted into the common duct, facilitated almost complete closure of the duct around it and easy removal. Bile spilling from the remaining rent in the duct was conducted to the exterior by a series of drains brought out through the skin, and the near complete closure was an improvement. Although he rarely performed gallbladder surgery, it was never far from his mind, and he would continue to work on devices to assist and improve its performance.

In the operating room Halsted was famous for his unshakeable cool and detachment. At moments of surgical crisis he was known to reprimand his assistants and order them to "act like surgeons."

Even the direst of surgical reversals did not change his tone or wet his brow. With his hands wrist deep in fresh blood pumping from a ruptured aorta, he murmured quite evenly to his resident, "Heuer, I fear we are in trouble." With that, he gained control of the situation, apologized to the room full of German observers for his difficulties, tied off the aorta, and completed the operation. The patient died 48 hours later. Halsted could have done no more, and he remained unshaken and unapologetic.

Halsted believed that crystal-clear thinking and a decisive and unemotional approach were the duty of the surgeon. He could calmly operate on both his mother and his sister as they lay before him in extremis, he maintained his composure when the ether anesthetic caught fire as he was cauterizing Sam Crowe's throat, and he showed no emotion when another ether explosion killed an anesthetized dog.

Physically, Halsted's hands were wide. He had thick, graceless fingers and thumbs foreshortened enough to appear deformed—certainly not the picture one conjures up of the hands of a master surgeon or a pianist spanning octaves. Despite his short stature, odd posture, and physically ungainly hands, Halsted's surgical ability was confirmed with every difficult dissection he performed. He rarely entered uncharted territory, studying and practicing until the anatomy was indelible in his memory. He never operated without a plan, demanded numerous experienced, attentive assistants who knew their jobs, spoke little, and focused. Nothing else existed but the work at hand.

He was detached, austere, and direct. In the operating room at least, he lived by the rules, and demanded no less of others.

Willis Gatch, a former resident, echoed the sentiments of many when he said, "Dr. Halsted had a long line of devoted assistants because of his austerity and not in spite of it."

CHAPTER TWENTY-NINE

Addiction

HALSTED WAS A SURGICAL phenomenon during his New York period, when his technique, daring, and imagination set him apart from others. Cocaine crippled him, and that heroic stage of his career ended abruptly. Intimations that the subsequent morphine use altered his surgical personality seem far-fetched, but nothing about his behavior remained as it had been. Certainly the drug inhibited his ability to live anything close to a transparent existence and was responsible for changes intrinsic to his persona. His social reticence and his lifestyle in general can be attributed in large measure to serving his addiction, while chronic absenteeism and some level of disorganization and detachment resulted from it.

In a number of instances cited previously, Halsted claimed illness and was unable to operate. But if drug-related disability drove him from the operating room, there is no evidence of his being at all impaired at surgery. With the sole exception of Cushing, none of the assistants or residents so closely associated with him over the years expressed an inkling of the influence of drugs on The Professor's life.

Willis Gatch, wrote, "I have been often asked whether I think Dr. Halsted conquered his cocaine habit. I never saw him do anything that would make me think otherwise. I knew nothing of this habit until I read MacCallum's *Life,* nor had anyone I knew at Hopkins ever heard of it."

Clearly, they knew nothing of the continuing morphine use, which had largely supplanted cocaine. The facts came as a shock when Osler's *The Inner History of the Johns Hopkins Hospital* revealed the secret in 1969.

Alfred Blalock, the next great professor of surgery at Hopkins, graduated from the medical school in 1922. It had been his intention to follow his hero, William Stewart Halsted, into surgery, and train under him at the hospital. In letters exchanged during his senior year he requested an internship on the surgical service. He was denied by Halsted, who died that same year. Wishing to stay at Hopkins, Blalock did an internship under Young, in urology. Then he contracted tuberculosis and left Baltimore to recover in the sanatorium at Saranac, New York. With his health regained, he returned as assistant resident in surgery but was not appointed resident. Disappointed, he left Hopkins and was briefly at the Peter Bent Brigham Hospital, in Boston. Once saying he wasn't there long enough to unpack, he left Boston precipitously to become the first chief resident at Vanderbilt, in Nashville. Blalock stayed at Vanderbilt and distinguished himself with his work on shock, pioneering the use of blood volume expanders to prevent circulatory collapse. He returned to Hopkins in 1941, as professor and chief of surgery. Three years later he performed the lifesaving "blue baby" operation, which effectively began the era of cardiac surgery.

Blalock held Halsted in great esteem. He knew Halsted as his teacher, followed him as chief, and was a student of his life and accomplishments. In a letter to the surgeon Allen O. Whipple, Blalock wrote, "I think it is all to Dr. Halsted's credit that he was able to overcome this habit, and I think it is probably very fortunate for American surgery that he acquired it."

This thought, echoed by Halsted scholars, can be very confusing. It is generally agreed that the cocaine episode in 1885 effectively ended Halsted's period as a hardworking, successful New York surgeon. But it was the prelude to his scientific awakening in the laboratories at Johns Hopkins, and the school of safe surgery, which then developed. It is incorrect to interpret this as validation of Halsted's lifelong morphine use as a source of inspiration, moderation, and personality change. It is not clear what details of the drug saga were available to Blalock, beyond the New York cocaine history, as Osler's notes became public years after Blalock's death. Welch's 1930 revelation of Halsted's continued episodic use of cocaine may or may not have been available to him.

Halsted was uncompromised in the operating room, analytical and productive in the laboratory, and able to spend long hours at intellectual pursuits. And yet he was undoubtedly addicted to morphine throughout his career at Johns Hopkins. A minority of Halsted scholars believe he may have abandoned morphine in his final years, but there is no hard evidence for that position. We must consider that he lived with a 35-year morphine habit and that he was never fully free of cocaine, in which he indulged only far from home and far from acquaintances with whom he would have to interact. After absenting himself and indulging his addiction for weeks at a time, he very likely tapered off by substituting morphine for cocaine, as he had learned at Butler. Then he returned home and routinely purged himself by confessing to Welch. Welch was initially unaware of what had been going on, and in fact had not even been suspicious. But since Halsted believed he knew the nature of his solitary holidays, Welch listened and did not betray his ignorance. The pattern was established: Halsted isolated and far from home, indulging his habit, confessing to Welch, and then dosing himself with morphine and resuming life as usual in Baltimore.

Halsted's summer travel puzzled everyone else. He did pay brief visits to surgeon friends, usually in Germany and Austria, visited their clinics, and kept up a lifetime of relationships. He collected honorary degrees and delivered papers, but for the most part he was alone. Osler wrote from England in 1911, "I have not seen the Professor, when over here he keeps in seclusion in a very funny way."

Halsted rarely spent time in London, or visiting Oxford. Instead, he passed through on his way to Brighton or Folkestone, seeing no one. On one such trip he wrote one of his secretaries, Miss Stokes:

This is an ideal spot. En route for Bonn, I have been here for a week, unable to tear myself away. Go to bed at ten punctually, and sleep usually until six. My corner room on the fifth floor has an unobstructed view of the oceanfront, and of the downs on the side. At night, I can vividly see the flashlights on the coast of France, 27 miles away. On a clear day one can see the French coast, and steamers and fishing boats are constantly in sight. I have a soft coal fire constantly, much to the amusement, I fancy, of the servants, who do not quite approve of the combination of open windows and a fire, when the thermometer registers per-haps 60 degrees, and they are complaining that it is 'ot.

In Paris, Halsted favored the Hotel Continental. Most of his time was spent in his room, and when he exited the hotel he did so by the side door to avoid acquaintances in the lobby and hotel staff. He did, in fact, make most of the scientific pilgrimages planned for each trip, but the majority of his time was solitary, answering to no one.

WHAT, THEN, IT MUST be asked, was the effect of a lifelong drug addiction on this most unusual man? One cannot claim Halsted's potential was never realized. He maintained his mental and physical strength and was, throughout his life, an enormously productive individual. What really can be ascribed to the chronic morphine addiction and episodic cocaine use? Did it change his personality? Very likely so. The initial cocaine episode documents evidence of his response. Hyperactivity, rambling speech, inattention, and suspended decision-making ability were hallmarks of this period, and drove him to seek help. The later cocaine use was episodic, restricted to private time, hidden from view, and relieved by reversion to morphine as he reentered society, and it is doubtful that he shared this secret with Caroline.

The use of morphine as a cocaine substitute was learned early, but never fully laid the craving to rest. The euphoria and sedation of morphine were easier to live with on a full-time basis, and he juggled the demands of daily existence and the drug quite well. But with the development of systemic tolerance, these effects become blunted. The need for "reward" offered by the drug does not diminish, and tolerance requires ever-larger dosage to sustain the same sense of well-being. The morphine sedative effect became less pronounced and increasingly integrated as a personality trait. Reticence gradually supplanted a more social alter ego, but only those familiar with the extrovert Halsted were aware of the dramatic change. Secrecy was a variable best managed by withdrawal, and the combination transformed a socially outgoing young man into the isolated and insulated individual that Halsted had become.

Managing drug dosage is an unpredictable art. Numerous factors including purity, route of administration, and metabolism vary, but usually within an acceptable range. Occasionally, the balance is disturbed and early signs of withdrawal or overdosage are manifested. Halsted on rare occasions suffered one or the other of these debilitating syndromes. At those times he was "ill," or "had a terrible Headache," and was forced to retire from surgery, or was taken with tremors and perspiration, as when Osler came upon him. The episodes, while unusual enough to gain notice, were insignificant within the span of a brilliant, 35-year career. Did the morphine make him more thoughtful, careful, and insightful? Unlikely. Halsted's evolution as surgeon and scientist was just that, an evolution. He was able to work with the morphine, not because of it. His insights into the direction that surgery should take were formed early, and the path through which they were achieved followed a logical progression.

The idea that the father of modern surgery could be addicted to morphine and cocaine throughout his long career is plainly counter-intuitive. More unsettling still is the level of performance he was able to maintain during those years. Surely the course of his life would have been far less convoluted without it, and perhaps his relation-ships a bit more traditional. But in all, he was unbent, healthy, able to function in civil society, accomplish more than most men could ever dream of, and set off no alarm bells. While hardly typical, the story belies the conventional wisdom concerning long-term drug use. What destruction the morphine wrought was served solely to William Stewart Halsted. There was little or no collateral damage.

CHAPTER THIRTY

Vascular Surgery

THIRTY YEARS AND 20 surgical papers passed between the startling surgery performed on Levin Waters and Halsted's final work on the subject of arterial aneurysms. Untold hundreds of dogs, dozens of patients, and numerous residents contributed to the journey, which was applauded for its fine scientific underpinnings by the National Academy of Science, whose membership had been disdainful of the idea of pure science associated with the craft of surgery. Halsted's work had forced the rethinking of that outdated position, and he took great pride in being accepted into the family of scientists. He had approached the great vascular unknown with the mind-set of a scientific explorer. While the wide range of his work was ultimately inconclusive, it cleared the way for some of the most dazzling medical achievements in history.

THE AORTA IS THE largest artery in the human body. The heart pumps the entire blood volume, some six liters, through it every minute. Rupture of the aorta is a cataclysmic event. The abdomen or chest fills with blood escaping from the rent in the great vessel, veins returning blood to the heart collapse as the circulating volume suddenly depletes, and shock and death result in minutes. The aorta is subject to the shearing force of trauma. It can be torn by penetrating injury, rupture at the site of an aneurysm or weakness in its wall, or in the hands of a surgeon attempting to repair it or prevent rupture. More frequently a weakness, distortion, or an internal tear manifests itself painfully, dangerously, and potentially lethally. There is no room for error.

Halsted was not the first to work in the area. It had always tempted surgeons as the most obviously dramatic time bomb presented to them. Wartime surgery brought opportunities for intervention. Larger arteries, wildly spraying blood, were crushed in clamps and tied off, usually resulting in amputation but sometimes in a warm, functional salvaged limb. Injuries to the aorta were a death notice, and reports of the occasional positive outcome stimulated thought. The great success in Waters's case raised the question of how one could interrupt flow through the major artery to a limb without resulting in gangrene of the limb. Halsted studied previous reports of ligation of the common iliac artery, the main blood supply to the leg, and came to the conclusion that the larger the artery, and the closer to the heart, the less the impairment that resulted from its occlusion. The salvation of the limb beyond the roadblock was due to collateral circulation, or arterial detours around the roadblock, which expanded and provided circulation.

The pathophysiology is a bit more complicated than the above description implies, but it did become clear that aneurysms of the larger vessels in the limbs could be safely tied off if one respected the collateral vessels arising before the aneurismal sac. Progressive occlusion of the vessel proximal to the aneurysm promoted collateral circulation. To encourage this, Halsted applied an aluminum band around the artery, which could be manually tightened to increase occlusion.

In March 1905, he summarized 90 experiments on the great vessels of dogs. The objective was to find a way to compress the aorta, which had never been successfully performed in man or beast. The aorta in humans was subject to marked degeneration over the years. Brittle cholesterol deposits in the wall of the aorta rendered it weakened and fragile, and syphilitic granulomas, which were not infrequent, ate away at the wall. Experimental studies showed that after complete occlusion, the vessel wall became atrophic and paper thin. Mont Reid, who worked with Halsted on the experiments, showed that though thrombosis and thinning of the wall occurred when the aluminum band was applied tightly enough for complete occlusion, loosely applied bands did not cause visible injury to the arteries. This was heartening news, since Halsted had been discouraged by an early case in which the pulsations of the dog's aorta against the aluminum band had caused it to cut through the wall, causing a hemorrhagic death for the dog. In other cases the aortic wall had become dangerously thin after three months of pressure. From 1904 to 1906, he applied the band to the large arteries of 100 dogs, with excellent results, and only one instance of the band cutting through the wall. It seemed safe enough to consider partial occlusion of the aorta in a human.

In 1909, Halsted reported, "The aluminum band has now been successfully applied in man to the common carotid artery twelve times, and once each to the thoracic aorta, the abdominal aorta, the common iliac, the femoral, and the innominate arteries."

Later that year he attempted three cases of banding the aorta. One was the first successful partial occlusion of the thoracic aorta to treat an enormous aneurysm of the upper abdominal aorta. In the second case, a band was first placed around the thoracic aspect of the aorta. Three weeks later the aorta was banded below the aneurysm in the abdomen. Ten days later the aorta ruptured. The third patient was operated on for a large abdominal aneurysm. The mass caused technical difficulties in reaching the band, and Halsted removed his gloves in order to more easily grasp the band and tighten it. The patient developed an overwhelming postoperative infection and died. Halsted was devastated. He had coolly dealt with losing patients before, and not infrequently while attempting to alter the explosive course of an expanding aneurysm. But this patient died from an infection as the result of a deviation from aseptic technique, which, as Halsted guiltily noted, was "the first in the annals of the Johns Hopkins Hospital in a clean abdominal case." To the ultimate detriment of his patient, even William Stewart Halsted suffered costly lapses.

Work on aortic aneurysm continued. Halsted's residents took up the mantle and helped establish additional benchmarks in surgery of the great vessels. It took half a century before the work finally bore fruit. Halsted spent thousands of hours in the Hunterian Laboratory facing off with the basic mysteries of the vascular system. So complex and consuming are the dynamics of blood flow and vascular integrity, and so deadly were surgical missteps, that Halsted may have devoted more time and energy to this subject than to any of his other interests. Among his collected surgical papers, 274 pages are devoted to a topic he was unable to master.[1]

---

1 In 1952, Michael DeBakey, then a young Texas surgeon, excised an aortic aneurysm and replaced it with a section of cadaver aorta. The following year he nudged the revolution a step further by replacing an aortic aneurysm with a tubular Dacron graft he fashioned on his wife's sewing machine.

CHAPTER THIRTY-ONE

Scientist

1904 HAD BEEN A YEAR of significant change at Johns Hopkins, and not all of it good. At 10:48 on the windy Sunday morning of February 7, the Great Baltimore Fire ignited in the city's commercial district. Baltimore's 51 horse-drawn, steam-powered pumpers taxed the ancient system of hydrants and proved inadequate to fight the blaze. Emergency equipment was rushed up from Washington, but that city's hose couplings did not match the Baltimore hydrants. Makeshift patching resulted in the loss of valuable water pressure, leaving the city to burn unchecked for 34 hours. Miraculously, no lives were lost to the fire, but among the material casualties of 1,343 buildings in 80 city blocks was considerable income-producing real estate provided by Johns Hopkins's bequest. The loss inflicted a great strain on the operating budget of the hospital.

William Osler, now the most famous physician in the world, was feeling wanderlust. It was no secret that the Canadian-born Osler was an unabashed Anglophile, and as early as 1894 he had told Kelly it was his dream to be knighted. In 1904, he was offered the Regius professorship of medicine at Oxford. It was a great honor, and the Hopkins community was not surprised when Osler accepted. By his own estimate he had been working too hard. That summer, at age 55, William

Osler prepared to leave for Oxford. Dinners and tributes were being planned everywhere in the months before his departure. Osler became increasingly emotional as his time at Hopkins drew to a close. In his farewell address he shook things up by reiterating his refrain on age: a man's great accomplishments occur before the age of 40; and at 60 he is useless to his profession, and should be put out to pasture. The new position would offer a quieter life, time to read and write, and the opportunity to educate his children in English schools. Much as he would miss the Hopkins social life that orbited about him, he believed an academic life required change to ward off going stale.

ON THE POSITIVE SIDE of the ledger, the new surgical building opened in the fall. For the first time since its inception, the Department of Surgery would be housed in comfortable, modern facilities. Halsted had toiled for 15 years in the afterthought of an operating suite in the basement under Ward G. As early as 1899, he had charged Cushing with drawing up preliminary plans for the new operating suite.

The construction of the surgery building was the first in a series of events after the fire that would have far-reaching effects on the institution. After the fire, the hospital trustees requested financial help from the Rockefellers, and John D. Rockefeller responded with a much-needed gift of $500,000. Over the ensuing years the relationship would grow, culminating in Rockefeller financial support for the establishment of the full-time system. Welch was already the president of the Board of Scientific Directors of the new Rockefeller Institute for Medical Research, in New York. Frederick Gates, Rockefeller's trusted adviser on philanthropic matters, was a great admirer of Osler. He had already read *The Principles and Practice of Medicine* and had become well acquainted with Welch.

The new building housed Baetjer's X-ray department on the second floor, Bloodgood's surgical pathology laboratory on the third floor, and on the top floor a large surgical amphitheater flanked by two sizeable operating rooms. Halsted and the resident staff used the west-facing operating room, and Cushing, Young, and the other subspecialists used the east room. The surgical amphitheater was used by Halsted for his "dry" clinics, and by Finney for his Friday-morning operative clinics. The Professor's office suite was on the operating floor as well. It consisted of an office, where he kept a substantial surgical reference library; an examining room; and a dressing room. But he rarely saw patients there. The office was occasionally used for meetings with visiting surgeons or for conferences, but he preferred to work at home, away from the interruptions and hospital chatter.

The opening of the new facility was celebrated with an "All Star" operation on October 5. Halsted chose a patient with osteomyelitis (bone infection) of the femur and was assisted by Cushing, Finney, Bloodgood, and Young, with Mitchell administering anesthesia. By all accounts, Halsted was in fine form that morning and enjoyed the tribute paid by his former residents in gathering around him. The surgeons, fully dressed in white, and gowned, had not yet begun wearing surgical masks, and the intense concentration on Halsted's face was plainly visible as he hammered away at the bone cavity with his favorite wooden mallet. There was no audience in the amphitheater, which wasn't a surprise, since little could be seen beyond Halsted's broad back. Sunlight streaming through the enormous window facing the benches blinded observers and silhouetted the action at the operating table. The only way to see anything was to stand with one's back to the window and face Halsted. Few dared that without an invitation.

BY THE START OF the 20th century, Johns Hopkins was unchallenged as the premier medical school in the country. "The very happy band" had pulled together and truly redefined the state of the art of medical education. The hospital had achieved international renown on the strength of the incomparable clinical work of Osler, Halsted, Kelly, and their stellar residents. Important visitors were commonplace at clinics, laboratories, lectures, and in the operating room, and a barrage of papers and bulletins chronicled their deeds and saw to it that the word got out. Texts by Osler and Kelly became required reading, and Halsted's monographs reinforced the position of the Halsted school of surgery.

The medical school had set absurdly high standards for admission and drew the best students in the country. A decade later, they, too, took their place at the forefront of medicine and science. Mall, Halsted, MacCallum, Cushing, and the others kept the experimental laboratories operating at full throttle, and the combined institutions were cranking out great works at a breathtaking pace. Things were moving ahead marvelously, but change was in the air.

By the time Osler was preparing to leave for England in 1905, a schism had developed in the previously unified approach to the new medicine, and the departing Osler had already taken a side. The heated power struggle between the basic scientists and the clinicians was coming to a boil. What had long been a philosophical argument now had practical implications. Welch and Mall were the primary proponents of a research-based faculty. Welch, forever the politician, continued to straddle the fence. He truly believed academic medicine belonged in the laboratory, but he wouldn't defend the position with all the power he could wield. Mall was probably the most significant and sought-after scientist on the faculty. He was strident in his advocacy of research as the highest academic calling, even at the expense of teaching, of which he had given evidence time and time again. Mall was the great prize won by Welch, when he lured the anatomist back from his professorship at the University of Chicago. He was a brilliant researcher, his lab was opening the world of embryology, and he was always available to help his colleagues think through their projects. Detested by students in the basic anatomy course he taught, he was beloved by those whose intellectual curiosity led them down the path of independent investigation. Those few young people Mall gently taught, in a manner Fleming described as not with a guiding hand but by "jogging the elbow," and looking in and offering words of advice from time to time. He intended to build a tradition of scientists, and he had no interest in teaching clinicians.

Osler did not shy away from the laboratory, but he was first and foremost a clinician and teacher. When asked what he would choose for his epitaph he had responded, "He taught medical students." So the lines were clearly drawn: Osler the clinician versus Mall the pure scientist. Welch valued both and took care not to openly take sides. The differences, while deeply held, did not suffuse the environment with animosity. The faculty members were in constant contact with one another, and despite the tension over the direction in which Hopkins should go, the overriding sense remained one of community. But at the last faculty meeting that he attended before leaving, Osler said to Mall, "Now I go, and you have your way," exposing his fear that the balance of power over Welch would now shift in Mall's favor.

William Stewart Halsted, a pivotal figure in the philosophical shift to pure science over clinical medicine, sat out the arguments and voted with his actions, which had been steadily drifting away from clinical practice and into research. Cushing summarized Halsted's attitude as "... caring little for gregarious gatherings of medical men, unassuming, having little interest in private practice, spending his medical life avoiding patients, even students, when possible, and when health permitted, working in his clinic and laboratory at the solution of a succession of problems which aroused his interest."

By 1905, Halsted was operating infrequently and had all but lost interest in private practice. But his stellar reputation and vast experience in surgery of the breast, hernia, and thyroid continued to attract well-heeled patients from around the country. Increasingly, the resident performed the routine procedures on Halsted's private patients. His fees could sometimes be outrageous, but most often they were not very different from those generally held in the community. One of the functions of the local medical societies was to fix fees at a comfortable level for the practitioner, and the guidelines were generally adhered to. The money was good, and he certainly knew how to spend it, but increasingly, his heart was in problem solving.

For Halsted, experimental surgery did not end at the Hunterian Laboratory. Private and charity patients alike were there for learning and teaching. Halsted's huge reputation and frosty manner projected supreme confidence, and he was able to convince patients to submit to procedures of little value to them, in the name of science.

At a thyroid surgery conference in Atlantic City, Professor Albert Kocher of Berne, son of the great surgeon Theodore Kocher, read a paper on his recent finding of increased numbers of circulating lymphocytes in patients with Graves' disease. Halsted had earlier shown the presence of masses of lymphoid tissue in the thyroid specimens removed from patients with the disease. It was too much of a coincidence to be ignored, and he set out to attempt to correlate the two findings. In his protocol, blood samples from his patients would be studied before and after surgery. But the patients were scattered throughout the country. Not trusting local facilities to study the samples, Halsted wrote his patients and asked them to return to Johns Hopkins to participate in the study. Though the text of the request has been lost, it must have been persuasive. The response astounded George Heuer, who helped coordinate the project.

"They came from long distances for a procedure which required but a few moments. One woman came from a remote place in Texas and spent four days on the train coming to Baltimore. Dr. Halsted saw her, thanked her for coming, remained while a drop of blood was removed from a prick in her finger, wished her a pleasant journey home and left her. Eight days on the train and the expense of coming and going for a five minutes' visit!"

Heuer remarked about it to Halsted, who replied, "How better could she spend her time than contributing to the problem of this disease."

Another example involved the work of Alexis Carrel,[1] a French surgeon working at the Rockefeller Institute for Medical Research, in New York City. Carrel had found that if a fixed amount of skin was removed from a dog, and the wound remained clean, the time to complete healing could be plotted, and the resulting curve could be converted to a formula that predicted the time required for healing.

Halsted set out to reproduce the results in humans, reasoning that it would be easier to keep the wounds clean in human subjects, and the result would have a more direct application. If humans were the most reliable subjects, then, he reasoned, private patients should be the most reliable humans to study. He assumed, of course, that the patients would cooperate. Heuer was witness to Halsted explaining to one woman the scientific journey on which they were about to embark. He told her that during her operation he would remove "precisely one square inch of skin" from her abdomen. "And then together we will study the healing of the wound."

Precise measurements of wound size were recorded, wounds were carefully dressed and kept scrupulously clean, and bacteriological samples of the healing wound were taken daily. As with virtually all the other subjects, the patient was as excited as Halsted about the ongoing experiment, and his daily visit was eagerly awaited. The wound from the surgery, for which she had entered the hospital, had long

---

1 In 1912, Carrel won the $39,000 Nobel Prize in Physiology or Medicine based on his work on suturing and transplanting blood vessels. He developed an antiseptic technique to sterilize healing tissue, which was very useful during World War I, and collaborated with Charles Lindbergh on a perfusion pump that was the precursor to the bypass machine. In an interesting sidelight, Carrel was brought to Rockefeller from the University of Chicago, by Simon Flexner. Flexner was a Jewish pathologist trained by Welch and one of the scientific directors of the new institute. The two became fast friends. During World War II, Carrel worked with the Vichy government, espoused many of the Nazi beliefs in eugenics, and was thought by many to have been the source of much of the bigotry associated with Lindbergh in later life. Carrel died in disgrace in France in 1944.

since healed, and the woman happily continued to pay private patient hospital charges as she remained the subject of his little experiment. Halsted saw nothing unusual about the arrangement.

* * *

WITH OSLER LEAVING, the strongest clinical influence on Welch disappeared, and Mall assumed undisputed control of his ear. Mall believed the departmental chairs should abandon practice and devote themselves to science, leaving patient care, and the attendant compensation, to others. It was Carl Ludwig who planted the full-time seed in Mall when he studied with him in Leipzig, in 1886. Ludwig believed the ideal system would have the clinical as well as preclinical professors devoting full time to research and abandoning private practice.

Mall had no interest in clinical medicine and wished to see Osler replaced by someone who could move the department "to a higher level." By this he meant a full-time research scientist. This was an audacious proposition, for Osler embodied everything that was good in medicine. With support from Mall and Halsted, Welch chose Lewellys Barker as professor of medicine. Barker was a Canadian trained by Osler at Hopkins. He had never been in clinical practice and was professor of anatomy at the University of Chicago. Primarily a researcher, he had spoken out in a 1902 address in favor of the full-time system. Osler had favored his longtime assistant William Thayer for the job, but Thayer was purely a clinician, and Mall, Welch, and Halsted had other ideas.

While the debate over full time smoldered, Halsted and the department of surgery marched forward. He no longer cared much for private practice but continued to charge the occasional outrageous fee, as did Kelly, and their actions added fuel to the trustees' dissatisfaction with the system. With Welch and Mall whispering in their ears, the trustees wondered out loud whether the hospital would not be better served by billing for these services and putting the chiefs on salary. But they didn't push too hard. Kelly already had a private hospital and could easily do without admitting patients to Hopkins at all. The heads of the newly formed surgical sub-departments had similar outside arrangements, and Halsted did as he pleased. The last thing the trustees wanted was to lose Halsted and Kelly, particularly while still licking their wounds over the departure of Osler.

HALSTED WAS NOW 52 years old. His face had become a bit fuller and flushed with color, and he was quite bald. The drooping mustache and patch of beard he wore beneath his lower lip were not yet fully gray, he continued to wear rimless glasses pinched on his prominent nose, and his protruding ears were accentuated by his short, sparse hair. His neck had thickened, and he appeared slightly stooped and shorter, but his muscular arms and upper body appeared unchanged. He worked at his own pace, slowly compiled his papers, and maintained active correspondence with surgeons around the world. He traveled to medical meetings with some regularity, usually favoring the East Coast, particularly New York, where he sometimes visited with his sisters. He spent considerable time at clinics in Europe but never bothered to do so in America, fearing there would be nothing to learn and he would waste precious time. His extended absences continued without excuse and with less resistance from the trustees. He was a valuable property, and they had learned to accommodate his idiosyncrasies. Laboratory experiments were terminated in the spring so that The Professor could leave, and during his absence experimental surgery ground to a halt. For Halsted, the Johns Hopkins season was a seven-month affair.

* * *

THE HOSPITAL HAD been in operation for 15 years, the medical school for 11 years. Welch, Osler, Kelly, and Halsted had established well-deserved, worldwide reputations, and Hopkins had become the most forward thinking medical institution in the world.

Welch had all but abandoned research, wrote almost no scientific papers, and continued to shirk teaching responsibilities. But he had become the country's most potent force in the advancement of medical science. He was consulting, supporting, counseling, and helping great minds and institutions make the decisions, which would move medical science, and public health, forward.

Halsted, alone among them, had reinvented a discipline. At every crossroad he had made decisions that changed the way surgery was performed, taught, and expanded. He had transformed the shunned black sheep of the medical world into a specialty offering the promise of mightily alleviating the suffering of the human condition.

Kelly was the greatest technical surgeon of his day, and a prolific writer and innovator. Osler, master of bedside medicine and teaching, brought clinical and laboratory disciplines together. But Halsted had quietly shown the way through the dark as he invented modern surgery. In time, he would be measured by the work of his disciples, and Cushing, Bloodgood, Finney, and Young were growing in stature.

Everything was going better than imagined at Johns Hopkins, but Osler's departure signaled the end of an era.

CHAPTER THIRTY-TWO

A New Paradigm

FEW NONSCIENTIFIC ISSUES HAVE stimulated as much heated debate among physicians as the controversy over full time. Should medical professors be full-time salaried employees of the university, restricted in outside earnings, or should they be permitted to earn income above their salaries in private practice? One could easily argue both sides if the issue were only that simple. At Johns Hopkins a new philosophy was gaining a foothold, which further complicated the issue. Tucked quietly under this simple question was the idea that once professors became "full time," they would be pure scientists, and abandon clinical practice altogether. That was a revolutionary premise which would prove more difficult to sell.

Medicine is a full-time job, and patients think of their doctors as clinicians. They are internists, surgeons, obstetricians, gynecologists, or pediatricians. While medical scientists are correctly perceived as another breed entirely—full time, but different. No patient in his right mind would choose a surgeon to repair his hernia simply because that surgeon had worked in the laboratory to uncover the function of the parathyroid glands. But in 1910 they were the same man, William Stewart Halsted. And he would figure prominently in the struggle.

For the first two decades of its existence, Johns Hopkins was the living embodiment of that gray area. It thrived, and grew, and became famous the world over based on the excellence of its clinician/scientists. When the line was drawn between Mall and Osler, it raised the question of dominance in the academic setting. Who should take the lead in the education of medical students? Should precedence be given to the pure medical scientist or the bedside teacher? At first it was a nonissue. The pure scientists like Mall, Martin, and Abel taught students in the two preclinical years. Halsted, Osler, and Kelly took over as the students were introduced to patients in the last two years of the program.

The lines became somewhat blurred as Halsted, never a great teacher of medical students, gave over much of this responsibility to his assistants, spent less time operating, and more time in the laboratory. Ludwig's dream of clinical professors devoting all their energies to research struck a chord in Mall, and he became a fierce advocate of the full-time system in its purest form. For the others, led by a relatively quiet Welch, it was a softer and more realistic concept: relieve the clinical professors of the need to engage in private practice to supplement their incomes, and allow them the luxury of teaching, research, and patient care, with the monies earned accruing to the university.

At the opposite pole from Mall was William Osler. The man who chose for his epitaph "He taught medical students" was a staunch defender of the status quo. Osler was outraged by the idea of laboratory scientists teaching medicine to future physicians. He believed his private practice, which he conducted mainly after 2 P.M., did not detract from fulfilling his duties. He apologized only for out-of-town consultations, which took him away from the hospital. But these cases, he believed, burnished the Johns Hopkins reputation, as the private practice fostered interaction between the Hopkins staff and important individuals in the community, and established the authority of Hopkins physicians. Halsted was silent.

ABRAHAM FLEXNER WAS a teacher and school principal in Louisville. He was a Johns Hopkins University graduate and the brother of Simon Flexner, Welch's former assistant who was now a director of the Rockefeller Institute. In 1908, Abraham Flexner's interest in educational philosophy brought him to the attention of the Carnegie Foundation for the Advancement of Teaching, where he was charged with preparing a report on the state of medical education in America. The American Medical Association, then a largely impotent organization, had championed the study, which gained importance with the backing of the Carnegie Foundation. Simon Flexner idolized Welch, and the pathologist had no small influence on the thinking of his brother. Two years later, the report found all medical colleges in the United States deficient, with a single exception: The Johns Hopkins School of Medicine. Welch's dream had become the prototype for proper medical education. The report quoted chapter and verse on the inadequacies of the proprietary medical schools: libraries without books, absence of laboratories, inadequate clinical instruction, lack of research, and the absence of teaching hospitals controlled by the medical school. Only 50 of 155 medical colleges were associated with universities. Only Johns Hopkins and Harvard required a college degree. Cornell required three years of college, 20 other required two years, and 132 medical schools required a high school education, or less.

The death knell had been sounded for proprietary medical schools. The country was scandalized, and the empowered AMA refused to certify schools that were deemed inadequate. More than half of the medical schools in the country were soon shuttered. But the winds of change had preceded the report, and at the better schools, change had already begun. Harvard, the University of Pennsylvania, P&S, and other medical schools associated with universities had already taken heed of the successful Hopkins model and were moving ahead. University-affiliated schools were given the benefit of the doubt and advised to address deficiencies. Some were made to consolidate with other schools in the community. Everything considered, the landscape was markedly changed for the better.

Critics point out that many necessary, though admittedly marginal, schools were forced to close, including several of the Negro medical colleges.

With the success of his report, Abraham Flexner gained considerable influence. He was not a physician, and he was of the firm conviction that medical education should be a laboratory science at the expense of clinical experience. The ball was rolling in the direction of full-time medicine, and Mall, having Flexner's ear, reinforced the need for that change. As John D. Rockefeller's wealth grew, Frederick Gates, his point man for philanthropy, focused his efforts on medicine, resulting in the Rockefeller Institute for Medical Research. When Gates asked Flexner what he would do with a million dollars to improve medicine, the response was, "I should give it to Dr. Welch."

Gates got the idea and sent Flexner to talk to Welch. A dinner was arranged at the Maryland Club, with Halsted and Mall in attendance. Mall saw his moment.

"If the school could get a sum of approximately a million dollars, in my judgment, there is only one thing we ought to do with it—use every penny of its income for the purpose of placing on a salary basis the heads and assistants in the leading clinical departments, doing for them what the school did for the underlying medical sciences when it was started."

Welch did not jump at the opportunity, and Halsted said little, but the issue was out in the open and the wherewithall to implement it was at hand. By June 1911, the trustees had endorsed Welch's plan for full-time professors, with fees from practice reverting to the university. The plan required the consent of the medical faculty, which was not quickly forthcoming.

Osler checked in from Oxford. "I did not take away from B a dollar made in practice." He defended the need to practice medicine.

"Would whole time men have the same influence on the profession at large—I doubt it." In an open letter to university president Ira Remsen, he angrily took issue with errors in Flexner's report to Gates and the aspersions cast upon Kelly, who earned hugely and donated a great deal of his income back to his department and his charities. Now the "happy band" were taking sides.

In 1912, Osler wrote that full time would lead to "a faculty of Halsteds. A very good thing for science, but a very bad thing for the profession."

In January 1913, Remsen resigned for health reasons, and Welch temporarily assumed the position of president of The Johns Hopkins University. Now he was truly in charge, but he stepped lightly. The idea of full time rested on providing adequate income for the professors, which, in turn, would be provided by the Rockefellers' General Education Board. By October, Welch had a consensus among the governing board of the medical school, and the Rockefellers honored him by naming the fund the William H. Welch Endowment for Clinical Education and Research.

There were two issues that needed to be addressed. First, was the full-time system going to separate the doctors from their patients? Physicians weighed in from everywhere, and the general consensus was that it would insidiously do so. Patients, too, felt uneasy about the fees rightfully earned by their doctors going to the university. Many Hopkins graduates were skeptical of the wisdom of the plan, and some bitterly opposed it. Leading members of the medical faculty, including Kelly and the psychiatrist Adolf Meyer, were unhappy with the decision and felt it was being foisted upon them by outside interests, meaning Gates, Flexner, and the all-powerful Rockefeller company Standard Oil.

The second issue was the need to establish a salary comfortable enough to attract significant individuals to the chairs.

Initially, the new rules would affect pediatrics, medicine, and surgery. For the time being gynecology would be exempt, as would the newly born subspecialties such as urology. John Howland, recently enlisted as professor of pediatrics, knew what to expect when he accepted the job and offered no resistance. The big surprise was Lewellys Barker. Barker had been primarily a laboratory man. When he replaced Osler in 1905, he was so uninitiated in the art of clinical medicine that he had to be instructed in the bedside techniques of patient examination. But Barker was smart and personable, and found he loved being a doctor. And he loved being in private practice. In the end he refused to give up the lifestyle, and the income, of his private practice and resigned as physician in chief. He took the title of clinical professor and built a thriving practice. Barker's second in command, William S. Thayer, who had been passed over for the job when Osler left, was offered the full-time position. He, too, declined.

Halsted had more or less cast his lot with the laboratory men, Mall and Welch, but he remained concerned that his residents have the opportunity to become the finest clinical surgeons and teachers of surgery. One of his criteria for choosing a resident was an interest in independent research, but his primary goal had always been creating well-rounded surgeons who would become professors of surgery and spread the gospel of excellence according to William Stewart Halsted.

Halsted sent a series of notes to the trustees to illuminate his thinking. In archive document #1207, in pencil on his personal stationery, Halsted writes:

1. The clinical men tend to deteriorate in certain directions. & the laboratory men are prevented from developing in others.

2. The world over the laboratory men are of a higher order than the clinicians; & among the clinicians the physician out-ranks the surgeon & the surgeon outranks the gynecologist.

3. As a rule the more intellectual men & those with the highest ideals select the laboratory branches ... The reward for the greater talents & higher achievements should be advance in

position & not increase in wealth . . . I am free from preju-
dice in trying to take a position in this matter, because it
would now make, as far as my income is concerned, very
little difference to me whether it (my income) was limited
to a $10,000 salary or not. The assurance of such an income,
which is perhaps a few thousand dollars less than what I am
presently making, would quite compensate for the uncer-
tainty of making so much in the future.

The ideal simple life is that which is not enforced.

The simple life is not ideal unless arrived at by voluntary
renouncement of luxury.

These last two sentences reflect a philosophy totally unlike the
manner in which the 61-year-old Halsted had lived his life. With every
financial advantage, Halsted surrounded himself with enormous personal comfort—a grand town house, a country estate, numerous personal employees, closets full of the finest custom-made clothing, and
unlimited first-class international travel—all of which would seem
anathema to the "simple life."

True, he had already shifted his focus to the laboratory and
restricted the number of private patients under his care. Ten years
previously he had been billing private patients thousands of dollars
for his services. But the evidence supports his lack of commitment to
private practice. He never established a private consulting room, and
he kept the ample work space allotted to him as a place to hang his
hat, study, and write. When he did see private patients it was either at
their home, in a hotel room, or in the hospital. His colleagues were far
more consumed with the effort and dedicated comfortable surroundings to their private enterprise.

In the beginning, pursuing private practice was not only the norm
but was the implied preference of the hospital trustees. Private income

would allow the doctors to live well without adding the burden of large salaries to the budget. The coming of full time, and the Rockefeller money to support it, eliminated the need for this pragmatic solution and obviously played into the hands of the Mall faction.

In the years following the institution of full time, Caroline Halsted often complained of the financial constraints the system imposed upon them. A $10,000 salary in 1913, the year the federal income tax law was ratified, would be about the equivalent of $300,000 in 2009. Not poverty level by any means, but less than Halsted was earning at the time. Their actual financial circumstances are unknown. It is unclear what, if anything, remained of his inheritance, but Halsted had never made an issue of lack of money, just as he never made an issue of having money. Suddenly he could no longer avoid the topic. In the end, he realized that at the heart of the "full time" debate was the money, and "that there were men who needed the stimulus of money making to compel them to work, but that these are not the desirable men."

"But," he added, earnestly, "wish men who have learned to work for work's sake, who find in it and in the search for truth, their greatest reward."

Halsted warmly endorsed the idea, but he had not romanticized it. He wrote to the trustees: "We should utterly fail as surgeons were our staff composed chiefly of laboratory workers who could not be given patients for treatment."

He felt that the surgical service was too small for the growing resident staff, and the "majority of patients occupying surgical beds cease to be of particular interest after operation, for their convalescence is uneventful." This very significant sentence stands as evidence of the sea change in surgery in the two decades with Halsted at its helm, as the struggle against postoperative infection had largely been won by his demand for strict asepsis, hemostasis, and gentle technique.

"In a word, for the success of the surgical department on its new basis it is necessary that the clinical facilities be greatly increased, for, if not, we shall fail to attract to this service men of the type not only ardently desired but essential to the carrying out of the plan to which we have pledged ourselves to adhere."

In 1913, it was an experiment meant to apply only to the leaders of the major departments: surgery, medicine, pediatrics, gynecology, and psychiatry. As things stood initially, only the professor would be affected. Proponents at Hopkins were strident in their views, but even supporters, such as Halsted, could paraphrase Osler's old refrain, that without clinical medicine there would be no medicine at all. Mall's position not withstanding, patient care did count. To be an effective leader, the professor had to be expert in the clinical practice of his specialty.

In the quarter century after it was instituted, the full-time system was expanded to include junior faculty members. The primacy of laboratory scientists rose and fell in a parabolic course over those 25 years. Sometime before World War II, the medical establishment came to its senses and recognized the importance of clinicians. If the goal was to help humanity, the physicians on the front line needed more appropriate role models and teachers than the laboratory men could offer.

Within the wide range of university full-time systems, some professors would be on straight salary, and others in complex financial arrangements with the university, which allowed them to recapture a percentage of their earnings. Some adopted an arrangement sometimes referred to as geographical full time, where professors were required to practice at the university hospital, but financial arrangements varied widely. Some doctors headed departments and taught medical students and residents for the honor of doing so, and supported themselves solely on patient fees, often quite handsomely.

Increasing financial pressure on hospitals and universities soon found the full-time physicians, from professor to young practitioner, had become profit centers for the institution. The paradigm had shifted from scientists freed from the constraints of practice, to clinician-teachers working as practitioners and subsidizing medical schools. All manner of arrangements exist today. Medical schools and hospitals pay multimillion-dollar salaries to star clinicians who fill beds and attract wealthy potential donors. They subsidize new, "full-time" practitioners with comfortable salaries and a promise of patient referral, and generally operate in the manner of large corporations, far removed from the ideals of Mall, Welch, and Halsted.

CHAPTER THIRTY-THREE

A New Era

A T AGE 61, HALSTED'S nicotine-stained mustache had gone white, his ice blue eyes appeared more forbidding than ever, and the skin of his jaw and neck had loosened. He was not sickly, but he wasn't quite well. Abdominal and chest discomfort had become a regular part of his life, and like most physicians, Halsted diagnosed and treated himself. Convinced his ailment was angina, he often took to his bed, but for the bulk of the time he was energetic and once again reinvented.

The older Halsted was generally more at ease and able to maintain a genuine interest in his juniors. With the coming of full time he was morally free of what he had come to increasingly dislike: the operating room. Always intense, and increasingly tired at surgery, his great joy had become the experimental laboratory. Halsted felt his duties were now clearly delineated as scientist and teacher. He still spent hours studying particular patients, and was no more communicative than he had been in the past. Patients whose problems interested him were, by unspoken rule, his patients, but they were considerably fewer in number. The resident took great care to follow and prepare these patients, but would never dare take them to surgery. This presented a problem, as Halsted often became otherwise engaged and neglected the patient for weeks. The resident dared not do the surgery, and feared reminding The Professor that his patient was languishing on the ward. When the patient finally came to his attention, Halsted would say he had been studying the proper treatment, and the issue would drop.

Formality remained the rule. Halsted never referred to colleagues by their given names. It was Kelly, Cushing, and Finney, never Howard, Harvey, or John. Initially, it was Dr. Kelly, Dr. Cushing, and Dr. Finney. Omitting the title was a sign of collegiality. Medical students were mister, or miss, and never called by their first names. No one at Johns Hopkins ever dared call Dr. Halsted "William."

The formality was rigidly applied to patients, though all were treated with respect. There was no personal banter or small talk with patients, particularly with ward patients, as Halsted felt the intellectual gap between them made such talk inappropriate. A patient's elevated social status carried no weight, for in his view it was a privilege to be treated by him, and he expected the relationship to carry on thusly.

One patient, a very well known woman, had a chronic condition that required repeated surgery over a period of years.

Halsted announced her arrival over the telephone to the resident.

"Heuer, is that you? I just wanted to say that we are in for a bad winter. Good night."

Ensconced in a private room made up with her own bed linen, and a telephone line to conduct long-distance business, she routinely ordered the staff about. On his first visit he was told, "Dr. Halsted, I have no time to waste, I am a very busy woman, I expect you to operate on me tomorrow."

"Yes, Miss A." And then to the waiting Heuer, "Gracious, Heuer, we are late for that very important operation. Good-bye, Miss A."

He returned to the irritated woman two days later, and again she demanded immediate surgery. This time he stayed away for five days. Miss A finally got the point, and she humbly requested that Dr. Halsted take care of her as soon as he could find the time.

"Now, Miss A, you are in a proper frame of mind to discuss your problem."

Halsted was far more strident in his expectations of private patients than the ward population. This attitude obtained in everything from intelligence to personal hygiene. When another socially prominent woman was examined in the hospital prior to surgery, he left the room visibly unhappy with her.

"Why, Heuer, she has a dirty umbilicus."

* * *

HALSTED NOW OPERATED only a day or two each week, and rarely did more than a single case each day. On operating days he would arrive at the hospital at 9:00 for 10:00 surgery. He took a taxicab from Eutaw Place to the surgical building, and the elevator to the fourth floor. In his dressing room he shed his black derby, his cane and gloves, and changed from his impeccable, dark three-piece suit, white shirt, and dazzling black leather shoes to the white duck operating costume, which now included a cloth face mask and white tennis shoes. He had abandoned the scrubbing and dipping routine in favor of washing with alcohol and a sterilized cloth, and did so before donning the sterile rubber gloves. The gloves were finely made and stood up well to multiple sterilizations. Sterile gloves were now in use everywhere. Other hospitals had already adopted the more convenient dry method, in which gloves were covered with a sterile, dry powder, which made for easier insertion of the hands and less irritation. Halsted stood by the wet method, dipping the sterile gloves in permanganate solution after sterilization. Halsted's belief in the impossibility of fully sterilizing the hands was unshaken. Sterile gloves were the only safe barrier between wound and surgeon, and he insisted on a change of gloves and instruments if the gloves were pierced, a technique rigidly followed today.

On the days he did not operate, Halsted worked at home until noon, lunched with Caroline, saw a few patients with the resident, and spent the afternoon at the lab. Some days he didn't appear at the hospital at all, and when he was feeling poorly he didn't appear for weeks at a time. During the school year he made formal ward rounds with the students, and conducted a "dry clinic" at which patients were examined and discussed. These sessions took place in the amphitheater on the fourth floor of the surgical building. The rest of the time he was free to dream up projects and concentrate his time at the Hunterian Laboratory across the street from the surgical building.

Cushing had moved on to Boston, leaving the surgery course without its inspired instructor. Rather than assign another assistant, Halsted resumed teaching the course himself. Or, more accurately, began teaching the surgery course. The first time around he had barely met his responsibilities. This time he enjoyed the experience, and threw himself into it. Over the next decade he would establish far closer relationships with the medical students and junior residents, and would be remembered quite differently by later graduates than he had been by their predecessors.

His thyroid, parathyroid, vascular, and intestinal surgery projects were in full swing for seven months of the year. Once May arrived, all work stopped just as abruptly as it always had, and vacation beckoned, but from October to May, Halsted was working full time at being "full time."

* * *

IF HALSTED CHANGED appreciably with the new system it was seen in the vigor with which he approached his experimental work. Lifting the restraints allegedly hampering the flowering of the academic lives of the professors had little more than symbolic effect on him. Halsted, more than anyone else at Hopkins, had done pretty much as he pleased. He had already cut back on surgery, but the constant talk about laboratory science touched everyone. Even Kelly, whose department was not included in the initial move to full time, announced his intention to spend more time in the laboratory. The topics that interested Halsted remained largely unchanged, but his residents and assistants became more deeply involved in laboratory problems than ever before. His relationship with the residents became somewhat more relaxed, and several of them were welcomed to the fringes of his private world.

Perhaps the first of the young people to see The Professor in a purely social setting had been Sam Crowe, then a medical student, in the summer of 1904. Over the years, Crowe got a lot of mileage out of the story of his ill-fated summer camping trip to the Black Mountains of North Carolina. The week he spent at High Hampton, the kind hospitality, the personal, time-consuming attention to the sick horse, the beauty of the surroundings, the elegance of The Professor strolling among his dahlias in white flannels and silk shirt, and the contrasting simplicity of Mrs. Halsted's homespun dress all made an indelible impression on the young man.

Crowe had the good fortune to have gained Halsted's attention as a medical student. Later, his work in the Hunterian Laboratory exploring pituitary function under Cushing led to an interest in neurosurgery. He hoped to accompany Cushing to Boston, but The Professor thwarted his plans by assigning him to head the department of otolaryngology. In the years from the opening of the hospital in 1889 until 1912, when Crowe was enlisted, diseases of the eye, ear, nose, and throat were treated in the dispensary. Distinguished specialists from the Baltimore medical community volunteered their time at no salary. If patients required surgery they were admitted to the hospital and assigned to Finney, Bloodgood, or the resident. The otolaryngologists serving in the dispensary had varying levels of training, and had never been granted operating privileges at Hopkins.

Halsted felt the time had come to organize the specialty of otolaryngology under a director within the hospital. The task fell to Crowe, who, like Young in urology, professed ignorance of the subject. Halsted would have none of it, and brought the topic to the medical board. Under questioning, he acknowledged that Crowe had no training in the specialty but was an able man, and would have time to travel to Germany to study. He went on describing his plan, including the proposal of a small salary for Crowe, when he was interrupted by Howard Kelly. The righteous Kelly demanded to know whether the proposed reorganization had been discussed with the men who had been serving so loyally in the outpatient department.

Halsted responded that he was embarrassed, but no, they had not been consulted. Kelly banged his fist on the table, outraged.

"Halsted, I am opposed to this. Everything we do here must be open and above board."

Halsted flushed.

"Kelly, you are absolutely right. How could I have perpetuated such an offense? It was an awful thing for me to do. I am ashamed, and I apologize for bringing such a recommendation before this dignified Board ... " Halsted continued to castigate himself and beg forgiveness, but he never withdrew his suggestion. Finally, Kelly had had enough.

"Halsted, stop it. I'll vote for it."

And another subspecialty of surgery had been created.

Crowe and his wife took up residence around the corner from the Halsteds, and despite the 30-year disparity in their ages, a friendship grew between the two couples. Mrs. Crowe found Mrs. Halsted interesting, and Caroline seemed to relish the company of the young woman. Halsted, while he liked and respected Crowe, continued to occupy his time with his work, his reading, and occasionally the old group from the Maryland Club.

* * *

GEORGE HEUER WAS Halsted's 13th resident surgeon and had come to think of him as his second father, hardly the description most would associate with the unreachable Professor. Medical school, assistant residency, and three years as resident had taught Heuer what he needed to know about how to approach an issue, when to make suggestions, when to make his own decisions, and how to become invisible when The Professor's neck turned red. Pleasing The Professor was a role he mastered, as had the residents before him. And Halsted, through the last decade of his career, came to appreciate, enjoy, and depend on the talented Heuer, who had mastered the disciplines of neurosurgery, general surgery, and thoracic surgery.

In the fall of 1914, Heuer returned from a surgical tour of Europe. Halsted invited him to stay at his home until he got settled. Caroline was still away, and Heuer was installed in her apartment on the third floor. Halsted's hospitality and generosity rained on the young surgeon. He personally carried logs for Heuer's fire up three flights of stairs and saw to it that fresh water and flowers were always at his bedside. After breakfasting in his suite, Halsted spent a few minutes in the dining room with Heuer as he was served. Scrutinizing every detail, he would not allow the famished Heuer to eat the boiled eggs in front of him, sending them back to the kitchen several times until they were properly coddled. Halsted even traveled across town to the Lexington Market to choose the grapefruit for the breakfast table.

The kindness and attention embarrassed the retiring Heuer, who tried to be as unobtrusive as possible. "I had been writing in my room on the third floor and my pen 'went dry'; and not finding any ink I went down to his room to fill it."

The fountain pen–obsessed Halsted asked to see Heuer's pen, examined it carefully, then opened a drawer in his secretary and produced three boxes of fountain pens. Each box contained a dozen pens, and each of the 36 pens was filled with ink and ready to use.

"You might like to try another," Halsted said, handing a box of a dozen to Heuer. "A perfect fountain pen is not easy to find."

The simple excess carried over to cigarettes and the inexpensive cigarette holders Halsted was rarely seen without. Heuer wrote that there were great quantities of cigarettes everywhere in the house, and Dr. Halsted "heaped upon me, many more than I could possibly smoke. There were boxes of cigarette holders, one of which containing 100 he gave me on my arrival with the statement that I should call on him for more when I had used them."

The atmosphere of disorganized pampered profusion was not lost on the household servants, who took advantage of the situation. Heuer overheard a conversation on the house phone in which large quantities of ham, pork chops, and other meats were being ordered, none of which ever appeared on the table. Halsted responded that he was probably "feeding the entire colored population of the neighborhood," but in the absence of Caroline, he didn't know what he could do about it.

After dinner the two men took coffee in the library. The ritual was an event in itself. After sorting the beans for size and color, Halsted ground them slowly and carefully, and then prepared the thick, black coffee. Conversation over coffee was heavily weighted toward surgery, and Halsted offered that Heuer's career should take him to New York. It was a prescient moment, for long after his mentor's death, and following a decade as professor at Cincinnati, Heuer became professor and surgeon in chief at New York Hospital–Cornell Medical College, where he established the institution's first residency program on the Halsted model.

* * *

WALTER EDWARD DANDY, the son of recent English immigrants, showed up at Johns Hopkins as a second-year medical student in 1907. He had forgone a Rhodes scholarship to begin his medical studies with advanced standing. Dandy and Mall found each other, and the medical student was assigned the daunting task of describing a two-millimeter human embryo, at that time the smallest specimen studied. The work became a benchmark in embryology and the specimen became known as The Dandy Embryo.

After graduation, Dandy worked in Cushing's lab for a year, trying to determine the vascular and nerve supply of the pituitary gland. His work proved important, and Cushing made Dandy his clinical assistant. Dandy was a driven, self-confident, and difficult individual. He and Cushing clashed loudly and often, yet Cushing invited the young man to go with him to Harvard. Thinking Dandy was leaving, Halsted filled his position in the program. Cushing then changed his mind and refused to take him along, and Dandy was without a job.

As usual, Halsted was gone for the summer. Dandy threw himself on the mercy of Winford Smith, Hurd's replacement as hospital director. Smith took pity on Dandy, and provided room and board for him, saying, "Sometime during the next year you will probably find out from Doctor Halsted what your status really is." It hadn't taken Smith very long to figure out how Halsted operated.

Dandy set to work in the lab and in short order produced a monumental piece of work. He was interested in the nature of cerebrospinal fluid, the liquid that bathes the brain and spinal cord. Hydrocephalus, originally meaning "water on the brain," actually refers to the production or accumulation of excessive amounts of cerebrospinal fluid. Within the skull the cerebrospinal fluid, or CSF, circulates around the brain in the subarachnoid space, where it floats the brain and acts as a shock absorber. The fluid circulates through the ventricles within the brain, and equalizes pressure between the brain and spinal cord. Hydrocephalus in children can cause, among other symptoms, enlargement of the not-yet-fused skull. In adults, all manner of symptoms from vomiting and dizziness to mental retardation and convulsions are associated with the condition.

Of particular interest to Dandy was the cause of hydrocephalus, and with Kenneth Blackfan, a resident in pediatrics, he was the first to produce hydrocephalus in experimental animals. Dandy developed a method to block free communication between the third and fourth ventricles by occluding the aqueduct of Sylvius, an anatomical canal between the ventricles, and hence circulation of CSF to the subarachnoid space. The resulting hydrocephalus suggested that little or no CSF was absorbed through the ventricles. If it could be absorbed, hydrocephalus would not result from blocking the aqueduct. Dandy then tested the theory by injecting the dye phenolsulfonphthalein into the ventricles of nonhydrocephalic patients. Within minutes the dye appeared in the CSF and urine. Using the same test in patients with hydrocephalus secondary to a blocked Aqueduct of Sylvius, the appearance of the dye was delayed for hours. Dandy had devised a test for blockage of the aqueduct and explained many of the mysteries of CSF absorption. Subsequently, Dandy and others performed studies confirming his findings.

Halsted said, "Dandy will never do anything equal to this again. Few men make more than one great contribution to medicine."

He was wrong.

If one needs to be reminded how very much an infant neurosurgery was at the time, consider that when Harvey Cushing left for Boston in 1912, Halsted replaced him as neurosurgeon with the resident George Heuer, who had risen to the position only the previous year. Heuer's experience was limited to a year as Cushing's assistant. Dandy worked with Heuer in the clinical practice of neurosurgery and continued his laboratory investigations on his own. From 1916 to 1918, Dandy was Halsted's resident. During that time he continued working in neurosurgery and became increasingly critical of the policy of decompressing the brain for palliation alone. Cushing had popularized the procedure and with his extraordinary care, made it easy to perform. Dandy thought there had to be a better way. Brain tumors, he felt, should be identified and removed like any other cancer. Anything less was doing the patient a disservice. But localizing the site of brain tumors was virtually impossible unless specific symptoms spelled out their site, or they were encountered upon opening the skull. In most cases the symptoms were only those of increased intracranial pressure. Headache, seizure, and loss of consciousness did nothing to locate the site of the tumor.

The eureka moment occurred when Dandy was looking at the chest X-ray of a patient undergoing an abdominal catastrophe. He could see at the top of the film that the liver was separated from the diaphragm by a layer of gas due to the intestinal perforation. The free air had clearly outlined the surrounding organs. Dandy began injecting air into the spinal column and the ventricles of the brain, and taking X-rays of the result. The injected air was less dense than cerebrospinal fluid and would show a blockage of the flow or a change in the position of the ventricles. This helped localize the space-occupying mass in the silent areas of the brain. If brain tumors could be localized, they could be removed earlier, and the patient offered a chance for cure rather than only palliation.

Dandy's development of pneumo-ventriculography was probably the greatest single advance ever made in neurosurgery. Halsted was happy to note that Dandy had done it again. In 1920, he wrote, "I know of no contribution to surgery since the opening of the Johns Hopkins Hospital which might rank with Dandy's . . . already it has made possible the precise location of cerebral tumors, the situation of which was not even suspected by competent men." Not a statement that would please Cushing.

Publication of the technique brought surgeons flocking, once again, to Johns Hopkins, this time to Dandy's operating room. Many of the visitors informed the Baltimore press of their presence in the hope of having the item picked up by their hometown papers. The publicity stunt was not lost on Halsted, who popped his head into Dandy's operating room, and was told what the neurosurgeon proposed to do. Halsted nodded and said, "Dandy, that's fine. If you hurry you can get it in the afternoon papers."

The animosity between Cushing and Dandy accelerated with Dandy's increased prominence. Cushing, the diminutive aesthete, had little time for anything but his work. Dandy was a larger man, round-faced and thick-waisted, with an intense personality. He was as devoted to his family as he was to his work, deriving great joy from both. He rarely attended medical meetings, believing they were social gatherings, and wasted time. A well-prepared, master technician, Dandy was fearless in expanding the boundaries of neurosurgery, often distressing or angering others along the way. In describing complicated and dangerous techniques, Dandy often wrote, "In safe hands this is a very safe procedure," which did little to win friends.

The feud was memorialized in irate letters from Cushing, and considerable grumbling on both sides, but a mutual admiration persisted amidst the rivalry. Cushing accused Dandy of being ill mannered, and of slighting him. Dandy intended from the beginning to be the best, not second best after Cushing. Though he felt no need for his approval, he was deeply hurt by Cushing's vitriol.

Dandy went on to make many memorable scientific and clinical contributions. In 1911, he addressed a more common ailment when he discovered the cause of what we now call a slipped disc, and devised the first treatment for it. Prior to Dandy, there had been no knowledge of the true nature of the spinal cord "tumor" that caused the symptoms bundled into the term *sciatica*.

Dandy's diagnostic skills were such that after yet another intuitive success, a neurologist who had been observing the phenomenon was driven to say, "Doctor, I think God must whisper in that man's ear."

Halsted was devoted to Dandy and had the highest regard for his abilities, but was continually frustrated by his inability to write a comprehensible paper. Halsted, who was anything but a gifted writer himself, made the issue a personal project. Books, poems, and a private English teacher could do nothing to turn the tide. Eventually, Halsted gave up and edited many of Dandy's early papers himself.

When Cushing made plans to leave for Harvard, Halsted wished him well. When Dandy was offered the professorship at the University of Cincinnati, Halsted did not want him to leave and suggested Heuer, Reid, or Carter in his stead.

Dandy was brilliant, loyal, hardworking, and arguably the most important neurosurgeon in the world. He spent his entire career at Johns Hopkins, but during Halsted's lifetime he never rose above the rank of associate professor of surgery. At Johns Hopkins there was only one professor of surgery.

* * *

GEORGE HEUER WAS RESIDENT from 1911 to 1914. He stayed on as Halsted's assistant and was in charge of neurosurgery until 1922, when he left to become professor of surgery at Cincinnati. During these formative years of his career he may have became closer to The Professor than any previous resident. For most of that decade, Heuer, Mont Reid, and Richard Follis were the surgery team. William Stevenson Baer led orthopedic surgery, Hugh Young urology, and Sam Crowe otolaryngology. Joe Bloodgood ran surgical pathology, and J. M. T. Finney was the reliable backbone of the department, as he had been since the hospital opened.

Heuer, like Dandy and Crowe, was seduced by Cushing and became his special assistant, thereby relinquishing his position as assistant resident on the surgery service. In 1909, when he hoped to return as assistant resident, there were no openings. Henry Hurd was still director of the hospital. In his usual grumpy fashion, he always saw to the welfare of the residents, and allowed Heuer to live at the hospital until an opening materialized on Halsted's staff. Working with Cushing never turned out the way one had envisioned.

CHAPTER THIRTY-FOUR

The World Changes

FRANKLIN P. MALL WAS a small man. Short, fine boned, and ascetic looking, he had light brown hair that he wore parted on the left and a faraway gaze. Neither his hair nor his bushy mustache appeared tamed, and he always looked younger than his years. He was a physician who didn't practice medicine, an anatomy teacher who refused to demonstrate anatomy to his students, perhaps the foremost proponent of medical science at the expense of clinical medicine, and the leading embryologist of his day. Mall's inquiring mind and soaring intellect made him one of the most celebrated of medical researchers, and his impatient and dismissive nature made him the most universally disliked professor on the faculty of The Johns Hopkins University School of Medicine.

Mall required junior lecturers to teach his courses, and survived generations of complaints about his acid tongue, simply because he was too valuable an asset to shed. The scope of his work was vast, and despite being thought of otherwise, he nurtured intellectual discourse and helped fellow researchers wherever he could. In addition to holding the chair of anatomy at Hopkins, he was the director of the embryological department of the Carnegie Institution in Washington. But Mall was not widely known beyond the most exalted scientific circles. His work was the bedrock of basic science, and far too arcane to make him a hero of the average physician. He was unknown to the lay public.

Mall, the prodigy, had studied embryology and pathology in Germany and was 23 years old when he arrived at the old pathological laboratory as Welch's first fellow. Halsted had already done a great deal, and certainly had been through a lot, when he arrived in December 1886. They were thrown together in the large south room at the Pathological, where it was impossible to be unaware of what was being done at the next bench. Halsted quickly found that Mall's work on the intestinal submucosa could have great implication in his work on intestinal anastomosis. They joined forces, lunched together in the gritty back room of the old beer saloon across from the Pathological, and enjoyed each other's company.

They were an intense pair. Both were fond of joking at the expense of others, and neither was particularly gracious on the receiving end. Once, in the saloon, after Halsted passed some amusing remark, the barman passed his dirty hand over the seated Halsted's bald head and said, *"Du hast deine Haare nicht umsonst verloren."* (You are bald for good reason.) In what his residents would soon recognize as the first sign of his anger, Halsted's neck and ears got red. Then his face flushed, and everyone but he had a good laugh.

These days Halsted lunched on milk, bread and butter, and cold meat, taken alone in his office on the top floor of the surgical building. When he found himself in the hospital staff dining room, he joined the table kept for the department heads and senior staff. But despite the fact that he chose to sit with his colleagues, he was uncomfortable in large groups and was always just on the outside of the friendly laughter—not at all like the quick wit Mall knew him to be.

Their early work on the submucosa was well received, and their friendship blossomed. Both were regular diners with the initial, little group at the Maryland Club, and spent a great deal of their time together during the early years. When both men married, their relationship continued in the laboratory, at lunch and the occasional dinner, and in regular Sunday visits to Halsted's home. Neither Mrs. Mall nor Mrs. Halsted was included in the socializing.

Mall had suffered with indigestion for years, but complaints of bloating and heartburn were far too common to be taken seriously. In late October 1917, he developed severe abdominal pain. His skin and eyes became yellow with jaundice, there was bile in his urine, and he was vomiting and hiccoughing uncontrollably. A low-grade fever developed, and his white count jumped to 24,000. The diagnosis of acute cholecystitis, with gallstones blocking the common bile duct, was obvious.

Halsted had just returned from his long summer holiday, and Finney, who was the ideal surgeon for the case, was away on his. No one dared tell Halsted he was second choice, nor call Finney back from vacation. On October 28, Halsted operated, assisted by Richard Follis. He found what he had expected: a gallbladder full of pus, stones, and gravel, much like the findings at his mother's operation. It was a recurring theme in his life.

Bile and pus drained from the tube in Mall's common duct, but the symptoms didn't abate. Mall continued to do so poorly that Halsted operated again on November 7. More stones were found in the duct, and another lodged in the entrance to the duodenum, which required the intestine to be opened, and resulted in peritonitis.

In April of that year, America had joined the war that had been raging in Western Europe for nearly three years. The celebrated surgeon Alexis Carrel, of the Rockefeller Institute, had recently returned from the front. Carrel had been treating war wounds with an irrigating technique. Utilizing an infusion apparatus he pumped Dakin's solution into the wound. Carrel claimed great success in sterilizing wounds thoroughly enough to allow the growth of new blood vessels in the form of granulation tissue to invade the area and begin the process of healing. Surgeons in the hospitals of the British Expeditionary Force conducted a six-month field experiment and confirmed

Carrel's results. The technique was hailed as a great advance. Coverage in both medical journals and the lay press, including the *New York Times,* hailed the achievement.

Halsted, at a loss for something to help Mall combat the infection, dispatched his assistant resident, Adrian Taylor, to the Rockefeller Institute, in New York. Halsted had a good relationship with Carrel, and instructed Taylor to question him about the use of the Carrel-Dakin treatment in an open abdominal infection. It is unclear why Halsted did not telephone Carrel himself and get the information firsthand, although the trip very likely also involved procuring the solution and observing the apparatus at work. Carrel advised Taylor that it would be safe to use in the abdomen and taught him the elaborate technique.

The rubber tubes were installed in Mall's abdomen, and a flushing routine was begun using Dakin's solution, which is a neutral 0.5 percent hypochlorite of soda—essentially, Clorox. The irrigations continued over the following week, closely overseen by Halsted. In the particularly bitter November week, he arrived by taxicab several times each day, formally dressed as always, and visited with Mall. He sat by Mall's bedside for hours and thought through the problem as his friend weakened. The Carrel-Dakin's flush eroded Mall's duodenum, and it perforated in several places. Mall lost a great deal of fluid and electrolytes as gastric juices and bile poured out of his intestine. The infection worsened when fecal contents from the perforations poured into his abdomen.

Franklin P. Mall died at The Johns Hopkins Hospital on November 17, 1917. He was 55 years old. Halsted blamed himself for the loss of his friend, but in truth, events were stacked against the anatomist, and his death was hastened by what was thought to be the newest in scientific treatments.

Carrel's casual approval of the intraperitoneal use of the caustic agent had been wrong. Others had similar experiences with Dakin's eroding the pleural lining of the lungs and causing fistulae, and it had become clear that the full ramifications of its use were yet to be known. Those who bore witness to the acceleration of Mall's free fall held Carrel in very low esteem. Halsted was never heard to blame the French/American surgeon. In conversations with others touching on Mall's death, Halsted limited himself to how much he missed his friend. He never openly disparaged Carrel, and though he never mentioned the incident, he wrote in the *Journal of the American Medical Association,* "I would warn against the use of Dakin's solution in so fresh a sinus lined with intestine."

Halsted returned to work, but an important link connecting him with Johns Hopkins had been lost. He wrote Councilman, at Harvard, "I shall never cease to mourn the death of the incomparable Mall." Only Welch and Councilman remained from the original group at the Pathological, and Halsted's correspondence with the latter became more poignant, but always slyly amusing. In one letter, he wrote, "I confess to having been not a little apprehensive lest the heat and insects of the equator might give a twist to your peerless disposition. [Councilman had planned a trip to the Amazon.] You say that inasmuch as a trained nurse is to be in the party you are not looking for trouble. Evidently you are not a clinician."

As he grew older, Halsted had become an even more prolific letter writer, and increasingly employed uncommon words. When he wrote, his favored *Century Dictionary* was always open on his desk. His medical prose was dense and the ten-dollar words made it even less enjoyable to read. Councilman wrote, "I find words which to me are new but which I suppose are commonplace in your conversation with the intellectual giants around you. For instance, 'temerous' which is fine, but I think you are the only one who has ever used it."

Tegmen, deligate, and *defract* found their way into his scientific papers. Halsted kept a notebook of unusual words and phrases and their derivations. After he created new medical terms to describe a procedure, he feigned horror that others were unfamiliar with them. He responded to German surgeons questioning the meaning of the term *ultraligation,* used in his paper on thyroid surgery, "Ligation of the thyroid artery at a point beyond that at which the branch to the parathyroid glands is given off." Who knew?

Some may have found this an annoying affectation, or perhaps deliberate obfuscation. Councilman certainly found it amusing. It was not a late folly, for Halsted's interest in etymology was long-standing. He and Caroline often discussed the derivation of words over dinner. And some of the pranks the "old gang" at the Maryland Club played on one another were word games, occasionally even based on classical Latin.

Obsessed with words, Halsted worked and reworked his scientific papers until they conveyed precisely what he wished his message to be, and encouraged the use of what he believed to be the single most critical word for scientific discourse: "If you put 'perhaps' before a statement and the statement turns out to be true, you will get credit for making it; if it turns out to be false you will not be blamed."

As Halsted considered his own mortality, he remained convinced that he would perish at 70, of gallbladder disease. With so much yet to be done, he focused his energies once again on the unsolved problems of intestinal anastomosis, aneurysm, exophthalmic goiter, and the swelling, or lymphedema, of the arm after radical breast surgery, which he called elephantiasis chirugica. He compared it to other forms of massive swelling of the extremity, which he believed to be caused by infection; after radical breast surgery, he believed the "dead space" created in the axilla filled with fluid and provided a perfect environment for infection to thrive. The operation was modified to eliminate the dead space and the medium for bacterial growth. This was largely successful, though even in the antibiotic era lymphedema was not totally eliminated.

In 1914, Halsted published his 650 cases of exophthalmic goiter. The bloody operation was always a test for the surgeon, and one he continued to perform. As his experience increased, he set about the daunting task of compiling the definitive monograph on the subject.

In 1915, he devised a method for draining the common bile duct through the stump of the cystic duct. The technique allowed closure of the common bile duct, and prevented the debilitating weakness caused by constant loss of bile. The first application of his innovation took place in March 1917. It was successful in every way, and the patient had a quick and uneventful recovery. Halsted was impressed, and advised, but did not insist upon, its adoption by his staff, which would come to have personal implications.

* * *

IN APRIL OF 1917, America declared war on Germany and joined the campaign which had been raging in Western Europe for nearly three years. The first troops of the American Expeditionary Force had shipped out for France in June 1917. By the following July there were more than a million American soldiers in Europe, and by November, the last month of hostilities, the number had doubled to two million men.

The rapid deployment of large numbers of troops into the escalating fight required massive medical and surgical support. To meet the need, many of the leading American hospitals mobilized their staffs and manned A.E.F. base hospitals as dedicated units. Base Hospital #18 was the Johns Hopkins Unit. With American casualties amounting to more than 300,000 dead and wounded, there was a great deal to do. Doctors and nurses around the country put their careers on hold to accept military commissions. The mobilization of the Hopkins unit, while generally applauded, and necessary, greatly reduced the manpower remaining at the hospital. Thirty-two Johns Hopkins medical students volunteered as well. Thirty of them had completed three years of medical school, and would earn their MD degrees for their service. The other two students had completed only two years, one of whom was the eldest son of J. M. T. Finney.

Volunteer Baltimore women made dressings, gowns, sheets, pillowcases, and towels, and local businessmen contributed $30,000 to equip the unit. In October, Base Hospital #18 took over a 1,000-bed hospital from the French. The surgical unit distinguished itself mightily by working night and day through those horrible final two months of the war.

Halsted was 65. Too old and infirm to serve overseas, he picked up the pace of his work at home, resuming a more arduous teaching and surgical schedule. He corresponded with many of the Hopkins men in the service, particularly his trusted assistant George Heuer, often letting him know how much he was missed and needed. In a letter dated April 29, 1918, he added the sentiment many of those stateside shared: "I fancy that by the time you return to America operative surgery will have no more thrills for you."

Heuer commanded the surgical unit of Base Hospital #18, and Baer was an orthopedic consultant to the A.E.F. Both men distinguished themselves at war and returned with experience that translated well to civilian service. Heuer, whose primary interest had been neurosurgery, became a leading expert in the treatment of penetrating chest wounds and trauma.

HUGH HAMPTON YOUNG, mustered as a colonel, was tapped by General John Pershing to command the urological unit of the A.E.F. and became intimately involved in public health measures. Before the advent of antibiotics, venereal diseases spread rampantly and plagued the armies. Young's knowledge, his particular interest in bacteriology, and his intense level of organization contributed greatly to the control and treatment of these diseases.

Baer, who founded the orthopedic department at Hopkins, rediscovered an efficient old treatment for cleaning chronic open wounds: maggots. Having examined two starving, wounded soldiers, Baer was thoroughly disgusted to see their week-old wounds crawling with maggots. Sweeping the worms away, he found the wound lined with clean granulation tissue, and healing. The method for cleaning wounds followed him home, but other more aesthetically acceptable methods of treatment, such as the Carrel-Dakin's irrigation, won the day.

Finney had assumed a position of great importance as a colonel and chief surgical consultant to the A.E.F. He had known President Woodrow Wilson for years, both as his doctor and as a member of the board of trustees of Princeton. General Pershing was aware of the connection and sent Finney from his assignment in France to Washington, D.C., to convince the president to choose the proper man as surgeon general at a critical moment for the army. Wilson heeded his doctor's advice, and Finney's stock with Pershing rose sharply.

Late in the horrible war, Finney shared a lunch and reminiscences with an old Hopkins friend, John McCrae, who died in a battlefield hospital shortly thereafter. McCrae was best known for his haunting poem,

In Flanders fields the poppies blow
Between the crosses, row on row,
That mark our place; and in the sky
The larks, still bravely singing, fly
Scarce heard amid the guns below.
We are the dead. Short days ago
We lived, felt dawn, saw sunset glow,
Loved and were loved, and now we lie
In Flanders fields.
Take up our quarrel with the foe:
To your firm failing hands we throw
The torch; be yours to hold it high.
If ye break faith with us who die
We shall not sleep, though poppies grow
In Flanders fields.

CHAPTER THIRTY-FIVE

"My Dear Miss Bessie"

I N NOVEMBER 1918, the war was winding down. Halsted, at 66 years old, was tired. He had endured two busy and uncomfortable years at a stage of his life when he should have been more at his ease. European travel had been impossible since the outbreak of hostilities in 1914. Though he and Caroline fully supported the war effort, he still had many close friends in the German scientific community. Contact was difficult, but he did what he could to soften the economic hardships inflicted on them toward the end of the war. Coping with the manpower shortage at the hospital was trying, but the Hopkins unit was doing its duty and was a source of pride to those remaining behind. Heuer, who had been carrying so much of the surgical and teaching burden of the department, would not return until the spring, but at least the end was in sight.

As weighty events were unfolding overseas, the enigmatic Halsted was beginning a relationship with Elizabeth Randall, a woman 40 years his junior. Well accustomed to hiding private matters, Halsted kept no diary, sought no confidants, and quietly carried out a relationship that had all the earmarks of youthful romance. Whether the relationship was consummated, or if such was even contemplated, is unknown. The story, patched together from a series of letters

Halsted wrote to the young woman, reveals a gentle, touching, and often humorous flirtation.

Elizabeth started the exchange, which spans a period of three years. The flirtatious letters speak only Halsted's words. Elizabeth's letters to him have not been found, but from his responses one can easily infer a mutual infatuation first communicated by her. Halsted and Elizabeth Randall seem to have known each other through Baltimore social circles. In his initial letter, in response to the first from her, he wrote:

My Dear Miss Bessie,

I am charmed by your letter which even in its expurgated form is much too 'lurid' for my deserving, but not 'fur mein Fahigkeit,' respective 'geraumigkeit zu verschlucken,' which, as young ladies so well know, is the infinite capacity of old men to swallow the lurid words of a young woman.

Wonderfully distressed to hear of the 'malade' and the boiling oil and fearing you may succumb before Christmas I am sending the enclosed card and nervously scanning the obituary notice columns . . .

Faithfully Yours,
William Halsted.

Three weeks later, after receiving a gift from Elizabeth before she was meant to go to France with the Red Cross, to join Base Hospital #18, he wrote, "Verily only a trained psychiatrist could have derived from such meager data that copious tears were flowing on the corner of Eutaw Place and Dolphin Street."

And then a telegram, sent to her at the Vanderbilt Hotel in New York, as she waited for deployment, said, "Letter follows on recovery of equilibrium sad case of love at first sight please consult alienist abroad in my behalf and advise W.S. Halsted."

Base Hospital #18 was disbanded before her departure, and Elizabeth served the Red Cross at a base in New Jersey. When she was about to return to Baltimore, Elizabeth invited Halsted for a drive in the country. He accepted, and wrote to suggest she invite her father as chaperone.

Other plans were made and letters and notes passed, and from the content it seems likely that the ten surviving letters were merely representative of the correspondence. The true nature of the relationship remains unknown, but an undated letter speaks for itself: "Please picture me every morning at eight o'clock, unchaperoned awaiting your arrival and preparing, flinging consequences to the winds, to float southwards on and on . . . Ever your devoted adorer."

The last of his letters was written some eight months before she married Harry Slack Jr., an otolaryngologist who had trained under Sam Crowe. It was sent from High Hampton on September 12, 1921, when Elizabeth had already begun seeing her future husband. The initial reference in the letter is unexplained, but the tone is obvious.

I carry it around with me everywhere—on fishing excursions, on mountain trails, on moonlight stills through "panthertown," to Sunday school and the dahlia garden. I wonder if the Paris creations in which you are presumably soaring can be so becoming and enticingly lovely as the pink costume you wore the afternoon you so graciously entertained my friends, the Leriches from Lyon, and my adored assistant G.J.H.—if he leaves us I shall be desolated and altogether inconsolable except in the delicious and fleeting moments of Cloud–Capped. (The Randall family estate)

* * *

IN THE CONSTANT company of illness and discomfort, Halsted began to spend more time at home. He was increasingly convinced that the pain he was experiencing in his chest and abdomen was caused by angina pectoris, due to inadequate oxygenated blood supply to the heart muscle. The usual cause of angina is progressive occlusion of the coronary vessels by cholesterol plaques, then called arteriosclerosis. In most instances the tipping point is exercise, when the heart muscle requires more oxygen than the compromised coronary arteries can deliver. Although the pain that drove him from the operating room was never definitively diagnosed as anginal, some element of it may well have been. The electrocardiogram, universally relied upon for diagnosis, was not yet invented, and there is no evidence of Halsted being treated with nitroglycerine, which had been available for the relief of the symptoms of angina since 1879. Morphine and rest could mask the pain and relieve the symptoms in moderate cases, and one might deduce this to have been his choice of action.

In the winter of 1919, he was confined to the house for two months, with severe bronchitis. Packets of Pall Mall cigarettes were available beside him wherever Halsted worked. A cigarette burned in one of his disposable, white holders for the solitary hours of the day, as he read and wrote. There is little doubt that his heavy cigarette consumption contributed greatly to his pulmonary problems and perhaps his chest pain as well, but he did not abandon the habit. The chest and abdominal pain became something of an obsession. He was certain that each attack would be his last. And then a particularly severe attack was surprisingly followed by jaundice, and the rules changed.

Halsted consulted with Dr. Thomas Boggs, who advised him of what he already knew. He had gallbladder disease, just like his mother and other relatives before him. He very likely had a stone blocking his common duct, and would need surgery. It was not what Halsted wanted to hear, but it was preferable to angina.

HE PUT OFF THE fateful day as long as he could. By spring, when he was well enough to travel, he went directly to High Hampton, forsaking the unaccompanied trips that had been so much a part of his routine.

By late August he once again felt the full fury of gallbladder disease, suffering painful bouts of colic from stones in the common bile duct. This time the great diagnostician needed no one to identify the source of his distress. It was his fate as he had envisioned it, and he immediately telegraphed Johns Hopkins to make preparations for his surgery. Halsted was admitted to the hospital on September 1. At the time of admission his temperature and pulse were normal, but his blood pressure was significantly elevated at 170/100, accounting for the florid complexion so often ascribed to his healthy appearance.

Finney was on vacation, and Richard Follis performed the surgery. Follis had followed Mitchell as resident, and was in private practice in Baltimore as well as on the staff at Hopkins. At operation the gallbladder, which was full of stones and gravel, was removed, and a single large stone was found obstructing the common duct.

Halsted had suggested that Follis employ his newly devised method of draining bile via the stump of the cystic duct, which had resulted in a remarkably smooth course for the patient for whom it was employed. Unfortunately, Halsted's cystic duct was located in an anomalous and inaccessible position, behind the common duct, and Follis felt drainage would be best carried out through a tube placed in the rent in the common duct. The tube was brought out through the skin, surrounded by six rubber cigarette drains. Within 48 hours after surgery bile began pouring out through the drainage tube, taking with it essential electrolytes and digestive enzymes. On the sixth day the tube was removed, but enormous volumes of bile continued to drain from the sinus tract.

Halsted suffered. Food and drink repelled him. He lost weight rapidly, and became weak and debilitated. Fearing for his life, the surgeons treated him with 300 cubic centimeters of salt solution by rectum every six hours to maintain his body fluids. Mont Reid led the group of doctors who stood vigil at his bedside and tried to force The Professor to eat.

The sinus tract gradually dried up, the flow of bile returned to the intestine, where it belonged, and the crisis was over. With that, Halsted's appetite returned with a vengeance. His attitude improved, and he soon began to write notes to friends and contemplate his next meal. The delight of eating, talking about eating, and savoring every delicious bite thoroughly occupied the latter days of his convalescence. Having personally experienced the ravages of the uncontrolled loss of biliary secretions, Halsted ordered his staff to institute closure of the common duct and utilize cystic duct drainage whenever possible.

He left the hospital on October 19. By January 1920, he was well enough to work, but the four-month illness had extracted its toll. The ferocious, indefinable energy of his personality was muted, his steely gaze had softened, and Halsted looked older. Prominent veins and gnarled fingers had transformed the large, powerful hands, and the slight stoop in his walk had become more pronounced. He had lost weight, and his face appeared pained even when it was not. Halsted became increasingly philosophical. He operated occasionally, worked in the lab, wrote his papers, and even managed to attend medical meetings in the spring. He spent the summer of 1920 happily in the country, returning to work in October as usual.

That December, Halsted was incapacitated with gastritis, generalized abdominal pain, and nausea. Again acting as his own physician, he diagnosed pancreatitis, secondary to obstruction of the pancreatic duct by a gallstone. This time he was correct, but happily the symptoms abated, and he resumed work. It was a remarkably productive period in which he produced two lengthy monographs, *The Operative Story of Goitre* and *Ligations of the Left Subclavian Artery in Its First Portion*. Both appeared in 1920 and were very well received, as was his paper on lymphangitis. In the lab he continued the decades-old struggle to develop a clean technique for intestinal anastomosis, coming up with several complicated and not wholly satisfactory solutions.

Halsted's strength never fully returned. The summer of 1921 was passed pleasantly with family and friends at High Hampton, but upon returning in October he suffered a series of painful skin infections, severe gastroenteritis, and then, in November, episodic symptoms of biliary colic returned. In the weeks between attacks he managed to work, but the healthy intervals became shorter. His declining health was as evident to his colleagues as it was to Halsted, and his urge to complete his work was met by an equal desire by those he touched to pay proper homage to him. Few had had the opportunity to speak of his significance to surgery and his influence on their lives. It was not something Halsted encouraged, and his imperious demeanor had forced even those with the warmest feelings for him to keep their proper distance. His work was its own reward. Honors and accolades were not necessary for The Professor's self-esteem, and he shunned them whenever he could.

But in April 1922, a gold medal had been struck by the National Dental Association "In recognition of his original researches and discoveries upon which the technique of local and neuroregional anesthesia in oral and dental surgery now rests." A grand dinner to present the award was thrown in Halsted's honor by the Maryland State Dental Association. Strawberries, lobster thermidor, breast of chicken, and Virginia ham were served. Tables were supplied with several brands of cigarettes, including Halsted's favored Pall Mall. Among the many speakers were Welch, Finney, Barker, and Frank Goodnow, the third president of The Johns Hopkins University.[1] Those close to Halsted threw reserve to the wind. They spoke freely of his great insight and surgical leadership, and

---

1 Goodnow tried to recruit Nobel Prize winner Albert Einstein to teach at Hopkins in 1927. The offer of $10,000 for the academic year was gratefully declined by Einstein, who said the sum was more money than he was worth. Einstein claimed difficulties in traveling to America and health concerns, neither of which stopped him from moving to Princeton to escape the Nazis. The sum of $10,000 was also the salary for "full-time" medical professors at Hopkins in 1913.

all he had done to alleviate suffering and advance medical science. Few had ever spoken of his accomplishments to his face, and perhaps had ever been forced to step back from years of daily interaction and assess the full impact of the odd giant in their midst.

Rudolph Matas, professor of surgery at Tulane University and the leading surgeon in New Orleans, shared many of Halsted's professional interests, including thyroid and aneurysm surgery. He was a student of surgical history, fully understood Halsted's role in creating modern surgery, and held The Professor in the highest esteem. They corresponded often, and Matas was a frequent visitor to Baltimore. On one such visit, Halsted operated on Matas at his home on Eutaw Place. Halsted, as usual, was exceptionally solicitous of his guest, and his concern made an indelible impression on Matas: "As I was convalescing in his home I learned to love the sound of his cautious footsteps as he approached my room late at night to assure himself of my comfort . . ."

It was Matas who made public his friend's enormous contribution and clear primacy in the discovery of local and regional anesthesia. Many in both dental surgery and general surgery had no clear knowledge of the origins, and the terrible cost, of local anesthesia, and Halsted had been reticent to tell the whole story. The wounds he incurred remained open 37 years later.

To Matas, Halsted wrote, "You are indeed a sturdy friend. I wrote very little on the subject of my cocaine experiments which for a year were carried on vigorously. Then my health gave way and for more than a year I was incapacitated, and thereafter for two years worked in the Pathological Laboratory of Dr. Welch at the Johns Hopkins. Thus my misfortune has its bright side as well as its gloomy side."

After the dinner he wrote Matas again: "My dear friend: How can I ever express my gratitude to you for this act of unparalleled kindness . . . Not a wink of sleep did I get during the night of Saturday—I was too exhilarated for repose. Once before in my life I was kept awake by great happiness—this was the night I passed successfully the examination for Bellevue Hospital in 1876. Then it was in contemplation of the future, now in reflection upon the good fortune which led to our friendship."

Halsted deserved the nation's appreciation for a contribution that had greatly relieved suffering and transformed a profession. The public acknowledgment was that much sweeter for coming through no lobbying, chest thumping, or hinting on the part of the recipient, all of which would have been unconscionably out of character.

For the first time in his life, Halsted felt unabashed joy at being celebrated, but he had not exorcised the demon, and time was running out.

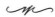

CHAPTER THIRTY-SIX

The Final Illness

HALSTED DID NOT LEAVE for High Hampton that year until mid-June. Attacks were now coming daily, and he was loath to leave Baltimore. When the frequency abated he chanced to make the trip, and for some weeks he felt better. On August 3, he responded to Welch's request for biographical material. His excuse for not having written sooner was "a furuncle on my firmament." On August 9, pain and jaundice returned. This time the diagnosis was not at all in doubt. For the next ten days he suffered severe chills, fever, nausea, and vomiting, and finally he telegraphed that he was returning to Baltimore. As luck would have it, Finney was once again out of town. Halsted requested that two of his favorite former residents, George Heuer and Mont Reid, rush to Baltimore for his surgery. Both men had been in Cincinnati, where Heuer had recently become professor of surgery.

On August 23, after a long, hot, and very uncomfortable trip, the Halsteds arrived at The Johns Hopkins Hospital. Halsted was yellow-green in color, dehydrated from vomiting and not eating, and clearly very ill. Rienhoff and Carter were the residents in charge of the ward when he arrived, and Reid immediately had them begin rehydrating their patient with large volumes of salt solution injected under the skin. After 12 hours of this therapy, his rapid pulse rate decreased and his kidneys began to function.

Caroline Halsted understood the gravity of the situation and spent much of each day at her husband's bedside. During her moments at home she dispatched a steady stream of status reports in the form of short letters dictated to one of Halsted's secretaries.

On August 25, George Heuer, assisted by Reid and Rienhoff, operated on his mentor. This time a single stone was found and removed from the common bile duct. Drainage was carried out through a tube in the stump of the cystic duct, by the method Halsted described. The incision in the common duct was carefully sutured closed, and two drains were placed alongside the tube from the cystic duct. By all obvious measures the operation was a success. Halsted's pulse and temperature returned to normal, and on August 26, he sent a message to Welch, in Atlantic City, that his condition was "very satisfactory."

Reid and Heuer nursed The Professor night and day. On August 29, Halsted passed a very uncomfortable night and was unable to hold down food. On August 30, which was the fourth postoperative day, he was able to eat oatmeal, cantaloupe, and tea, and retain all he had eaten. His condition remained weak but stable. Then, on September 3, he suddenly vomited a large quantity of blood and began to pass black, bloody-tarry stools. He was bleeding into his digestive tract. The bleeding continued over the following days, and blood transfusions were obtained from several donors, including Mont Reid. When the frustrated Rienhoff could find no more veins for the transfusions, Halsted, moribund but unchanged, calmly asked if he had ever considered putting the needle into the brachial artery. The idea was a brilliant revelation to the young Rienhoff, but The Professor had performed the same arterial puncture for lamp gas poisoning more than 40 years before.

On September 5, Caroline telegraphed precisely the same short, formal message to Halsted's sisters Bertha and Minnie, his brother Richard, and his nephew W. Halsted Van der Poel:

Doctors consider Dr. Halsted's condition very critical.
Caroline Halsted

Over the next four days, Halsted weakened further. He became feverish and developed lobar pneumonia, and an already critical course rapidly accelerated downhill. On September 7, 1922, on his surgical ward at The Johns Hopkins Hospital, William Stewart Halsted died.

CHAPTER THIRTY-SEVEN

Afterward

W ITH A FULL RESERVE of scientific detachment, Mont Reid and William Rienhoff attended the autopsy on the body of William S. Halsted, in the dead house of The Johns Hopkins Hospital. Examination of the internal organs revealed a well-healed incision in the common bile duct. The entire small intestine, from pylorus to ileocecal valve, was cherry red with blood under the mucosa. There was no evidence of abdominal infection. A pint of turbid fluid was found in the chest cavity and pleurisy surrounded the right upper lobe of the lungs, which had been consolidated by pneumonia. There was severe arteriosclerosis, especially in the coronary arteries.

Halsted had brought with him, on his final admission to the hospital, a daily record of the dilute morphine solution he had been taking for pain during the months of July and August. The amounts charted were unusually small, typically no more than ten milligrams in 24 hours—a remarkable, and unlikely, dose for a man who had been using almost ten times that for more than 35 years. Halsted brought this dilute morphine solution to the hospital and it was administered by injection as he needed it. One suspects that either the "dilute" solution was not all that dilute or, as some postulated, he had finally broken the chokehold of his addiction. Had this been true, it would have been a properly dramatic conclusion to a battle of epic proportions.

Nothing was written to clarify the situation by the only two knowledgeable survivors, William Welch and Caroline Halsted, but Welch, on his deathbed, said in reference to cocaine:

> Although it has been widely reported that Halsted conquered his addiction, this is not entirely true. As long as he lived he would occasionally have a relapse and go back to the drug. He would always go out of town for this and when he returned he would come to me, very contrite and apologetic, to confess. He had an idea that I could tell what he had done. I couldn't, but I let him go on thinking so because I felt it was good for him to have somebody to talk it over with.

* * *

A FUNERAL SERVICE was held in the library at Eutaw Place on Saturday, September 9. Ranks of chairs were provided for the guests in the book-lined room. Everywhere, small tags of blue paper stood from the volumes like flags of tribute to the man who spent so much of his life among them. The Reverend Samuel Bushnell officiated. Among the four readings was a poem by W. K. Wallace, another member of the Yale class of '74.

William Stewart Halsted's body was cremated at the Loudon Park Cemetery in Baltimore, and his ashes were transported to the Greenwood Cemetery in Brooklyn. On September 17, they were interred in the large family plot overlooking New York Harbor. Caroline Halsted was exhausted from the month-long ordeal, and did not accompany her husband's remains on his final trip. She was not at all close with the Halsted siblings and did not wish to spend this sad time with them. Richard Halsted, Bertha Halsted Terry, Minnie Halsted Van der Poel, and their families attended the small ceremony. One of Bertha

Terry's sons-in-law was a clergyman, and he said a brief prayer, following which they adjourned to her apartment on Park Avenue. Only William Welch attended both services.

Caroline Halsted stayed in constant contact with Welch. On October 11, she wrote, "Dr. Halsted once said of them [his sisters], 'they have not the least grasp of what the word science means.' I was not going to interfere in any way with what they wanted. You know how people feel about their brother's wife." She was grateful for the help Welch had given her, and went on to tell him of Halsted's feelings for him:

> I sometimes wonder if you have any idea of the great love and admiration that Dr. Halsted had for you. He never mentioned you without praise. Most of us meet with adverse criticism from those who love us best but I never heard him say anything but what a true friend you have always been to him and how much you and all your work meant to the Johns Hopkins. He often said 'Welch is the Johns Hopkins. Without him it would be nothing. He has been the best friend to me that any man could ever be.'

Welch suggested a simple inscription for the flat, granite grave marker:

William Stewart Halsted, M.D.
September 23, 1852–September 7, 1922
Professor of Surgery in the Johns Hopkins University

Caroline Halsted was overwhelmed by the death of her husband, and frightened for her future. Despite a groundswell of support from her family, her few friends, and the senior hospital community, she was rudderless and depressed. Unable to fully comprehend her finances, Caroline busied herself preparing to sublet the house at 1201 Eutaw Place. On November 20, Sam Crowe called Dr. Boggs and asked him to look in on her. She had been complaining of a headache and fever, and Boggs's examination revealed a rapid, irregular pulse as well. He suggested hospitalization. Caroline refused. The following day her condition worsened, and against her wishes, Crowe took her by ambulance to The Johns Hopkins Hospital. There she was diagnosed with left upper lobe pneumonia. At noon on November 27, Caroline Halsted died, barely two months after her husband.

WILLIAM HALSTED'S DEATH was mourned throughout the surgical world. The Baltimore community felt the loss acutely at all levels of society. He was memorialized in a laudatory tribute in the *Baltimore Sun*, in which H. L. Mencken recognized his contributions and contradictions, his icy countenance and his humanity, what he had done to modernize surgery and how he stood out among the great men of Hopkins.

The American public was generally unaware of William Stewart Halsted. He was not as famous as Osler, Welch, or Cushing, nor as prolific as Kelly. He didn't make speeches or befriend the powerful, and the fruit of his seminal work would not fully ripen for at least a generation. At the outset of Halsted's career, fewer than a dozen doctors restricted their practices to the unsustainable, barbaric, and off-putting practice of surgery. Over his 33 years at the helm of surgery at Johns Hopkins, Halsted not only invented an entire surgical philosophy, he instituted a system to inculcate in surgeons this philosophy, which spawned several generations of the finest teachers of surgery in the world.

His goal was to train "not only surgeons but surgeons of the highest type, men who will stimulate the first youth of our country to devote their energies and their lives to raising the standards of surgical science." In this, his success is everywhere to be seen. Of Halsted's 17 residents, 12 became professors of surgery, associate professors, assistant professors, or surgeons in chief. Forty-six of his 55 assistant residents held academic titles, and the residents of his residents came to lead major surgical faculties throughout the country.

Direct and indirect Halsted disciples became professors of surgery at Johns Hopkins, Harvard, Yale, Cornell, the University of Virginia, Columbia, the University of Cincinnati, George Washington, Stanford, the University of California, and a host of other places. Halsted-descended clinical professors, associate professors, and assistant professors are too numerous and far flung to enumerate. Virtually every academically affiliated surgeon can trace his or her teachers, and his teacher's teachers, to William Stewart Halsted.

Far more impressive is the fact that every well-trained surgeon in the world is trained in a Halsted-type system, and all still live by the Halsted principles of surgery. Aseptic technique, gentle handling of tissue, scrupulous hemostasis, and tension-free, crush-free, and anatomically proper surgery are the rules. And they are Halsted's rules. Although "Halsted" is not a household name, every individual in America who undergoes successful surgery owes William Stewart Halsted a nod and a deep debt of gratitude.

Scrub suits and sterile gloves began in Halsted's operating room. His imagination, innovation, and diligence brought the first successful operations for breast cancer and hernia. He made local and spinal anesthesia a reality, and was a pioneering vascular surgeon, a pioneering endocrine surgeon, and the encouraging godfather of neurosurgery, urology, and otolaryngology. And he created the humane, scientific, experimental laboratory, where medical students learn surgery, surgeons learn new techniques, and lifesaving surgical advances are born.

Halsted was a complex and isolated man, forbidding and nurturing; rigid, proper, and secretive; compulsive and negligent; stimulating and reclusive; addicted and abstemious; oblivious and solicitous; and always concerned with advancing the science of surgery. For many it remained inconceivable that he was other than the mentor who led them into a new era. For his equals he remained a strange disciple of another calling. For the few who knew of his ability to navigate uncharted waters while the siren song rang in his ears, his journey was nothing short of heroic. If a single person can be considered the father of modern surgery, the only contender is William Stewart Halsted.

* * *

HERBERT HOOVER, THE 31st president of the United States, wearing striped trousers and cutaway coat, silk top hat in hand, strode to the podium at Continental Memorial Hall. Sixteen hundred scientists, physicians, and government officials filled the seats. Hoover stood erect, looked out over the audience, and said, "William Henry Welch is our greatest statesman . . . and has contributed more than any other American in the relief of suffering and pain in our generation and for all generations to come."

It was 1930, and the occasion was the national celebration of Welch's 80th birthday. The hour-long festivities were carried by radio across America, and that week Welch's portrait graced the cover of *Time* magazine. The world had changed so much since the birth of bacteriology, since he had established the country's first pathology department at Bellevue and become a professor of pathology at The Johns Hopkins University, chief of pathology at The Johns Hopkins Hospital, founding dean at the medical school, first director of The Johns Hopkins University School of Hygiene and Public Health, and scientific director of the Rockefeller Institute for Medical Research. It was a new and healthier world, and Welch had been at its epicenter for half a century.

Humility and decency were hallmarks of Welch's character, and one can imagine his shrinking response to the national outpouring of admiration, to say nothing of finding his face on a magazine cover. His reticence about his own accomplishments was legendary. After discovering the causative organism of gas gangrene, Welch had insisted upon referring to the microbe by the descriptive name, *Bacillus aerogenes capsulatus,* never joining the rest of the scientific world in honoring its discoverer with the name Clostridium Welchii.

It has been said that bacteriologists, not surgeons, made surgery safe. Intellectually, Welch followed Pasteur, Koch, and Lister into the operating room, teaching surgeons that aseptic surgery was safe surgery. Wound infections did not materialize spontaneously. Bacteria could be identified and avoided, and patients could be protected by simple aseptic precautions. Scrupulously clean operating rooms, sterilized instruments, proper hand decontamination, sterile gloves, and ultimately, face masks and sterile gowns made the difference between life and death. It was as simple as that.

Welch came to understand the importance of sterility in surgery; Halsted had arrived at the same conclusion on his own.

Welch took it a step further. He recognized that prevention of disease was possible on a grand scale by identifying the agents of disease, and insulating the population from them, and founded The Johns Hopkins School of Public Health. Halsted founded an equally far-reaching safe school of surgery.

Himself a follower of Koch and Cohnheim, Welch passed the baton to a new generation of students who set about changing the world. Among them was a U.S. Army doctor named Walter Reed. Reed identified mosquitoes as the vector for yellow fever, instituted mosquito control, staunched the loss of life in Central America, and made the building of the Panama Canal possible. That is the true meaning of public health, as was identifying the need, and the means, to contain tuberculosis prior to the advent of antibiotics. By the application of simple public health measures to prevent airborne transmission of the disease, annual deaths from tuberculosis dipped from the millions to the thousands in the early 20th century.

Over a span of 40 years, Welch had been the buffer and filter between Halsted and the academic world in which he functioned. In his fatherly manner, Welch had managed to defuse the fallout from his friend's lifetime of erratic behavior and fastidiously concealed drug use, and only in his final years, a decade after Halsted's death, did he finally reveal that he had never been fully cured of his cocaine habit.

Welch recognized greatness, allowed for weakness, and encouraged a singular talent to flourish. William Stewart Halsted, and the birth of modern surgery, had been part of his legacy.

In his last years, indulging his interests as a bibliophile, Welch founded and directed The Johns Hopkins University Institute of the History of Medicine.

It is difficult to quantify his influence on American medicine, but the recognition he received was not misplaced. The story of Johns Hopkins pivots about Welch's role in the critical, early stages. His influence on the transition to scientific medicine far exceeded his own specific accomplishments, and William Welch was the essential catalyst for an era of great progress in medicine.

Disorganized and perhaps overburdened, Welch had spread himself thinly, but he never relinquished the role of reliable friend and mentor to Halsted. Welch remained active through his 84th year, and died of prostate cancer at his beloved Johns Hopkins Hospital on April 30, 1934.

EPILOGUE

THE WEST READING ROOM on the second floor of the Welch Medical Library is a quiet spot. It is sparsely furnished beneath double-height ceilings and hung with poorly lit portraits. In a place of honor on the far end of the room a massive, dark painting dominates the wall.

The painting, measuring 10 feet 9 inches by 9 feet 1 inch, is anything but joyful. It depicts the four doctors: Halsted, Welch, Osler, and Kelly. Mary Elizabeth Garrett commissioned the picture in 1905, and somehow convinced a reluctant John Singer Sargent to take on the task. Sargent had previously painted her portrait, which hangs in the room as well. The experience had been notably unpleasant for him. During the sittings he claims to have "felt like a rabbit in the presence of a boa constrictor."

Sargent was then the most renowned portrait painter in the world. His paintings were shown everywhere, and he was famed for his renditions of Robert Louis Stevenson, Claude Monet, Theodore Roosevelt, and the scandalous Madame X. The artist was losing interest in portrait painting and skeptical about the project. But, as usual, Mary Elizabeth Garrett prevailed.

In early June, the great men were gathered at Sargent's Tite Street studio in the Chelsea section of London for a joint sitting. Osler had recently relocated to Oxford, Halsted was passing through London on a summer journey, and Welch and Kelly made their schedules agree.

The studio was composed of two adjoining row houses, and the workroom itself was quite large and had good northern light from double-height mullioned windows. Sargent was a burly man with a full beard, enormous appetites and interests, and very much unlike the four austere men before him. Not at all restrained, he prowled the room grumbling as he worked and tried to provoke them.

Unable to achieve a satisfactory composition, Sargent struggled with the painting for nearly a year. After an early attempt, he had thrown up his hands in frustration and left the studio. Volatile, and unwilling to compromise his art, he struggled with himself and his subjects. Upon evaluating Osler for the first time, the artist shook his huge head and muttered that he had never before been asked to paint a man with green skin. Session after session he paced, chain-smoked cigars, complained, disparaged his subjects, and freely aired his displeasure whenever the mood struck him.

Osler, proud to have recently assumed the chair at Oxford, had dressed in his red university robes. Sargent was outraged and rebuked the gentle Osler with a diatribe on the horrors of that particular British Red-Coat shade, a color he insisted caused seamstresses to go blind.

And so it went. The more difficult the creation of the picture became, the more unease permeated the group.

Sargent disliked the standoffish Halsted. Famously distant with strangers, Halsted's intolerance and sarcasm were quick to surface, though most annoyingly, he never deviated from his soft, gentlemanly delivery. He would sit quietly, smoking his expensive Pall Mall cigarettes through his cheap white cigarette holders, and observe the process. His comments, when he made them, were withering, and not at all appreciated by the artist. Legend has it that Sargent took his revenge by painting Halsted poorly, and in colors that would soon fade. Much was made of the depiction of Halsted's thumb as short and graceless and the blue shadow painted under his eyes, but both were accurate.

Then, as often happens at the darkest moment, inspiration struck. The artist ordered delivery of a huge Venetian globe from his Fulham Road studio. When it arrived, the globe proved too large for the doorway.

Now convinced he had found his way, he ordered the door jambs chopped away and his precious prop installed behind the berobed foursome. Having won the moment, Sargent sketched the new arrangement and announced, "Gentlemen, now we have got our picture."

Sometime later he enhanced the vertical focus of the background by adding a painting from his collection. The dark addition was a copy of *St. Martin and the Beggar,* by Jorge Manuel Theotocopouli, the son of the Spanish master El Greco, who had painted the original. A painting of a painting of a painting, but it seemed to do the trick.

The group portrait was a great success in both Britain and America. Welch and Osler were unhappy with the likeness of their friend, and it was said that the picture told more of the dynamic between them than a glance at four men in ceremonial robes would imply. Halsted said nothing, but his actions spoke for him. Notoriously camera shy, he used a photo of his bust as his official likeness for a decade. The solemn portrait of the four doctors of Johns Hopkins was greatly admired, and the fame of the painter and his subjects grew.

Finally installed where it now sits in the library, the painting darkened over the years. After a major restoration in 2001, it now appears as it was originally painted. Of the four doctors, only William Stewart Halsted appears to be posing happily, and from every angle he seems to be wearing a sly smile as he looks over the room.

ACKNOWLEDGMENTS

THE STORY OF William Stewart Halsted is the story of modern surgery, replete with larger-than-life personalities and dangerous bumps in the road. Researching this book meant frequently coming across names that rang with personal memories or recognition, and brought to life the transition of my teachers to their teacher, George Heuer, and through him to Heuer's teacher, William Stewart Halsted. After leaving the Air Force, I spent two years as a surgical resident under Roscoe S. Wilcox, at the Kaiser Foundation, in Southern California. As skilled a raconteur as he was a surgeon, Dr. Wilcox's stories stayed with me, and Heuer and Halsted became more than just names. Later, at the New York Hospital, other Heuer's residents kept the flame alive. Within a few degrees of separation most surgeons can establish their own link to Halsted, and his story is part of theirs.

I was lucky enough to finally bite the bullet and write the tale. Many others have done similar work in journal form. Their work has made mine easier.

James L. Gehrlich, head of archives at the New York Hospital, made his peaceful, twenty-fifth floor aerie a place for research, and was generous with his help. Andrew Harrison, Material Cultural Archivist at Johns Hopkins Medical Archive, was guardian of a treasure trove of Halsted Material.

Michael Bliss wrote two wonderful books on the period, on which I leaned shamelessly. Entitled *Harvey Cushing, a Life in Surgery* and *William Osler, a Life in Medicine,* they stand as the definitive works on the period, and I recommend them to any who my work has not already soured on the subject. William MacCallum's, 1930, biography, *William S. Halsted, Surgeon,* tells the story as one who lived those historic times alongside his subject. The same can be said for the autobiographies of J. M. T. Finney and Hugh Young, both great sources of Halsted material. Harvey Cushing's Pulitzer Prize–winning biography of William Osler also provided insights and a personal point of view. Here too, it has been interesting, knowing so many of Cushing's descendants, and so little about the man until reading Bliss's work. There are too many papers and addresses to mention. Many of these and related books are cited in the references, and I tried to give credit where credit was due. All errors in citation, facts, and otherwise are solely mine.

Much of the early research for this book fell upon my son Jason Imber, himself a writer, who enthusiastically found time when I could not. Many thanks, Jason. My agent, the exceptional Amanda Urban, was the most insightful of readers — unstinting of praise and criticism, usually right on the mark, and always a dream to work with. Political columnist-turned dramatist Michael Kramer is more than just my friend; he willingly read through an early draft and was generous with his editing skills and unpleasant comments. My wife, Cathryn Collins, deep in her own world of business and film-making, offered help and support throughout, and survived the process. Elizabeth Stein helped greatly with the editing process. At Kaplan, executive editor Don Fehr saw merit in the book and took on the project. Unfailingly intelligent, he and Kate Lopaze have been encouraging, thoughtful, and have made this a most pleasant experience.

REFERENCES

THIS BOOK WAS WRITTEN to tell the important and interesting story of a singularly influential man. Although it was never intended to be the ultimately scholarly biography of Dr. William Stewart Halsted, no liberties were taken with the facts, as they are known. Over the years, Halsted biographers have been hampered by the reticence of the subject, and particularly his unwillingness to share the details of his epic struggle. In the face of his exaulted position in the medical world, early biographers did not actively confront the issue. Later biographers no longer had access to his contemporaries, and were forced to rely on a collage of vignettes to flesh out the man and his story. The books and articles listed below provided insight into Halsted and his times, and were a great source of information for this book. Specific references to statements or disputed issues are found in notes on the chapters to follow.

Bibliography

Andrew, Rob Jr. *Wade Hampton, Confederate Warrior to Southern Redeemer.* Chapel Hill: University of North Carolina Press, 2008.

Barren Island. 1939 WPA Guide to New York City.

Bliss, Michael. *Harvey Cushing, A Life in Surgery.* New York: Oxford University Press, 2005.

Bliss, Michael. *Willam Osler, A Life in Medicine.* New York: Oxford University Press, 1999.

Burns, Ric, and Sanders, James. *New York: An Illustrated History*. New York: Alfred A. Knopf, 1999, pp. 88–102.

Burrows, Edwin G., and Wallace, Mike. *Gotham, A History of New York City to 1898*. New York: Oxford University Press, 1999.

Crowe, Samuel James, M.D. *Halsted of Johns Hopkins, The Man and His Men*. Springfield, IL: Charles C. Thomas, 1957.

Cushing, Harvey. *The Life of Sir William Osler, Vol. I*. Oxford at the Clarendon Press, 1926.

Cushing, Harvey. *The Life of Sir William Osler, Vol. II*. Oxford at the Clarendon Press, 1926.

Dunbar, David S., and Jackson, Kenneth T. *Empire City: New York Through the Centuries*. New York: Columbia University Press, 2002. "Murray Hill Reservoir," Nov. 25, 1849, pp. 206–208. "The New Colossus," Emma Lazarus, 1883, pp. 314–315.

Finney, J. M. T. *A Surgeon's Life: The Autobiography of J. M. T. Finney*. New York: G.P. Putnam and Sons, 1940.

Fleming, Donald. *William H. Welch and the Rise of Modern Medicine*. Baltimore, MD: Johns Hopkins University Press, 1954.

Flexner, Simon, and Thomas, James. *William Henry Welch and the Heroic Age of American Medicine*. Baltimore, MD: Johns Hopkins University Press, 1941.

Franz, Caroline Jones. "Johns Hopkins: How a Farsighted Quaker Merchant and Four Great Doctors Brought Forth, with Maddening Slowness, One of the Finest Medical Centers in the World." *American Heritage Magazine*, February 1976, Vol. 27, Issue 2.

Freeburg, Victor O. *William Henry Welch at Eighty: A Memorial Record of Celebrations Around the World in His Honor*. New York: The Milbank Memorial Fund, 1930.

Freud, Sigmund. *Cocaine Papers*. New York: Stonehill Publishing Company and Robert Byck, 1974.

Garrison, Fielding H. *John Shaw Billing: A Memoir*. New York and London: G.P. Putnam and Sons, The Knickerbocker Press, 1915, pp. 181–212.

Gonzalez-Crussi, F. *A Short History of Medicine*. New York: Random House Publishing, 2007.

References

Green, Ann Norton. *Horses at Work*. Cambridge, MA: Harvard University Press, 2008.

Halsted, William Stewart. *Surgical Papers, Vol. 2*. Baltimore, MD: Johns Hopkins University Press, 1924.

Halsted, William Stewart. *Surgical Papers, Vol. 1*. Baltimore, MD: Johns Hopkins University Press, 1924.

Harris, Leslie M. *In the Shadow of Slavery*. The University of Chicago Press, 2002.

Heuer, George J. *Dr. Halsted*. Unpublished.

Homberger, Eric. *The Historical Atlas of New York City*. New York: Henry Holt and Company, 1994.

Jacob, Kathryn A. "Mr. Johns Hopkins." *The Johns Hopkins Magazine*, January 1974, Johns Hopkins University.

Larabee, Eric. *The Benevolent & Necessary Institution*. Garden City, NY: Doubleday and Company, 1971.

Lathrop, James R. *History and Description of The Roosevelt Hospital, New York City*. 1893.

MacCallum, W. G., and Welch, W. H. *William Stewart Halsted, Surgeon*. Baltimore, MD: Johns Hopkins Press, 1930.

National Library of Medicine. John Shaw Billings Centennial, U.S. Public Health Service, June 17, 1965.

Obituary for Johns Hopkins, *The Baltimore Sun*, December 25, 1873.

Rutkow, Ira M. *Bleeding Blue and Gray, Civil War Surgery and the Evolution of American Medicine*. New York: Random House, 2005.

Rutkow, Ira M., M.D. *Surgery, An Illustrated History*. St. Louis, MO: Mosby-Year Book and Norman Publishing, 1993.

Rutkow, Ira M. *The Surgical Clinics of North America, 75th Anniversary Issue*. Philadelphia, PA: W. B. Saunders Company, December 1987.

Vexler, Robert L. *Baltimore, A Chronological and Documentary History 1632–1970*. Dobbs Ferry, NY: Oceana Publishing, 1975.

Young, Hugh. *A Surgeon's Autobiography*. New York: Harcourt, Brace, and Company, 1940.

Notes

CHAPTER 1

Page

1   *All that is loathsome...* Charles Dickens, *American Notes* (Whitefish, MI: Kessing Publishing, 2004).

6   *Phillips Academy...* F. S. Allis, Jr., *Youth from Every Quarter: A Bicentennial History of Phillips Academy, Andover* (Lebanon, NH: University Press of New England, 1978).

8   *If you get an election...* Edwards A. Park, MD, "Pediatrician's recollections of Dr. Halsted," *Surgery* 32, no. 3 (September 1952): 474.

8   *did not go in for social activities...* Ibid.

CHAPTER 2

11   *In 1845...* "Surgery Before Anesthesia," *American Society of Anesthesiologists Newsletter* 60, no. 9 (September 1996): 8–10.

11   *Gilbert Abbott...* James W. May, Jr., MD, "Gain Without Pain: The Dawn of Elective Surgery," *Plastic and Reconstructive Surgery* 122, no. 2 (August 2008): 631–38.

12   *The state of lack...* Oliver Wendell Holmes, letter to William Morton, November 26, 1846.

12   *In 1896, the 50th anniversary...* Hugh Young, *A Surgeon's Autobiography* (New York: Harcourt, Brace, and Company, 1940), 69–70.

CHAPTER 3

24   *I had little expectation...* Letter from William S. Halsted to William H. Welch, August 3, 1922, Alan Mason Chesney Medical Archives, Johns Hopkins University.

25   *Lister's antiseptic technique...* William H. Welch, memorial meeting for Dr. William Stewart Halsted, Homewood, Sunday, December 16, 1923.

CHAPTER 4

Eric Larrabee, *The Benevolent and Necessary Institution* (New York: Doubleday and Company, 1971).

29   *Halsted always claimed to have taken a competitive...* James L. Gehrlich, Contextual Narrative for Halsted's Tenure as House Physician at New York Hospital, The New York Hospital Archives.

30   *Clinical progress notes...* New York-Presbyterian Hospital archives.

32   *Professor Emil Zuckerkandl...* Letter from William Stewart Halsted to William H. Welch, August 3, 1922, Alan Mason Chesney Medical Archives, Johns Hopkins University.

CHAPTER 5

42   *Wait a minute...* W. G. MacCallum and W. H. Welch, *William Stewart Halsted, Surgeon* (Baltimore, MD: Johns Hopkins Press, 1930).

42   *He was in Albany...* Letter from William Stewart Halsted to William Henry Welch, High Hampton, North Carolina, August 3, 1922.

42   *the first emergency blood transfusion...* MacCallum and Welch, *William Stewart Halsted, Surgeon.*

44   *Roosevelt Hospital...* James R. Lathrop, *History and Description of the Roosevelt Hospital, New York City,* 1893.

CHAPTER 6

47   *Shocked at the cost...* Sigmund Freud, *Cocaine Papers,* edited by Robert Byck, MD, notes by Anna Freud (New York: Stonehill Publishing Company, 1974), 6.

53   *In two minutes there was complete...* R.J. Hall, MD, letter to the *New York Medical Journal,* 1885. Reprinted in *Surgical Papers* I (1924), 167–77.

55   *Neither indifferent...* W.S. Halsted, "Practical Comments on the Use and Abuse of Cocaine Suggested by Its Use in More Than 1000 Minor Operations," *New York Medical Journal* 42 (1885): 495–510.

58   *the Captain's medicine locker...* Daniel B. Nunn, MD, "Dr. Halsted's Addiction," *Johns Hopkins Advanced Studies in Medicine* 6, no. 3 (March 2006), 106–108.

CHAPTER 7

Mr. Johns Hopkins... Kathryn A. Jacob, *The Johns Hopkins Magazine,* Johns Hopkins University, January 1974.

Caroline Jones Franz, "Johns Hopkins: How a Farsighted Quaker Merchant and Four Great Doctors Brought Forth, with Maddening Slowness, One of the Finest Medical Centers in the World," *American Heritage Magazine,* February 1976.

61   *In the fall of 1872...* Ann Morton Green, *Horses at Work* (Boston: Harvard University Press, 2008): 168–70.

61   "The Horse Plague," *New York Times,* October 25, 1872.

62   *At his death...* "Death of Johns Hopkins," *The Baltimore Sun,* Thursday morning edition, December 25, 1873.

64   *John Shaw Billings...* National Library of Medicine, John Shaw Billings Centennial, U.S. Public Health Service, June 17, 1965.

      Fielding H. Garrison, MD, *John Shaw Billings, A Memoir* (New York and London: G.P. Putnam's Sons, 1915), 181–212.

66   *Auerbach's Keller...* Simon Flexner and James Thomas Flexner, *William Henry Welch and the Heroic Age of American Medicine* (New York: Viking Press, 1941), 92.

70   *He attended a session...* Victor O. Freeburg, ed., *William Henry Welch at Eighty: A Memorial Record of Celebrations Around the World in His Honor* (New York: The Milbank Memorial Fund, 1930).

71   *I wish I had a picture...* Edwards A. Park, MD, "A Pediatrician's Recollection of Dr. Halsted," *Surgery* 12, no. 3 (1932): 447.

72   *That's too bad. Loomis...* Donald Fleming, *William H. Welch and the Rise of Modern Medicine* (Baltimore, MD: Johns Hopkins University Press, 1974): 70.

72   *I shall never forget the circumstances...* Freeburg, ed., *William Henry Welch at Eighty.*

CHAPTER 8

79   *In April...* Letter from W. S. Halsted to William H. Welch, August 3, 1922, High Hampton, North Carolina.

80 *Dr. Fred C. Shattuck...* Letter from Roy McClure to Heuer, October 22, 1948, Heuer papers, New York Hospital Archives.

81 Halsted at Butler. "A Pediatrician's Recollections of Dr. Halsted," *Surgery* 32, no. 2 (September 1952): 475.

82 *Nobody knows where Popsie eats...* Hugh Young, *A Surgeon's Autobiography* (New York: Harcourt, Brace, and Company, Inc., 1940), 55.

83 *two hundred pound eighty year old...* H.L. Mencken, *The Baltimore Sun,* April 11, 1935.

CHAPTER 9

92 *Halsted's heroic determination...* MacCallum and Welch, *William Stewart Halsted, Surgeon.*

CHAPTER 10

97 *Big crowd...* J.M.T. Finney, *A Surgeon's Life: The Autobiography of J.M.T. Finney* (New York: G.P. Putnam's Sons, 1940).

CHAPTER 11

101 *Between an hotel...* William Osler, MD, "The Inner History of the Johns Hopkins Hospital," *Johns Hopkins Medical Journal* 125, no. 4 (October 1969): 187.

102 *Osler recommended...* Ibid.

CHAPTER 12

105 *Welch believed...* William H. Welch to Emma Welch Walcott, October 23, 1888, Michael Bliss, *William Osler: A Life in Medicine* (New York: Oxford University Press, 1999), 172.

105 *Billings had visited...* Osler, *The Inner History,* 186.

106 *It makes one's blood boil...* Harvey Cushing, *The Life of Sir William Osler, Vol. I* (Oxford: Clarendon Press, 1926), 307.

CHAPTER 13

112 *The operating room...* Hugh Young, *A Surgeon's Autobiography* (New York: Harcourt, Brace, and Company, 1940), 60.

114   *Operating table...* Young, *A Surgeon's Autobiography,* 59.

114   *Nurse Caroline Hampton...* Finney, *A Surgeon's Life,* 89.

CHAPTER 14

117   *Thirty-eight years old... Surgical Papers by William Stewart Halsted* (Baltimore, MD: Johns Hopkins Press, 1924), 16.

122   *250 clamps...* Michael P. Osborne, "William Stewart Halsted: His Life and Contributions to Surgery," *Lancet Oncology* 8 (2007): 256–65.

123   *a mistaken kindness to the patient...* Ibid.

CHAPTER 15

127   *duty bootie... Johns Hopkins University Gazette,* May 15, 2006: 2.

128   Description of tea party. MacCallum and Welch, *William Stewart Halsted, Surgeon,* 82.

130   Letter from Halsted to Mall. Alan Mason Chesney Medical Archives, Johns Hopkins University.

131   Letter from Caroline Hampton to Lucy Baxter. Alan Mason Chesney Medical Archives, Johns Hopkins University.

133   *There I was alone...* Samuel J. Crowe, "Personal Recollections of Dr. Halsted," *Surgery* 12, no. 3 (September 1952): 464.

134   *Halsted has taken a large house...* Neil A. Graven, *Annals of Hopkins,* Winter 2007.

135   *a great student... white oak or hickory...* MacCallum and Welch, *William Stewart Halsted, Surgeon.*

CHAPTER 16

141   *This was the first intimation...* William Osler, MD, "The Inner History of the Johns Hopkins Hospital," *Johns Hopkins Medical Journal* 125, no. 4 (October 1969): 184–94.

CHAPTER 17

147   *William T. Bull... Surgical Papers by William Stewart Halsted* (Baltimore, MD: Johns Hopkins University Press, 1924): 266.

150 *Just one question, Kelly...* James F. Mitchell, MD, "Memories of Dr. Halsted," *Surgery* 32, no. 3 (September 1952): 456.

152 *Give him morphia...* James F. Mitchell, MD, "Memories of Dr. Halsted," *Surgery* 32, no. 3 (September 1952): 451–60.

152 *second hernia patient...* Surgical Papers by William Stewart Halsted, 276.

153 *Mitchell, I have an awful headache...* Ibid.

154 *Dear Mitchell. I telephoned...* Ibid.

CHAPTER 18

161 *Ah, but we are...* Finney, *A Surgeon's Life.*

CHAPTER 19

167 *The White Owl of High Hampton...* "William Stewart Halsted," lecture by Dr. Peter D. Olch and J. Scott Rankin, *Annals of Surgery* 243, no. 3 (March 2006): 418–25.

168 *land purchases...* Letter to Halsted from Frank R. Frost, December 22, 1902, Alan Mason Chesney Medical Archive, Johns Hopkins University.

170 *Halsted's pajamas...* George Heuer, unpublished biography of Halsted, 74.

173 *salouchy...* Daniel B. Nunn, "Interview with Madge Dillard Merrel: Caroline Hampton, an Eccentric but Well Matched Help Mate," *Perspectives in Biology & Medicine* 42 (1998).

179 *"general talk"...* Ibid.

CHAPTER 20

184 *Mary Elizabeth Garrett...* Flexner, *William Henry Welch and the Heroic Age of American Medicine,* 219.

188 *Mall telegraphed...* Ibid., 226.

CHAPTER 21

189   *When a student complained...* Michael Bliss, *Willam Osler, A Life in Medicine* (New York: Oxford University Press, 1999).

CHAPTER 22

193   *Have you ever made a bloodcount?...* James F. Mitchell, MD, "Memories of Dr. Halsted," *Surgery* 32, no. 3 (September 1952): 452.

195   *When I went to the...* Joseph Colt Bloodgood, MD, FACS, "Halsted Thirty-Six Years Ago," *The American Journal of Surgery* 14, no. 1 (October 1931): 98.

196   *He made a few mistakes...* Ibid.

200   *Halsted and relieved Mitchell...* James F. Mitchell, MD, "Memories of Dr. Halsted," *Surgery* 32, no. 3 (September 1952): 451–60.

CHAPTER 23

210   *I wanted to write...* Letter from Caroline Halsted to William Halsted, Alan Mason Chesney Medical Archives, Johns Hopkins University.

212   *practical jokes...* Flexner, *William Henry Welch and the Heroic Age of American Medicine*, 172.

213   *referring to a chordee...* William Rheinoff, *Personal Reminiscence of JHMS*, 17.

213   *Finney tells of a telephone call...* Finney, *A Surgeon's Life*, 295–6.

216   *Crim...* Young, *A Surgeon's Autobiography*, 61.

CHAPTER 24

222   *When one of the three female students...graduate...* Bliss, *William Osler, A Life in Medicine*.

225   *On that armchair...* Young, *Hugh Young: A Surgeon's Autobiography*, 66.

CHAPTER 25

232   *The talk was of pathology...* Samuel James Crowe, MD, *Halsted of Johns Hopkins* (Springfield, IL: Charles C. Thomas Publishers, 1957), 66.

238 *Keep your mouth...* Michael Bliss, *Harvey Cushing: A Life in Surgery* (New York: Oxford University Press, 2005).

241 *Hunterian Laboratory...* Crowe, *Halsted of Johns Hopkins*, 70–71.

CHAPTER 26

248 Halsted bills.

251 *Among the Hopkins men were any number of fashion plates...* Finney, *A Surgeon's Life*, 95.

255 *Cushing believed both Halsted...* Bliss, *Harvey Cushing: A Life In Surgery*, 117.

CHAPTER 27

258 *Surgery would be...* Willis D. Gatch, MD, *Surgery* 32, no. 3 (1952): 168.

260 *Oh yes, Young...* Young, *Hugh Young: A Surgeon's Autobiography.*

260 *dilate the bladder...* Ibid.

261 *The following October...* Ibid., 76.

262 *Why can't I get over...* George Heuer, unpublished biography of Halsted, 52.

262 *a nod or a sly smile...* Ibid.

263 *which they named Mercurochrome...* Young, *Hugh Young: A Surgeon's Autobiography*, 245–55.

CHAPTER 28

271 *Levin Waters...* Surgical Papers by William Stewart Halsted, Vol. I (Baltimore, MD: Johns Hopkins University Press, 1924): 311–13.

275 *Heuer, I fear we are in trouble...* George Heuer, unpublished biography of Halsted.

275 *Dr. Halsted...in spite of it...* Willis D. Gatch, MD, *Surgery* 32, no. 3 (1952): 168.

CHAPTER 29

278 *Alfred Blalock...* The Allan Mason Chesney Archives, Johns Hopkins Medical Institute.

280 *I have not seen the Professor...* Harvey Cushing, *The Life of Sir William Osler, Vol. II* (Oxford: Clarendon Press, 1926).

280 *This is an ideal spot...* MacCallum and Welch, *William Stewart Halsted, Surgeon*, 192–93.

280 *Hotel Continental...* Ibid.

CHAPTER 31

287 *1,343 buildings...* Robert L. Vexler, *Baltimore, A Chronological & Documentary History* (Dobbs Ferry, NY: Oceana Publications, 1975), 70.

288 *As early as 1899...* Letter from Harvey Cushing to Hugh Auchincloss, December 13, 1937.

289 *The Professor's office suite...* George Heuer, unpublished biography of Halsted, 61.

291 *Halsted was operating...* Ibid.

292 *They came from long...five minutes' visit!...* George Heuer, unpublished biography of Halsted.

CHAPTER 32

297 *"full time"...* Donald Fleming, *William H. Welch and the Rise of Modern Medicine* (Baltimore, MD: Johns Hopkins University Press, 1954), 165.

298 *Osler was outraged...* David Dary, *Frontier Medicine* (New York: Alfred A Knopf, 2005), 307.

299 *Only 50 of 155...* Flexner, *William Henry Welch and the Heroic Age of American Medicine*, 307.

300 *If the school could get...* Flexner, *William Henry Welch and the Heroic Age of American Medicine*, 308.

300 *I did not take way...* Fleming, *William H. Welch and the Rise of Modern Medicine*, 177.

301 *a faculty of Halsteds...* Ibid., 178.

301 *Leading members of the faculty, including Kelly...* Bliss, *Harvey Cushing: A Life in Surgery*, 383–84.

304 *The coming of full time...* Letter to the trustees, Alan M. Chesney, MD, *Surgery* 32, no. 3: 482–84.

304 *that there were men...* MacCallum and Welch, *William Stewart Halsted, Surgeon.*

304 *We should utterly fail...* Letter to the trustees, Alan M. Chesney, MD, *Surgery* 32, no. 3: 482–84.

CHAPTER 33

308 *There was no personal banter...* George Heuer, unpublished biography of Halsted, 56.

308 *Heuer is that you...* Ibid., 57–58.

309 *Why, Heuer, she has a dirty umbilicus...* Ibid.

309 *Halsted now operated...* Ibid., 48–49.

312 *Halsted, I am opposed to this...* Samuel James Crowe, MD, *Halsted of Johns Hopkins* (Springfield, IL: Charles C. Thomas Publishers, 1957), 148.

313 Heuer at Eutaw Place. George Heuer, unpublished biography of Halsted.

313 *Walter Edward Dandy...* Crowe, *Halsted of Johns Hopkins*, 85–88.

318 *Dandy was offered the professorship...* William F. Rienhoff, Jr., MD, *Personal Reminiscence of the Johns Hopkins Medical School and The JH Surgical Service, 1915–1960.*

CHAPTER 34

322 *Once, in the saloon... and everyone but he had a good laugh...* MacCallum and Welch, *William Stewart Halsted, Surgeon*, 68.

324 *Halsted, at a loss...* Rienhoff, *Personal Reminiscence of the Johns Hopkins Medical School*, 9.

325 *I would warn against...* William Stewart Halsted, *Journal of the American Medical Association* 73 (1896, 1919).

325 *I shall never cease to mourn...* MacCallum and Welch, *William Stewart Halsted, Surgeon*, 199.

325 *I find words... who has ever used it...* Ibid.

325 *Tegmen, deligate, and defract...* Ibid., 188.

326 *If you put 'perhaps'... you will not be blamed...* Willis D. Gatch, MD, "My Experiences with Dr. Halsted," *Surgery* 13, no. 3: 467.

328 *Heuer commanded... chest wounds and trauma... Flanders Fields...* Finney, *A Surgeon's Life*, 157–58, 181, 193–94.

CHAPTER 35

331 *As weighty events were unfolding overseas, the enigmatic Halsted was beginning a relationship...* Cameron, Gordon, et al., "William Stewart Halsted: Letters to a Young Admirer," *Annals of Surgery* 234, no. 5 (November 2001): 702–07.

334 *Halsted consulted with Dr. Thomas Boggs...* Finney, *A Surgeon's Life*, 298.

337 Menu of dinner in Halsted's honor. George Heuer, correspondence, New York Presbyterian Hospital Archives.

338 *As I was convalescing... assure himself of my comfort....* George Heuer, correspondence, New York Presbyterian Hospital Archives.

338 *To Matas, Halsted wrote...* MacCallum and Welch, *William Stewart Halsted, Surgeon*, 224–25.

CHAPTER 36

341 *a furuncle on my firmament...* Letter from Halsted to Welch, August 3, 1922, Johns Hopkins Hospital Archives.

343 *On September 5, Caroline telegraphed...* Caroline Halsted, letter from Halsted Archive.

CHAPTER 37

345 *The entire small intestine...* Rienhoff, *Personal Reminiscence of the Johns Hopkins Medical School*, 28.

346 *Welch, on his deathbed...* Daniel B. Nunn, MD, "Dr. Halsted's Addiction," *Johns Hopkins Advanced Studies in Medicine* 6, no. 3 (March 2006): 108.

347 *Dr. Halsted once said of them... about their brother's wife...* Caroline Halsted, letter to William Welch, Halsted Archives.

347 *I sometimes wonder ... that any man could ever be...* Caroline Halsted, letter to William Welch, Halsted Archives.

350 *Herbert Hoover...* Ceremonies in Washington, D.C., in honor of the eightieth birthday of Dr. Welch, April 8, 1930, in Victor O. Freeburg, ed., *William Henry Welch at Eighty,* Millbank Memorial Fund, William H. Welch Medical Library, 22, 33–35.

INDEX

A

Abbott, Gilbert, 11
Abdominal aneurysm, 285
Abdominal surgery, 33, 34, 88
Abel, John J., 188, 190, 192, 201
Absence, 333–34
Absences, 207, 235, 310
Actinographer, 265–66
Addiction, 50, 55–58, 277–82
Admission requirements, 228, 290
Aequanimitas, 105
Alcoholism, 180–81
American Expeditionary Force, 327
American Medical Association, 299
American Surgical Association, 191
Amputation, 13
Anatomy, 22
Anderson, Sherwood, 224
Andover Academy, 6
Anesthesia, 12, 19, 48, 51–52
Animal experimentation, 86–90
Anthrax bacillus, 15
Antique collections, 216–17
Antisepsis, 18–19
Antiseptic soaks, 112
Antiseptic surgery, 25
Antiseptic technique, 18, 33
Aorta, 283–85
Aorta banding, 285

Appearance, 6, 295
Appendectomies, 26, 139
Appendicitis, 218, 234
Arterial aneurysm, 271–72
Artery forceps, 38
Aseptic surgery, 111–16, 139–40, 228
Aseptic technique, 109, 113, 272–73, 349
Astor Place Riot, 2
Astronomer, 172
Athletics, 6–7
Autopsy, 42

B

Bacteriologists, 351
Bacteriology, 10, 14–16, 68–6, 72
Baetjer, Edwin, 213, 252
Baetjer, Frederick Henry, 265–66, 288
Baltimore and Ohio Railroad, 60–62, 185
Baltimore Sun, 62, 211, 348
Barker, Lewellys, 198, 251, 294, 302, 337
Barnum, P.T., 3
Basedow's disease, 268
Bassini, Edoardo, 148–49
Baxter, Lucy, 131
Bedside chart, 30–31
Bedside teacher, 298
Bellevue Hospital internship, 24–26

Bellevue Hospital Medical College, 69–70

Bernays, Martha, 47–48

Bichloride of mercury, 111

Bilary colic, 337

Bile duct draining, 327

Billings, John Shaw
Baltimore, 91, 94
Big Four and, 142
early medical staff, 102
home surgeries, 248–49
Hopkins (Johns) and, 64–66, 68, 70–71
Johns Hopkins Hospital and, 96
Johns Hopkins Medical School, 186
Osler (William) and, 105
U.S. medical education and, 155, 163

Billroth, Theodor, 33, 38, 56, 119

Birth, 1

Black spot, 14

Blackfan, Kenneth, 315

Blackwell, Elizabeth, 184

Bladder, 261

Blalock, Alfred, 278, 279

Bleach, 324

Bliss, Michael, 241

Blood pressure
cuff, 241
monitoring, 30

Blood transfusion, 42–43

Bloodgood, Joseph Colt, 273, 289, 296
aseptic technique, 222, 226–27
Cushing (Harvey) and, 233
experimental work, 208, 213
new departments, 311
operating room, 115–16
residency, 193–96, 198, 200

Boggs, Thomas, 334, 347–48

Bonner, Rachel, 102, 129–30

Bradley, Douglas, 169, 170, 174–75, 179

Brady, James Buchanan, 263

Brady Urological Institute, 263

Brahms, Johannes, 33

Brain
dissection, 33
tumor, 230–31

Breast cancer, 81, 117–26, 140

Brewer, George, 57

British Expeditionary Force, 323

British Medical Journal, 195

Broadway, 2

Brockway, Fred W.
Baltimore, 134
breast cancer, 118, 123
Johns Hopkins Hospital, 99–100
residency, 194
U.S. medical education, 160, 162

Brown, Tom, 202

Brownstones, 2

Bryn Mawr School, 185

Bull, William T., 79, 147

Bushnell, Rev. Samuel, 7–8, 254, 346

Butler Hospital, 92

C

Cabot and Chandler, 65

Calcium metabolism, 269

Camille, 2

Carbolic acid, 17–18, 111, 112, 114, 199

Carnegie, Andrew, 71

Carnegie Commission, 228

Carnegie Foundation for the Advancement of Teaching, 299

Carnegie Institution in Washington, 321–22

Carrel, Alexis, 293, 323–25

Carrel-Dakin's irrigation, 329

Carter, Sally, 128, 214, 341

Cashiers Valley, 132–33, 167

Catgut sutures, 221–22

Central nervous system, 50

Centre Street Dispensary, 23

Centripetal transfusion, 43=44
Century Dictionary, 325
Cézanne, 224
Chamber pots, 2–3
Chambers Street Hospital, 44, 79
Charity ward patients, 227
Charvet shirts, 250
Chemical tests, 23
Chlorine hand wash, 39–40
Chloroform, 12, 151
Cholecystitis, ix, 323
Cholera epidemics, 1, 16
Cigarette smoking, 135, 198–99
Civil War, 5, 9, 14, 25, 30, 59, 179
Clark, Alonzo, 23
Clarke, George E., 99, 123, 162
Clark University, 130, 187
Clinical medicine, 304–5
Clinical Society of Maryland, 123
Clinics, 22
Clothing, 249–51
Cocaine, 47–58, 80
    addiction by Halsted, 91, 142, 191,
        278–79, 281, 346
    as anesthesia, 51–52, 93, 151–52
    as snuff, 55
Coeducation, 185–87, 224
Coffee, 251
Cohnheim, Julius, 68–69, 155, 351
College clubs, 7–8
College of Physicians and Surgeons,
    4, 21–22, 23, 30, 67, 70
College of the City of New York, 4
Columbia College, 21
Columbia University, 70, 349
Commonwealth Fire Insurance
    Company, 4
Complete blood count, 193
Compound fractures, 13, 17, 26
Cone, Claribel, 224
Cone, Etta, 224

Contaminated air theory, 64–65
Cook County Hospital, 102
Cope, Oliver, 125
Cornell, 264, 299, 349
Councilman, William T., 76
    in Baltimore, 89, 93
    breast cancer, 121
    experimental work, 207
    John Hopkins Medical School, 186
    Osler (William) and, 108
    U.S. medical education, 159
    World War I and, 325–26
Country life, 167–82
Craniotomies, 229
Crile Jr., George, 125
Crim, 216–17
Croton Distributing Reservoir, 3
Crowe, Samuel, 347
    Cushing (Harvey) and, 236
    experimental work, 214–15
    home surgeries and, 244
    new departments, 311–12, 319
    resident selection, 264
    thyroid research, 275
    in World War I, 333
Crystal Palace, 3
Cushing, Harvey, 82, 229–45, 348
    aseptic technique, 228
    in Baltimore, 130
    experimental work, 216
    hernia repairs, 150–51
    home surgeries, 247–48
    new departments, 308, 31`0, 315–19
    residency, 201, 257, 262
    scientist, 288–90, 296
Cystoscope, 261

D

D. Appleton and Company, 157
Dachsunds, 217–18
Dahlia garden, 168, 169–71

Dalton, John C., 22–23
Dalton's Physiology, 8
Dandy, Walter Edward, 314–19
Dandy Embryo, 314
Davis, Egerton Y., 157
Dead space, 203
DeBakey, Michael, 286
Delafield, Francis, 67
Demeanor, 81–82
Dennis, Frederick, 68, 70–71
Dentistry, 11, 52
Depression, 48
Detachment, 275
Dickens, Charles, 1
Dismissive behavior, 161
Dissection experience, 24, 32–33
Dixon, George, 34
Dog surgery, 173–74, 222–23
Donaldson, Frank, 211
Draft Riots, 5–6
Drawings, 235
Drug addiction, 79–80
Dumas, 2

E
Edison, Thomas, 41, 43
Eiffel, Gustave, 250
Einstein, Albert, 337
Elective surgery, 199
El Greco, 355
Embryology, 33, 34
Emery, L. Winder, 103
Empyema, ix
Endocrine glands, 93, 243
Endowment, 184–85
Engagement, 129–31
Entertaining, 215–16
Epididymis, 32
Epinephrine, 52, 190
Erie Canal, 3
Esmarch, Johannes Friedrich von, 34

Ether anesthesia, 11–12, 112, 151, 203
Etymology, 325–26
Evans, Herbert M., 269–70
Evans, Mrs. Herbert, 253
Excellence obsession, 252
Experimental laboratory, 166, 307
Experimental medicine, 76, 77
Experimental model, 23
Experimental surgery, 208, 292
Extended absences, 190–91

F
Faculty, 107
Faust, 66
Final illness, 341–43
Finney, J. M. T.
  aseptic technique, 227
  in Baltimore, 134
  breast cancer, 117, 123
  early medical staff, 102
  experimental work, 206–7,
    213–14, 218
  Halsted's gallbladder disease,
    335, 337
  home surgeries, 251
  Johns Hopkins Hospital and,
    95–96, 99–100
  new departments, 398, 311
  residency, 197–98, 260, 262
  scientist, 289, 296
  teaching and, 192
  U.S. medical education, 159, 160,
    162
  in World War I, 323, 327, 329
Fire building, 135
Fire logs, 251
First-aid bandage, 34
Fitzgerald, F. Scott, 224
Fleischl-Marxow, Ernst von, 48
Fleming, Donald, 71, 72, 291
Flexner, Abraham, 299–300

Flexner, Simon, 190, 198, 212, 225, 293, 299
Flint, Austin, 139
Follis, Richard, 262, 323, 335
Folsom, Dr., 80
Food preservation, 14
Formality, 308–9
Foster, Stephen, 3
Fountain pens, 252
Fractures, 13
Freshman Eating Club, 7
Freshman Society, 7
Freud, Sigmund, 47–48, 51, 57
Frost, Frank R., 168
Frozen sections, 196
Full-time professors, 300–306
Funeral, 346

G

Gallstones, 139, 334–35, 342
Gallstone surgery, ix–x, 44, 274
Gangrene, 14
Gardening, 8, 133
Garrett, Mary Elizabeth, 184–87, 353
Gas gangrene, 350
Gas poisoning, 43–44
Gastrectomy, 33
Gastritis, 336
Gatch, Willis, 275, 277–78
Gates, Frederick, 288, 300, 301
Geneva College of Medicine, 184
George Washington, 349
German language, 32, 252
Germ theory, 10, 39
Gilman, Daniel Coit
    in Baltimore, 91, 96–97
    early medical staff, 101–3
    Hopkins (Johns) and, 63–64, 66, 68, 70–71
    Johns Hopkins Medical School, 184, 186–87

Osler (William) and, 109
    residency, 196
    U.S. medical education, 155
Gonorrhea treatment, 38
Goodnow, Frank, 337
Goodyear Rubber Company, 114
Graduated responsibility residency, 107, 140
Graves' disease, 267–69, 292
Gray's Anatomy, 8, 42, 51, 77
Great Baltimore Fire, 287
Great Epizootic, 61
Greenwich Village, 2
Gwinn, Mary, 184
Gynecologic surgery, 142–44

H

Haines, Mary Louisa, 4
Haines, R. T., 4
Hall, Richard J., 52, 53, 79
Halsted II hernia operation, 149
Halsted Jr., William Mills, 4, 78–79
Halsted, Caleb, 3–4
Halsted, Caroline Hampton
    in Baltimore, 135–36
    country living preference, 169–82, 197, 209–10, 215, 217–18, 252–54, 259, 304, 312
    final illness and death of husband, 342–43, 346–48
    as nurse, 102–3, 114–15, 118, 128–32
Halsted, Minnie, 34
Halsted, Richard, 4, 79, 346
Halsted, Robert, 3–4
Halsted, Thaddeus, 4, 29
Halsted, Timothy, 3
Halsted, William Mills, 4
Halsted, Haines and Company, 4, 78
Hambleton, Francis H., 211
Hamilton, Frank, 25–26, 35
Hampton II, Wade, 128, 259

Hampton, Frank and Sally, 128

Hampton, Isabel, 102–3, 129, 197

Hampton, Wade, 128, 176

Hand decontamination, 37

Hand scrubbing, 18, 113

Harper's Weekly, 30

Harrison, Mrs. Benjamin, 184

Harrison Narcotics Tax Act
    (1914), 179

Hartley, 54

Harvard Medical School, 11, 89–90,
    92, 185–87, 245, 264, 299, 325, 349

Haskell, Lucy, 128, 129, 171, 252

Heaton, Hannibal, 167–68

Hemingway, Eernest, 224

Hemorrhage, 38, 43

Hemostasis, 34

Hernia repair, 116, 145–54, 191

Heuer, 308–9

Heuer, George, 170, 292, 312–14, 319,
    328, 342

Histology, 67

Hoag, W. E., 54

Holdorf, Geoge, 152

Holmes, Oliver Wendell, 6, 12, 16

Homans, John, 244

Homes, 134–36

Homeschooling, 5

Honeymoon, 132–33

Honors essay contest, 27

Honors graduation, 27

Hoover, Herbert, 350

Hopkins, Gerard, 60

Hopkins, Johns, 59–63, 65, 103,
    155, 227

Hopkins, Joseph, 103

Hopkins Brothers, 60

Horseback riding, 178

Hospital living, 127–37

Hospital stays, 247

Hotel operations, 101

House staff accommodations, 159

Howell, William H., 187, 201

Howland, John, 301–2

Human excrement, 2–3

Humor, 162, 212–13

Humors imbalance, 13

Hunter, John, 10, 241

Hunterian Laboratory of Experi-
    mental Medicine, 241–43, 245,
    286, 292, 311

Hurd, 185

Hurd, Henry M., 103, 109, 164, 185,
    194, 197–98, 225, 249

Hydrocephalus, 315–16

Hypodermic syringe, 179

Hypothyroidism, 269

I

Infection, 10, 203

Infraorbital nerve, 52

Inguinal hernia repair, 140, 145–54

*Inner History of the Johns Hopkins
    Hospital, The*, 278

Instrument sterilization, 111

Insulin, 190

Internment, 346–47

Internship, 24–26

Intestinal anastomoses, 88–90, 140

Iodoform ointment poultice, 32

J

James family, 129

James, Henry, 8, 85

James, William, 224

Jefferson, Thomas, 129

John Hopkins School of Medicine,
    223–24

Johns Hopkins Bulletin, 148, 149,
    164–65

Johns Hopkins Colored Children
    Orphan Asylum, 62

Johns Hopkins Hospital, 62–66,
    95, 107
    Medical Society, 148, 164
Johns Hopkins Medical Journal, 141
Johns Hopkins School of Medicine,
    66, 107, 187
Johns Hopkins University, 12, 31, 34,
    57–58, 62–63, 76
Joint and extremity surgery, 34
Journal Club, 164, 264
*Journal of the American Medical
    Association*, 325
Journal of Experimental Medicine, 225
Journal of Urology, 264
Junior Society, 7

K

Kelly, Howard Atwood, 273, 348, 353
    aseptic technique, 226–27
    in Big Four, 142–44, 150
    experimental work, 208
    full-time professor, 301
    Johns Hopkins Medical School, 185
    new departments, 308, 310–11
    Osler (William) and, 109–10
    scientist, 289, 295, 296
    U.S. medical education and, 155,
        157, 159, 165
King George III, 29
King, Elizabeth, 184, 185
King, Francis T., 66, 96, 101–2, 164,
    184, 227
King's College Hospital, 16
Klein Deustchland Riot, 2
Koch, Robert, 15–16, 67, 69, 72–73,
    155, 163, 351
Koch's postulates, 15–16
Kocher, Albert, 292
Kocher, Theodore, 292
Koller, Carl, 49–50, 51
Königstein, Leopold, 49

L

Laboratories, 228
LaFleur, Henri, 156, 158, 159, 207
Lancet, The, 17, 195
Land acquisitions, 167–74
Laryngectomy, 33
La Traviata, 2
Letter writing, 251–52, 325
Leukocyte, 67, 193
Lidocaine, 52, 151
Life of Sir William Osler, The, 239, 278
*Ligations of the Left Subclavian Artery
    in Its First Portion*, 336
Ligatures, 10
Limb amputation, 9
Lincoln, President, 61
Lind, Jenny, 3
Lindbergh, Charles, 293
Lister, Joseph, 16–17, 25, 33, 39, 98,
    111–12, 155, 194–95, 351
Lister's technique, 37
Local anesthesia, 233
Lockwood, William, 211
Long, Crawford W., 12
Loomis, Alfred L., 72
Lubarsch, Otto, 71
Ludwig, Carl, 68, 77, 298
Lumpectomy, 125

M

MacCallum, William, 269, 278, 290
    country, 174
    Cushing (Harvey) and, 241, 245
    experimental work, 215
    residency, 258
    teaching, 192
Macewen, Sir William, 98
Madame Cézanne, 224
Madame X, 353
Madison Square, 40–41
Magendie, François, 242

Malaria, 1
Malaria letter, 207
Mall, Franklin P., 77
  aseptic technique, 222
  in Baltimore, 87–89, 92, 130
  experimental work, 211
  full-time professors, 298, 300, 304
  home surgeries, 255
  Hopkins (Johns) and, 96
  Johns Hopkins Medical School,
    187–88
  new departments, 314
  residency, 198, 201
  scientist, 290–91, 294
  teaching, 189, 192
  World War I, 321–24, 325
Mammography, 119
Manhattan, 2
Manure piles, 2
Marriage, 132
Martin, H. Newell, 76, 187
Maryland Club, 211, 300, 312, 322
Maryland State Dental Association,
  337
Massachusetts General Hospital,
  10–11, 95, 97, 194, 231–32
Mastectomy, 124
Matas, Rudolph, 338–39
Maternal mortality, 39
Matisse, Henri, 224, 250
Mayo, Will, 122
McBride, Thomas, 23–24, 38, 40–41,
  44, 54–57, 70, 78–79
McBurney, Charles, 218
McCormick, Medill, 250
McCrae, John, 329
McDowell, Annie, 102, 103
McGill University School of Medi-
  cine, 105, 108, 186
Medical and Chirurgical Faculty of
  State of Maryland, 106–7

Medical education, 106–7
Medical Gynecology, 144
Medical literature, 209–10
Medical papers, 163–65
Medical school, 183–88, 289–90
  tuition, 21–22
Medical scientists, 298
Medical student education, 191–92
Medicine, 8, 108
Mencken, H. L., 83, 348
Meningioma, 231
Mephistopheles, 66
Merchants National Bank of Balti-
  more, 61
Merck Company, 47
Mercuric chloride, 113–14, 199
Mercurochrome, 263–64
Meyer, Adolph, 301
Meynert, Theodor, 33
Microtome, 196
Midwives, 39
Mikulicz, Johannes von, 33
Mitchell, James Farnandis, 152–54,
  193–94, 106–202, 227, 249, 259, 289
Mitchell, Joe, 232
Modern surgery, 350
Monet, Claude, 353
Morphine, 48, 80, 124, 152, 165,
  179–81, 345
  addiction, 91, 141–42, 191, 207, 279,
  281–82
Morse, Samuel F. B., 3, 6
Morton, William T. G., 11
Motor nerves, 50
Mountain people, 171–72

N

Nash, Dr., 52
National Academy of Sciences, 283
National Dental Association, 337
Neck arteries, 27

Neurofibromatosis, 67
Neuropathology, 48
Neurosurgery, 150, 229–45, 317–19
New Haven Railroad, 8
New York Hospital, 4, 29–30, 44, 65
    and Bloomingdale Asylum, 4
    —Cornell Medical College, 314
New York Medical Journal, 55
New York Odontological Society, 54
New York Public Library, 3
New York Times, The, 78, 250, 324
New York University, 70
Nightingale, Florence, 102
Nitrous oxide gas, 11
Novocaine, 151
Nurses' training school, 102–3
Nursing, 200–201

O
Operating room, 111–16
Operating room nurses, 197
Operative Gynecology, 144, 227
Operative Story of Goitre, The, 270, 336
Ophthalmology Congress (1884), 49
Opium, 179
Osler, William, 105–10, 181, 348, 353–54
    aseptic technique, 222, 226–27
    in Baltimore, 94, 127, 129
    in Big Four, 141–42
    breast cancer cure, 123
    Cushing (Harvey) and, 231, 238, 245
    early medical staff, 101–3
    experimental work, 207–8, 213
    full-time professors, 298, 301, 305
    Halsted's addiction and, 278, 280
    home surgeries, 247, 251
    Johns Hopkins Hospital, 97–98
    Johns Hopkins Medical School,
        185–86
    residency, 201, 259, 265
    scientist, 287–89, 294–96

U.S. medical education and,
    155–59, 162
Outpatient services, 38, 53, 158
Oxalic acid soak, 113

P
Pancreatitis, 336
Parathyroid glands, 269–70
Park, Edwards A., 80, 213
Park, Davis and Company, 51, 179
Parsons, Louisa, 102, 103
Pasteur, Louis, 14–16, 18, 39, 72–73,
    155, 351
Pasteurization, 16
Pathology, 67, 69–70, 76, 83
Pen, 313–14
Perfusion pump, 293
Peripheral nervous system, 50
Peristalsis, 88
Peritonitis, 14, 323
Perityphlitis, 26
Permanganate, 113
Pershing, John, 328–29
Peter Bent Brigham Hospital, 245, 278
Phenol, 18, 112
Phi Theta Psi, 7
Phillips, Dr. John, 6
Phillips, Samuel, 6
Phillips Academy, 6
Phippen, Hardy, 134, 194
Picasso, 224
Pituitary Body and Its Disorders,
    The, 244
Pituitary function, 240
Play performances, 8
Pneumo-ventriculography, 317
Postgraduate medical training, 107
Postmortem examination, 108–9
Pranks, 211–12
Preceptor, 22
Presbyterian Hospital, 44, 54

Prince Leopold, 12
*Principles and Practice of Medicine,
    The,* 157–58, 226, 288
Private practice, 302–4
Private tutoring, 21–22
Procaine, 151
Professor of surgery, 183–88
"Professor, The," 123
Progress notes, 30
Prostate cancer, 261–62
Psi Epsilon, 7
Psychiatrist, 103
Public health, 64, 351
Puerperal fever, 39, 40
Pulmonary edema, 69
Pure Food and Drug Act (1906), 179

Q

Quaker faith, 60, 61
Queen Victoria, 12, 114
Quizmasters, 41–42
Quizzes, 21–22

R

Rabies vaccine, 15
Railroads, 3
Randall, Elizabeth, 331–33
Randolph, Miss, 129
Rectal cancer, 33
Rectal examinations, 262
Redford, Lewis, 244
Redi, Francesco, 14
Reed, Walter, 351
Reid, Mont, 335, 341–43, 345
Remsen, Ira, 301
Research, 290
Residency, 193–204, 314
    questions, 160–61
    selection, 257–58
    successes, 348
    surgeons, 206–7

Revere, Paul, 6
Rienhoff, William F., 223, 258,
    341–42, 345
Riots, 2
Robb, Hunter, 226
Robeson, Paul, 176
Rockefeller, John D., 288, 300
Rockefeller Institute for Medical
    Research, 288, 293, 300, 324
Rockefellers' General Education
    Board, 301
Roentgen, Wilhelm, 231
Roosevelt, Franklin D., 176
Roosevelt, James, 44
Roosevelt, Theodore, 44, 229, 353
Roosevelt Hospital Dispensary, 158
Roosevelt Hospital in New York City,
    37–39, 44, 53, 218, 267
Rubber gloves, 114–15

S

Sabine, Thomas A., 25
Salary, 249, 253, 302–3
Saline solution, 203
Sands, Henry B., 22–23, 29, 37–38,
    44, 267
Sanitation, 2
Sargent, John Singer, 353–55
Sawyer, Dr., 80
Scarpa's space, 106
Schleich's solution, 153
Schooling, 5
Scientific Man and the Bible, A, 144
Scientific method, 86
Scientist, 292–96
Scrub suits, 18, 349
Semmelweis, Ignaz, 39
Sensory nerves, 50–51
Sewers, 2
Sexuality, 254–55
Shattuck, Fred C., 80

Silk sutures, 221–22
Simmons, Mrs. Thomas, 75, 86, 91, 127
Skin grafting, 34–35
Skull and Bones, 7–8
Slack Jr., Harry, 333
Sladen, 251
Slipped disc, 318
Smith, Kate, 176
Smith, Stephen, 25
Smith, Winford, 315
Smoking, 26
Socializing, 211–13, 311–12
Sophomore Society, 7
Southern Medical Journal, 12
Spaniels, 218
St. Martin and the Beggar, 355
Staining techniques, 196
Standard Oil, 301
Stanford, 349
Steam sterilization, 18
Stein, Gertrude, 224–25
Sterile gloves, 203–4, 205, 349
Stevenson, Robert Louis, 353
Stokers, Miss, 280
Stool, 88
Street gangs, 2
Surgeon-in-chief, 98, 133–34
Surgeon's sleeves, 18
Surgery, 9–10, 98
    abroad, 31
    building, 288–89
    residents, 99, 140–41
    routines, 156
    schedule, 136–37
Surgical attire, 309–10
Surgical clinics, 223
Surgical papers, 31
Surgical pathology, 195, 222
Surgical staff growth, 162–63
Surgical tourniquet, 34
Surgical training, 33–34

"Swedish Nightingale," 3

T

Tasters, The, 7
Taxis, 146
Taylor, Adrian, 324
Teaching, 157–58, 189–92, 259
Telegraph, 3
Telephones, 41
Temper, 200
Tent operating room, 45
Terry, Bertha Halsted, 346–47
Thayer, William S., 156, 158, 251,
    294, 302
Theotocopouli, Jorge Manuel, 355
Thiersch, Karl, 34, 35
Thomas, Allen M., 39, 40, 57
Thomas, Carey, 184, 185
Three Lives, 224
Thyroid gland, 93, 259, 267–70
    surgery, 33, 140, 153–54
Tool decontamination, 37
Toronto School of Medicine, 108
Trachoma, 49
Training system, 205
Transport, 208–9
Travel, 279–80
Trichloroethylene, 12
Trigeminal neuralgia, 54, 236
Trusses, 145–46
Tubercle bacillus, 16
Tuberculin, 163
Tuberculosis, 1–2
Tufts, Rev. Mr., 5
Tulane University, 338
Turner, John, 245
Typhoid, 35

U

Union Theological Seminary, 4
University-affiliated schools, 299–300

University of California, 63, 349
University of Chicago, 130, 188, 290, 294
University of Cincinnati, 318–19, 349
University of the City of New York, 3
University Club, 40
University of Maryland Medical School, 76, 110, 197, 201
University of Michigan School of Medicine, 77, 188
University of Pennsylvania, 194, 264, 299
University Place Presbyterian Church, 4
University of Virginia, 349
Urology, 259–64

V
Vanderbilt, 278
Van der Poel, Minnie Halsted, 346
Van der Poel, Samuel, 25, 32, 34, 42–43
Van der Poel, W. Halsted, 343
Vascular aneurysm, 140
Vascular surgery, 205, 259, 283–86
Venable, Richard M., 211, 212
Verdi, 2
Veterinary pursuits, 214–15
Vienna General Hospital, 39
Visiting physician, 39
Visitors, 214–19
Volkmann, Richard von, 34, 119
Voltaire, 162
Von Recklinghausen, F. D., 67–68, 69

W
Wagner, Ernst, 66, 68
Waldeyer, Wilhelm, 67
Wall Street, 3
Wallace, W. K., 346
Ward nurse, 161
Ward rounds, 160, 192

Warren, John Collins, 11
Waters, Levin, 271–72, 283
Welch, William Henry, 337, 350–52
    aseptic techniques, 225–37
    in Baltimore, 85–86, 127, 129, 132
    in Big Four, 142
    breast cancer cure, 115, 121
    choosing best men, 75–78, 81–83
    Cushing (Harvey) and, 237–38
    experimental work, 208, 211–12
    full-term professors, 299, 300
    Halsted's addiction, 55–58, 279
    Halsted's final illness, death, 342, 346–48
    Hopkins (Johns) and, 66–73
    Johns Hopkins Medical School, 185–87
    New York, 40–42, 44
    operating room, 115
    Osler (William) and, 105, 108–9
    residency, 195, 196, 261
    scientist, 295–96
    teaching, 190, 192
    U.S. medical education, 155, 157, 159, 165
    World War I, 322
Welch Medical Library, 353
Wells, Horace, 11
Whipple, Allen O., 278
Wiener Allegemeines Krankenhaus, 39
Wilde, Oscar, 250
William H. Welch Endowment for Clinical Education and Research, 301
William Welch and the Rise of Modern Medicine, 71
Williams, J. Whitridge "Bull," 165, 226
Wilson, Woodrow, 329
Wölfler, Anton, 33, 56–57
Women physicians, 222
Women's Fund Committee, 184

Women's Fund Memorial Building, 187
Wood, Leonard, 229–30, 245
Woodbury, John, 54
Word usage, 325–26
World War II, 305
World's Fair (1853), 3
Wound healing, 140, 293–94

X–Z

X-ray, 124, 231–32, 288
exposure, 265–66

Yale, 6–7, 67, 85, 235, 264, 349
Yellow fever, 1
Young, Hugh Hampton
aseptic technique, 226
Halsted's addiction, 278
new departments, 311
residency, 259–64
scientist, 289, 296
surgery's early days
World War I, 328–29
Zuckerkandl, Emil, 32

ABOUT THE AUTHOR

DR. GERALD IMBER is a well-known plastic surgeon and authority on cosmetic surgery, and directs a private clinic in Manhattan. He is assistant clinical professor of surgery at Weill-Cornell School of Medicine, and on staff at the New York-Presbyterian Hospital, where he served his residency, and learned a great deal of Dr. Halsted.

In addition to scientific papers and lectures, Dr. Imber has written numerous general-interest articles as well as books on plastic surgery. *Genius on the Edge* is his first biography.